CONTENTS

PART IV THE HEART: HOW TO KEEP IT FROM BREAKING

PART V CUTTING-EDGE ADVANCES IN ANTIAGING

A NEW WAY
TO AGE

OTHER BOOKS BY SUZANNE SOMERS

A NEW WAY TO AGE

The Most Cutting-Edge Advances in Antiaging

SUZANNE SOMERS

GALLERY BOOKS

NEW YORK   LONDON   TORONTO   SYDNEY   NEW DELHI

Gallery Books
An Imprint of Simon & Schuster, Inc.
1230 Avenue of the Americas
New York, NY 10020

First Gallery Books trade paperback edition August 2020

GALLERY BOOKS and colophon are registered trademarks of Simon & Schuster, Inc.

For information about special discounts for bulk purchases, please contact Simon & Schuster Special Sales at 1-866-506-1949 or business@simonandschuster.com.

The Simon & Schuster Speakers Bureau can bring authors to your live event. For more information or to book an event, contact the Simon & Schuster Speakers Bureau at 1-866-248-3049 or visit our website at www.simonspeakers.com.

Interior design by Jaime Putorti

Manufactured in the United States of America

10   9   8   7   6   5   4   3   2   1

The Library of Congress has cataloged the hardcover edition as follows:

Names: Somers, Suzanne, 1946– author.
Title: A new way to age : the most cutting-edge advances in antiaging /
    Suzanne Somers.
Description: First Gallery Books hardcover edition. | New York : Gallery Books, [2020] |
    Includes bibliographical references and index.
Identifiers: LCCN 2019036076 (print) | LCCN 2019036077 (ebook) |
    ISBN 9781982110949 | ISBN 9781982110956 (trade paperback) |
    ISBN 9781982110963 (ebook)
Subjects: LCSH: Older people—Social aspects. | Older people—Psychology. | Aging.
Classification: LCC HQ1061 .S6544 2020 (print) | LCC HQ1061 (ebook) |
    DDC 305.26—dc23
LC record available at https://lccn.loc.gov/2019036076
LC ebook record available at https://lccn.loc.gov/2019036077

ISBN 978-1-9821-1094-9
ISBN 978-1-9821-1095-6 (pbk)
ISBN 978-1-9821-1096-3 (ebook)

To my sexy husband, Alan Hamel, whom I've been with for fifty years.

What fun we are having together this "new way"!
We have love, and we have health.
Every day with you is a gift and a blessing.

The seven best doctors in the world are: God, sunlight, diet, rest, exercise, self-confidence, and friends. Maintain them in all stages and enjoy a happy life.

—Anonymous

PREFACE

You never know where the "lesson" is going to come from, the life event that causes the proverbial "shaking of the shoulders"—a wake-up call, if you will—that changes the course of your life. It happened to me many years ago: cancer, an event so sobering I knew I needed to make a major change in the way I had been taking care of myself. Clearly what I had been doing up to that point wasn't working, yet my breast cancer diagnosis was a negative that turned out to be a positive, a veiled gift that opened my eyes to how I had, unknowingly, actually been abusing myself. I had to make changes, and the choices I made to recover forced me to face my own mortality and to come to grips with my beliefs.

The idea of pumping my body full of poison as a means to heal did not jibe with my beliefs; it sounded crazy and still does. I decided to take charge of my health and my cancer—and win. I did it my way. It was not arrogant. I researched, met with cutting-edge, forward-thinking doctors who had stepped out of the comfort of their pharmaceutically driven practices to go for true natural healing. I took charge of my health. I became the contractor, and my different doctors were my subcontractors, but make no mistake,

I ran the show. I gained control!

Cancer changed my life and set me on a path of health and natural healing. I've never looked back.

My book *Bombshell: Explosive Medical Secrets That Will Redefine Aging* was published in 2012. It revealed the latest cutting-edge advances in medicine at that time. Today, eight years later, *everything* in the alternative and antiaging world is exploding. The information and discoveries on aging have moved even further forward with lightning speed. It's a fast-moving train, and you want to jump on it right now.

This book, *A New Way to Age*, goes further—much further—and is updated with brand-new information about "new thinking" integrative and alternative doctors and other professionals; aging without using drugs unless absolutely necessary; bioidentical hormone replacement (a true game changer); environmental toxins and their effects on our health; the miracle of stem cell protocols; new ways to care for the heart; plus gut health and its connection to brain issues and brain health and how to reverse the damage. Also, the new exciting frontier of targeted peptide treatments, cell rejuvenation, sexual rejuvenation, even the potential healing properties of non-THC cannabis. The information in this book can change the way you age in the most fantastic way. I live this life. It is mind-blowing. You are going to learn about slowing down and even *reversing* aging, allowing you to live longer with quality and full function, bursting with energy and vitality.

This book revisits a few of the doctors I've interviewed in the past: those who have never stopped learning, as well as today's new doctors, the movers and shakers shaping this "new way to age." Their updated, current cutting-edge information and protocols are going to astound you.

This is a nondrug book; a couple of pharmaceuticals are mentioned, but in those instances, I've also given the natural equivalents. This "new way" is attainable for all who desire optimal health and youthful aging. I'm proud to introduce you to

A NEW WAY TO AGE!

THE NEW WAY TO AGE

The goal of life is to die young—as late as possible.
—Ashley Montagu

The famed futurist Ray Kurzweil, dubbed by Bill Gates as "one of the smartest men in the world," once asked me, "Suzanne, how long do you see yourself living?" I thought about it and said, "Well, with the way I've chosen to take care of myself, I could actually envision living to be a hundred and ten." He said, "Okay, on your hundred tenth birthday, you've got your brain, you've got your bones, you're in great health. Is that the day you want to die?" I thought about it and imagined that if I could continue living in great health and happiness with a well-working brain and strong bones, living longer would be very appealing to me. And so my journey began.

The message of this book is that there is *a new way to age* without sickness and with clarity, energy, and virility created by the choices we make on a daily basis.

WHAT IS AGING?

Technically, aging is about worn-out parts. It was once thought of as something concerning only "old people," but it has now accelerated; in today's world we are experiencing a new and frightening phenomenon: young people who can't sleep, young people with hormone deficiencies, young people who can't absorb minerals from their GI tracts and who are so distressed by the toxic assault of today's chemicals that the once normal process of digestion and having an intact gut barrier wall (part of the immune system) is no longer functional; people are walking around with gut linings that are shredded like an old car tire. This is a disaster. Gut dysfunction leads to brain issues: ADD, ADHD, OCD, dyslexia, dyspraxia, autism, Alzheimer's disease. When did this happen—or better yet, *why* did it happen?

Unexplained weight gain seems to be plaguing everyone; it doesn't seem to matter how much you eat, it just won't go away. We go to the gym, we exercise until we can't sweat anymore, we diet with lousy results. What is happening? What is wrong? Certainly, our rising exposure to chemicals and overconsumption of sugar are contributing.

Some reasons for rising obesity rates are that people are eating way more processed carbohydrates (including simple sugar, such as fructose), causing an overall increase in calorie intake in recent decades (by approximately 400 calories per day compared to the 1970s), increased intake of commercially processed foods that are low in fiber, and a dramatic increase in vegetable oil consumption, resulting in a significant increase of harmful omega-6 refined vegetable fats.[1]

What if I told you that nowadays no one is born without a toxic body burden? Consider this fact: The Environmental Working Group did a study on the cord blood of infants across the economic spectrum, from the poorest to the richest. It tested for 287 different toxins (mind you, the babies had not yet even tasted breast milk); every single baby tested positive for a minimum of 180 toxins! Think about that: our first "room," our mother's womb, is no longer clean and safe.

Add to our toxic burden the impact of aging and how physicians treat each ailment in isolation, as opposed to systemically correcting the onslaught of biological deteriorations that occur as we grow older. But don't despair; whether you are young or old, optimal health and more are available. The rejuvenation of the body is now possible in ways never before thought of. The doctors in this book have dedicated their lives to finding a "new way."

"Back then," if any of us had appreciated our perfectly working, functional body we would have taken better care of it. I wish I had known about this new way in my twenties. I would have embraced it enthusiastically, and perhaps I wouldn't have gotten cancer. But we didn't know. We thought that chemicals, pesticides, and pharmaceutical drugs were the answer. Nirvana. Health made easy—but unbeknownst to us, they came with a big price, and now all of us are suffering the results. They *were* too good to be true.

You can "keep on keepin' on" and doing things the same way you have been—or you can go a different route: A NEW WAY.

It's what I am doing.

In this book, I lay out my program for delaying aging. I tell you what I do, the doctors I go to, every vitamin, every supplement, and every hormone I take, along with all the tests I have done to determine my deficiencies so you can get a clear idea of this "new way to age."

We all want to know if there is a way to:

· Live a long life of high quality and no illness

· Keep our "juice" through bioidentical hormone replacement to stay energetic, sexy, and sexual

· Save our memory, save our brains

· Detoxify our body and thrive on a toxic planet that is trying to do us in

· Prevent heart disease

· Prevent cancer

· Prevent Alzheimer's disease

· Prevent unwanted weight gain

· Discover new protocols for age reversal: senolytics, NAD+, targeted peptides, the healing potential of non-THC cannabis, and more

· Take advantage of the miracles of stem cells and the doctors who are in the vanguard in studying them

· Take advantage of telomere lengthening for longer, healthier life through the supplement TA-65

- Take advantage of energy medicine: ways to determine which organs and glands are working at optimum

- And of course, live longer, healthier, and with a high quality of life!

It's all in this book.

My role, as I see it, is to find and present to you information from the most up-to-date, cutting-edge doctors, scientists, and professionals on breakthroughs relative to aging and achieving greater longevity with optimal health—a "recipe" of sorts that when followed can take you on a journey of optimal health and long life. I will present the nondrug options and introduce you to the doctors who "get it." These doctors are your hope.

I've been laughed at, ridiculed, called a "health nut," criticized by the media, taken on by snotty newscasters calling me "another celebrity who thinks she's a doctor." I suck it up.

For me and the way I've chosen to approach my health and aging, I feel "right." I do it my way; I've educated myself, I've used my celebrity to get to the best and the brightest professionals in the field, and I've shared what I've learned with all those who have wanted to read or listen. I lecture all over the United States, in Canada, and overseas, and I am proud to have millions of my books in print globally. I have been given an honorary doctorate by National University because I've done my homework, plus I've done enormous research to come to two simple conclusions: (1) what we lose in the aging process must be replaced with the natural version as determined by lab work and your individual deficiencies and (2) we are under a massive environmental assault. In order to survive and thrive, you have to rid your body and your life of all the chemicals and toxins you possibly can, including pharmaceutical drugs unless *absolutely necessary*!

If your body is already toxic from the environment, does it make any sense to keep adding foreign molecules in the form of over-the-counter and pharmaceutical drugs?

Of course, there's more to it, but in order to take advantage of the new "recipe," the first step is to change your thinking and to realize that the new way to age is to:

1. Replace what has been lost in the aging process due to stress, toxicity, and aging itself with natural supplementation and natural bioidentical hormone replacement; find out and replace your nutritional and mineral deficiencies; and learn about cutting-edge science and how to source it.

2. Take advantage of as many of the new breakthroughs in natural health and age reversal as you can afford.

We will go through each step chapter by chapter. These steps require a qualified doctor, the "new doctors" who understand the "new way to age." Your best bet for finding the right kind of doctor is to consult the list in the back of this book or go to www.foreverhealth.com. It's a free service, and the people there will direct you to the right kind of forward-thinking doctor near you.

Aging is a fantastic experience if you approach it correctly. Remember that the big gift is the acquired wisdom, that "knowing," the "aha moments" when everything makes sense for the first time. Wisdom is something no young person can buy or have.

However, if indeed aging is about worn-out parts, your job, to age well and differently from your parents, is to listen to the language of the body and do what's necessary to change the paradigm; those aching joints, the fatigue that won't go away, weight gain, inability to sleep, and the first signs of conditions such as autoimmune issues, gut issues, and cancer, these things are all part of the language. Most people wait until they find themselves in a catastrophic state and then desperately search for a miracle. What is ahead of you in these pages are the new doctors who know how to decipher what is wrong based on lab work or new cutting-edge techniques such as bioimpedance (see the interview with Dr. Michael Galitzer in chapter 20), which can test the voltage of your various organs and glands to see what is not firing at full speed. What an advantage, heading problems off at the pass! Other common problems such as bloating, gas, and constipation are some of the hallmarks of aging and will be addressed in this book.

Bioidentical hormones are a game changer; hormones are the first thing to decline, so it's best to get that balance restored before you go further. All of the doctors in this book are experts in replacing hormones naturally. Bioidentical hormone replacement therapy (BHRT) totally changed the quality of my life. Then there are cutting-edge advances: medical breakthroughs such as targeted peptides (think natural skin rejuvenation), telomere lengthening, and cell rejuvenation (see the interview with Bill Faloon in chapter 16) to clean out cellular debris with once-weekly inexpensive senolytic activator supplementation, which promotes age reversal, and the great new advances with NAD+, which repairs DNA breaks!

There is so much more, and it's all exciting, enabling you to achieve greater longevity and quality of life.

The lab tests you should explore can be found at the back of this book. This kind of lab testing covers hormone levels, mineral and nutritional deficiencies, mold testing, stool testing, toxicity levels, and more. Life Extension has the most reasonably priced lab tests, and it has a large staff of doctors, scientists, and professionals to assist you with their interpretations.

The Dalai Lama, when asked what surprised him most about humanity, answered, "Man. Because he sacrifices his health in order to make money. Then he sacrifices money to recuperate his health. And then he is so anxious about the future that he does not enjoy the present; the result being that he does not live in the present or the future; he lives as if he is never going to die, and then he dies having never really lived."

PART I

CHOICES:
The Time Is Now

CHAPTER 1

CAN WE REVERSE AGING?

*Do not go where the path may lead, go instead where
there is no path and leave a trail.*
—Ralph Waldo Emerson

This book is about aging in the best possible way. I am vitally interested in living as long as possible, as long as that life is one of quality, as long as my brain is in perfect working order and my bones are strong and agile. Who wouldn't want that?

I have not assigned a "number" to my longevity. I'd like to stay alive as long as possible, but the caveat is that I want robust health until the last breath. This book and the interview below open the possibilities of living your life a different way: in good health, without all the afflictions that possess and plague humanity in the aging process.

Aging begins at the cellular level. But it took a long time to figure that out. For much of the twentieth century, biologists thought that cells were immortal, but in the 1960s, the microbiologist Leonard Hayflick discovered that some human cells divide forty to sixty times before stopping at what we now call the Hayflick Limit. The ability of cells to divide is important. It's what helps your body repair damage (for instance, after you cut your finger) or fend off attack (for instance, when your immune system defends against a virus).

Since then, researchers have discovered that even cells that keep dividing *do age*, and they become inefficient at performing basic functions such as repairing DNA and recycling proteins, lipids, and other key molecules. At that point cells are unable to maintain themselves; they accumulate damage, which impedes their ability to function normally or repair bodily tissues. It's like a car that falls into disrepair until one day, it just won't start.

As our cells die or degenerate, our senses diminish, our skin sags and wrinkles, our joints ache, our muscles collapse, and eventually the diseases associated with our older years creep in to finish us off: stroke, Alzheimer's, pulmonary fibrosis, diabetes, heart disease, cancer. Most people are programmed to accept this tragic paradigm.

One approach related to antiaging is to kill off old, "broken" cells that have hit their division limit; another is to restore or rejuvenate stem cells, which are needed to maintain our tissues and organs. In chapter 16, Bill Faloon explains this cutting-edge technology in detail—maybe you want to go to Bill Faloon's chapter right now to learn the newest cutting-edge advances in antiaging.

If you have an old car, you can keep it running and even rejuvenated by replacing old parts. Today, people who get a stem cell transplant find that there are additional benefits if the donor happens to be younger than they. In that scenario, the health of that stem cell recipient often improves.

> We've been wrong about what our job is in medicine.
> We think our job is to ensure health and survival. But
> really it is larger than that. It is to enable well-being.
> —Dr. Atul Gawande

It's very exciting that today a whole new way to approach health has emerged, and leading the charge are the "new doctors." They are all MDs, doctors who realized the limitations of traditional medicine, stepped out of their comfortable standard-of-care boxes, and reeducated themselves in the new way.

When you need allopathic (pharmaceutical) medicine, it's a godsend to cure an infection or alleviate pain after surgery, but for normal body upkeep and care of the ailments caused by *deficiencies*, allopathic medicine has hit a wall. Pharmaceutical drugs essentially put a "Band-Aid" on deficiencies; they will never cure a deficiency, just keep it at bay, and once the medication stops you return to a state of dis-ease. These new doctors practicing alternative and/or integrative medicine think differently.

Antiaging medicine listens to the language of the body; it is an opportunity for you to recognize that something is "off" when you experience things such as fatigue (feeling dog tired), lack of energy, a chronic illness, a lowered immune system, a high or low thyroid hormone level, "lazy" brain, "chemical" brain, leaky gut, hormonal imbalances, autoimmune disease, or cancer.

At some point we are all going to get the latest flu or whatever else is going around, but as a general rule people who practice antiaging medicine don't get sick.

Antiaging medicine builds up the immune system by putting back all the minerals, nutrients, hormones, and body deficiencies usually considered part of natural aging; in addition, it deals with the accelerated aging that is taking place in younger and younger people in today's world due to the massive chemical assault.

Read the interview with each doctor carefully. In this book, I give you a cross section of physicians in different parts of the United States and Europe, but www.foreverhealth.com also has a roster of qualified doctors across the country, so you will be able to find one near you.

The doctors featured in this book have their own unique approaches to health, mostly nondrug, embracing disease prevention rather than care. If you are reading this book, I know this matters to you.

MEET THE DOCTORS AND EXPERTS

DR. ALLAN MAGAZINER has been a fixture in the antiaging and alternative world for decades. His practice typifies what to expect when you embark on this new kind of medicine. He is knowledgeable and an expert in bioidentical hormone replacement therapy, among many other specialties. I have sent many of my East Coast friends to him, and they have all reported back that they *love* him.

DR. JONATHAN WRIGHT, a national treasure, gives supplement tips on things most doctors are not aware of: on aging well without drugs, for instance; which supplement can repair damaged cartilage; which supplements accelerate weight loss; and many more. Don't miss this one. Dr. Wright explains how to live a drug-free life using "nature's tools." In taking a natural approach, he believes we can avoid all over-the-counter and pharmaceutical drugs unless absolutely necessary. He believes that good working of the body "engine" depends on providing it with the correct "fuel."

Dr. Wright does testing to determine mineral and nutritional deficiencies through lab work. All the doctors in this book have this expertise. Working with a qualified doctor is important. Doctors who have not continued their educations to learn about the new ways are not equipped to handle the effects of the environment on the human body or to help you restore a good quality of life.

Dr. Wright also understands the importance of gut health, how the gut gets "sick" and how you can fix it, plus the importance of diet and good-quality food to longevity and optimum health. He also describes the health benefits of limiting your sugar and grain intake to avoid obesity, weight gain, and disease and how to conquer gut issues arising from chemicals, toxicity, and genetically modified foods. He explains the puzzle of autoimmune diseases: how they originate and how to eliminate them.

DR. JEFFREY R. GLADDEN is another of the new kind of doctor. I was of mixed mind about his interview: Should I put him into the heart section, as he is a cardiologist, or with the "in the trenches," all-around integrative doctors? I decided to do the latter. He was trained as an interventional cardiologist, but in his practice, he came to realize that the heart is only a part of the body "system," and he wanted to create a new dynamic approach to treating the heart as a part of the whole. In other words, "Let's take care of the whole body."

All the doctors in this book understand the significance and importance of replacing missing sex hormones as well as thyroid hormone with bioidentical hormones, as determined by your deficiencies through lab work interpreted by a qualified doctor. Hormones are at the base of a new way to age.

JULIE CARMEN, my yoga instructor of nineteen years, explains the value of yoga as exercise for long life, strong bones, flexibility, and accessing your wisdom.

DR. THIERRY HERTOGHE explains new ways to age without wrinkles, how to keep your sex drive alive, and how to strengthen your body with peptide replacements as well as injections of human growth hormone (HGH), insulin-like growth factor 1 (IGF-1), and insulin, taken together, for results that have been shown to improve certain aspects of aging related to appearance (skin) and body composition (muscle and fat). Plus how to deal with all the issues and diseases normally accompanied with aging. His chapter is a mindblower and as he explains, rejuvenation is possible. You'll learn how to save your bones by understanding hormone replacement therapy, including with HGH, as determined by your deficiencies, as well as why this hormone is misunderstood. Plus, he teaches how to regain your energy and stay sexual, or keep your brainpower and "juice."

DR. ABRAHAM MORGENTALER of Harvard demystifies the issue of prostate health and testosterone. For all you men out there who have been scared into avoiding testosterone replacement, Dr. Morgentaler's chapter will put your fears to rest. Hormones are a game changer for men's health issues and aging.

DR. KENT MACLEOD is the founder and CEO of NutriChem Compounding Pharmacy & Clinic in Canada. An international thought leader, he is also an award-winning pharmacist with more than thirty years of clinical experience in delivering patient-centered health care.

DR. STEPHEN SINATRA in chapter 13 plus EECP Global Cardio Care in chapter 14 present a new way to take care of the heart without drugs unless absolutely necessary. The body has a language, and by listening to it carefully, you can practice prevention and avoid heart attack, lower your blood pressure without drugs, and avoid heart disease and stroke.

DR. WALTER PIERPAOLI explains the new cutting-edge antiaging protocols such as resetting your endocrine clock with thyrotropin-releasing hormone (TRH), the miracle hormone that wakes up a "lazy" brain and reverses aging. He explains how it is now very possible to keep your memory and keep your brain with discoveries like the newly discovered hormone TRH.

There is new information about the role the jaw plays in heart health. Yes, the *jaw*! Have you ever wondered about "sudden heart attacks" and where they come from? Read the interview with DR. LEONARD FELD in chapter 15, and you will be astounded.

BILL FALOON of Life Extension explains the advantages of boosting nicotinamide adenine dinucleotide (NAD+), turning down an obesity-promoting cell protein, and other age reversal discoveries including *senolytics*. You won't want to miss the interview with him in chapter 16.

Senolytics are exciting compounds that remove senescent cells from our bodies. With age, senescent cells linger and create metabolic havoc, which contributes to degenerative diseases and a shortened life span. Senolytic compounds selectively reduce our senescent cell burden. Put simply, it cleans out cellular debris. Cellular debris is toxic and accelerates aging, so this is an exciting breakthrough.

NOEL PATTON explains the new findings regarding TA-65 for telomere lengthening. It comes as a supplement and is a potential antiaging discovery.

DR. DIPNARINE MAHARAJ explains what stem cell therapy can do, how to access it, and how to use bone marrow stem cell transplants to renew your immune system. A strong immune systems equals less disease and degeneration.

DR. MARC DARROW of Los Angeles, a stem cell expert in the field of sports injuries, is hands-on when it comes to relieving pain. Surgeries for those with sports injuries are all but unnecessary as stem cell bone marrow transplants from their own blood can be used with remarkable results.

DR. JONATHAN M. FISHBEIN, a scientist and clinical trialist, gives his findings on non-THC CBD as a potential for pain control.

DR. MICHAEL GALITZER explains the steps to take to avoid cancer without drugs, new protocols if you do have cancer, and the fact that developing cancer is not inevitable. He can determine the balance between energy production and energy recovery through bioimpedance, a process that looks at body fat, body water, and, most important, something called the *phase angle*, which is a measure of regeneration. His theory is our bodies are always destroying old cells and creating new cells. The phase angle tells us how well we are regenerating and creating new cells. This is good health.

If you don't have health moving forward, you have nothing.

It's exciting to think that in most cases, we can now achieve great health without drugs. As you explore each step chapter by chapter, you will find the answers to your rheumatoid arthritis, your distended gut, your inability to sleep, your memory loss, your autoimmune diseases, your brain fog, your premature wrinkling, your hair loss, your brittle nails, your unexplained weight gain, and your fear of cancer, plus how to protect yourself from developing Alzheimer's disease.

By reading about what each of these cutting-edge doctors and experts have to teach and following their steps to healthy aging, you will be well on your way to experiencing the new way to age.

Most of the protocols are affordable, some are even free, and then there are some that are pricey. You can cherry-pick according to what you can afford. The more expensive protocols are the "kiss," the icing on the cake, but by no means does "the new way of aging" depend on wealth. You will find affordable interventions throughout this book.

What an advantage and what a gift to the world it would be to re-claim the "elders of the tribe": well-functioning brains allowing them to access their well-earned wisdom and become productive members of society. As I see it, the planet is crying out for wisdom, but at present our elders are so pilled up, they can't think. The doctors in this book and their followers are changing that paradigm.

In essence this information is about avoiding all the hallmarks ex-pected of aging. By making significant changes in the food you eat, the supplements you take, and the hormones you replace, and the products you use, you can expect a new and better life.

There is a new way to age. I'm doing it, and it's the best decision I've ever made. I love this stage of my life: I have health and "juice," joy, wisdom, and perspective; I have energy, vitality, clear-headedness, and strong bones. I am able to work with vigor and exercise as I wish. I write and publish a book most every year about cutting-edge health, things I want to share with my readers. Also, I am a Las Vegas headliner with a ninety-minute solo show nightly, and I'm ready for more each day. I am a productive member of society rather than a drain on it. ALL BE-CAUSE I AM HEALTHY! AND HAPPY!

Interview with

DR. ALLAN MAGAZINER

Let's begin our journey with Dr. Allan Magaziner. He has been a fixture in the antiaging and alternative medicine world for decades. His practice typifies what to expect when you embark on this new kind of medicine. He is knowledgeable and an expert in bioidentical hormone replacement therapy, among many other specialties. I have sent many of my East Coast friends to him, and they have all reported back that they *love* him.

Everyone asks me what I'm doing to maintain my good health. I take it as a compliment, and I have to say I have never felt better in my life. I have energy and excitement about life and a "rockin' " libido, and I'm enjoying my age. My new wisdom has infiltrated my thinking, and life seems much simpler. I believe that all of my optimism is due to the fact that I feel good and healthy. I wake up happy in the morning.

How can you achieve this? Dr. Magaziner is a good place to start. I am in complete agreement with him and his approach to healthy aging.

Dr. Magaziner is one of the new kinds of doctors, part of a courageous group of physicians who early on saw the limitations of allopathic (conventional) medicine. Dr. Magaziner looks for the cause of diseases, works to educate his patients, and shows them how to take steps to prevent a catastrophic event with the goal of living a long life without illness and ultimately (a long time from now) dying naturally. We have all become used to today's tortuous, long-drawn-out deaths, but he offers a new way to live with wellness; to optimize quality of life, live a long time, and then die naturally. In my estimation, his way is a better way. With Dr. Magaziner, you take a journey of wellness: you go to the doctor when you are well to stay well; drugs are a last resort. This kind of medicine puts back the things that have declined in the aging process, whether through bioidentical hormones or nutrients. This new way helps keep the brain, heart, immune system, and GI tract healthy and functioning properly, making your good food and healthy lifestyle choices work to your great advantage. Dr. Magaziner is a functional medicine specialist in Cherry Hill, New Jersey, and has been practicing for thirty-five years. He graduated from Chicago College of Osteopathic Medicine at Midwestern University in 1983 and specializes in integrative, functional, and preventive medicine.

SOMERS: Thank you for your time, Dr. Magaziner. We've known one another for quite a while, and I'm happy to present you in this book as "a new kind of doctor." Relative to today's medicine, did you become disillusioned, or did you always want to be involved in integrative and alternative medicine?

MAGAZINER: I graduated medical school in '83, thirty-five years ago, and I decided to go into this type of medicine right from the beginning. A lot of my colleagues, friends, and classmates were saying things like "What are you doing?," "How do you know what to do?," "Why are you going into this?," "Who's going to refer patients to you?," and "Are you sure this is what you want to do?" I decided to go into this type of medicine for a personal reason: my mother was very sick, and she had been helped by another doctor at that time who did practice some integrative or functional medicine, and it greatly improved her condition. She ended up opening a health food store when I was fifteen years old and still in high school. I worked nights and weekends to help the family business, and it was there my eyes opened up to a whole world.

SOMERS: Tell me about your patients and who they are.

MAGAZINER: The majority of them have already been through conventional treatments that have mostly failed. They're suffering from side effects, they're not getting any better, they're not improving, and their quality of life is going down the drain. They come to me because conventional medicine doesn't put enough emphasis on quality of life, and that's an area where we excel in our field. The majority of the people I see are genuinely open-minded, and they know they want a new approach.

The majority are very open-minded. I explain to them they got into trouble because of the environmental assault in today's world plus their bad diet and lifestyle habits but now we are going to approach things in a brand-new way to try to reverse their poor health.

One female patient who is diabetic and developing Alzheimer's wanted help. I said, "You really have to start by changing your diet. Start reducing sugar intake, eliminate processed foods, wheat, and let's see how you do, you may feel better." I saw her again today and she was feeling better, but she told me she's missing all those foods, so I explained how addictive and inflammatory these foods can be and I gave her alternatives and options. I explained if she keeps eating and doing the same things that she's been doing, she can't expect any different results.

SOMERS: How long does it take for sugar cravings to stop when you give it up cold turkey?

MAGAZINER: It depends on the individual and other personal factors, how sick the person feels to begin with. If some individuals are feeling lousy, they'll give up quicker. But then you have others that just aren't ready to make the transition. I've seen some patients recently diagnosed with cancer who give up their addictions cold turkey, whether it's sugar or cigarettes, whatever it is, whereas others aren't feeling lousy enough, so that often takes longer. We're all so biochemically different.

Every person's genetics, their triggers, their experiences, and their environments are so different that I have to individualize the treatment to each patient. Some are going to take several sessions with me to get them to begin tapering off some of their allergic or inflammatory foods.

SOMERS: As it relates to unwanted weight gain, do you think it's genetics, or is it just eating the same foods as those who have preceded us? In other words, are unhealthy food choices instilled at young ages that cause us to habitually grow fat over generations?

MAGAZINER: We are predisposed to conditions, but we can change what's called the expression of our genetics; it's called the phenotype versus the genotype. We can change the expression of these genes by how we live and the choices that we make every day.

Especially in regard to foods, because food is much more than just calories or macronutrients, the way we process our food is also information to our genes and information to our cells. The foods we decide to consume and the choices we make each day can turn on certain genes or turn off certain genes.

We can't change genes as of now, but we can change the expression of those genes, so we don't necessarily have to become diabetic or hypertensive or obese if we're willing to make those sacrifices. Even though someone may be genetically susceptible toward their predecessors' diseases, it doesn't mean they have to be expressed.

SOMERS: You mean we are actually in control so that if your mother was fat and your grandmother was fat, it doesn't necessarily mean you are going to be fat because you can override your genetic expression by your choices.

MAGAZINER: Exactly.

SOMERS: How do you go about looking for the underlying causes of disease?

MAGAZINER: Too often in traditional settings a doctor diagnoses a patient with a disease or condition—high blood pressure, diabetes—and they give them a pill: an antidiabetic pill and/or drugs to lower blood pressure, right? But instead of just treating the name of the disease, I look for the underlying causes of the disease. I developed something called My Wellness 360, twelve different major factors that commonly cause people to feel ill. It's things we've all heard of: our nutritional status and nutritional deficiencies, our detox pathways, our hormone balance, our inflammatory pathways, our stressors, our food intolerances and chemicals we're exposed to, and more than that. There's twelve of them.

SOMERS: Can you list all of them?

MAGAZINER: The twelve major factors that contribute to the diseases of today are:

- Nutritional imbalances

- Poor digestion and absorption

- Food intolerances

- Hormone and neurotransmitter imbalances

- Mitochondrial dysfunction

- Oxidative stress

- General stress reactions

- Electromagnetic stress

- Detox pathways

- Immune dysregulation and inflammation

- Environmental chemicals

- Genetic susceptibility

Those are the twelve major factors I've identified that I believe contribute to most of the diseases of today.

SOMERS: And you would be able to treat for these conditions at your clinic, right?

MAGAZINER: Correct. We investigate these conditions and believe these are common links for most of the chronic illnesses we see today. Patients give us their history; we conduct physical exams and a thorough evaluation through labs, which then allows me to prioritize these twelve different factors for each patient.

SOMERS: What's the average age of your patients?

MAGAZINER: It varies. I see children age two and up to people age ninety-five. The majority are ages anywhere from forty to seventy.

SOMERS: Those are the ages when we really start caring about failing health.

MAGAZINER: Yes. People think they're invincible when they're young. And as you get a little older, you start realizing your vulnerabilities.

SOMERS: When I got cancer, I decided I would eat as if my life depended upon it. I believe it's about the food. Do you?

MAGAZINER: That's the number one area to begin with; our food has become so adulterated, processed, transported, and devitalized in so many different ways in the last fifty, sixty years that today so many people have nutritional and various metabolic imbalances. Food is the key, but sixty to seventy percent of our calories today come from processed foods and simple sugars, and that alone doesn't leave a lot of space left for healthy foods.

SOMERS: What about genetically modified foods?

MAGAZINER: I talk to my patients about eating organic food whenever possible. GMOs have been linked to a lot of health problems. There are suggestions they may increase risk of various cancers, autoimmune disease for sure; leaky gut syndrome, which leads to more inflammation; and leaky brain, which can contribute to brain and memory problems. You can go on and on. There's enough evidence today that the genetic modification of our foods is causing great problems with allergies, learning disabilities, and we probably don't even know all the different conditions that GMOs might be contributing to.

SOMERS: The movie *Genetic Roulette* was a real eye-opener for me, that GMOs create an insecticide factory in your intestines. Do you get a lot of people complaining about their stomachs?

MAGAZINER: The GI tract is one of the most common problems I address: genetic modification of our food, the overuse of antibiotics and other medicines, antidepressants, antihistamines, they are all adversely affecting the microbiome, the bacterial balance of our gut.

SOMERS: Are gut problems becoming epidemic?

MAGAZINER: Yes, as a result of all of these things: GMOs, overuse of medications, antibiotics are all setting us up for inflammation, even depression and cancer progression.

SOMERS: Where does inflammation come from?

MAGAZINER: One of the key areas is the gut, and there are many more. Traditional medicine has neglected and ignored the gut for so long. My new patients are usually those who first went to a GI doctor, where he or she generally looks at the anatomy of your body, meaning endoscopy, colonoscopy, MRI. Those tests are looking for tumors and cysts and growths, but they have very little to do with the function of the body, so the gastroenterologist really isn't doing any analysis to assess the actual function of the GI tract.

Doctors in functional medicine frankly excel in this area, because we do so many functional tests that see deficits and problems. We then address those issues and are able to radically improve people's health because we're addressing the *function* of the body, not just the anatomy of the body.

SOMERS: When you say functional tests, do you mean lab tests?

MAGAZINER: Yes, various and unique lab tests.

SOMERS: My favorite is the stool test. I'm being sarcastic.

MAGAZINER: I warn them. I say, "Look, you did it once, you don't have to do it again for quite a while." You may do it again a few years down the line, but I agree, a comprehensive digestive stool test is not a pleasant one, but it's very informative.

SOMERS: How common and dangerous is leaky gut?

MAGAZINER: I think it's more common than we realize. There are so many insults today. Even the wheat is very different from the wheat that existed sixty or seventy years ago. The genetic modifications of our foods from 1990 on, coupled with all the medications we're taking, then add in the chemicals in our food, our water is contaminated as well with substances like heavy metals, pesticide residues, even traces of medications—you can go on and on.

All these things injure and damage the gut lining and the protective mucosa, and when that happens it sets up a whole cascade of potentially great amounts of inflammation. Leaky gut is real, but it's also very, very important to address because it leads to inflammation, and inflammation now has been associated with most of the chronic illnesses we see today—even things like heart disease, high blood pressure, cancer, diabetes, Alzheimer's, and depression are associated with inflammation. Conventional doctors aren't well versed in this arena, so they hand out all the anti-inflammatory medicines, then we mindlessly take them; we have a little pain, a little headache, people take ibuprofen or Aleve, not realizing all those medications also injure the protective lining of the GI tract.

SOMERS: So the "easy fix" of over-the-counter medications, which provide little more than a temporary Band-Aid, are actually exacerbating and injuring ourselves long term. Do you ever recommend simple old-world remedies like Epsom salts?

MAGAZINER: Yes. Epsom salt baths are great to help reduce aches and pains. I often recommend taking a little bit in water as a bicarb solution for gut issues. Epsom salts is also great for relaxation. Old-time remedies can be terrific. I mean, let's face it, up until seventy-five years ago or so, that's how we treated patients, using home remedies. We also used many more herbs and spices like ginger, castor oil compresses, cinnamon, all very effective anti-inflammatories that also reduce oxidative stress and pain. But today, instead, we jump to pharmaceutical agents as the first or even only choice, which is a shame. I read recently that over 128,000 people die every year because of prescription medications,[1] and I'm not talking about overdoses; rather, these are people taking the proper dose of medications, properly prescribed. It's become the fourth leading cause of death in the United States. We have to be cognizant and cautious and shouldn't just jump to pharmaceuticals as our first choice.

SOMERS: Are you trying to align with nature?

MAGAZINER: Nature certainly knows best, and we've deviated way too much in the last fifty years. But the pendulum is starting to swing back, and people are starting to return to nature. There is a rise in organic food supplies and sales, and more people are starting to use natural cleaning agents around their house and are also looking for farm-to-table restaurants. The pendulum initially went so far away, but it's starting to come back, and I hope it does.

SOMERS: Well, I think you're a big part of that.

MAGAZINER: We try. If everybody does their part, it would be great for the sum of the whole, and we'd all be on a better track toward good health.

SOMERS: Are you able to use CBD oil in New Jersey?

MAGAZINER: CBD [extracted from hemp] is not as legal in New Jersey as it is in California, but currently we have dispensaries, and doctors can give a patient, if they feel they have the right indications, a card allowing them to purchase medical marijuana. Non-THC CBD is legal to be sold in New Jersey and most states, as it is for pain and anxiety and it is nonhallucinogenic. We use a lot of CBD. We just have to be cautious, because some CBD is derived from industrial hemp, and that can sometimes have some high levels of heavy metals.

You should ask wherever you're buying it from for a certificate of authenticity, if possible, to show that it's organic and doesn't have any heavy metals. Also, for CBD to be most effective, it should have what we call natural-occurring terpenes. These are different substances from naturally occurring plants that allow for the full effect, the *entourage effect*. Terpenes are what give certain plants their aroma, and they can have powerful health benefits. CBD can be used orally or topically to take the edge off. It's good for sleep, depression, anxiety, and for pain. CBD is very safe and very effective.

SOMERS: Do you feel we're better off using a natural remedy than putting foreign molecules in our body?

MAGAZINER: Most of the time natural is best. Let's face it, there are very toxic things in the environment that are natural, so you have to be careful. Radon, for example: it's in the soil, but it can creep through the foundation of a house and cause lung cancer. There are certain toxic and poisonous mushrooms. I just mean, with a few exceptions, natural remedies should be our first choice; in other words, let's see what nature provided, because it generally won't have side effects or at least the intensity of the side effects.

I explain this to my patients when people have depression or anxiety, they don't have a deficiency of Prozac or they don't have a deficiency of Wellbutrin and Zoloft, right? But they may have a deficiency of certain B vitamins or certain neurotransmitters or certain hormones, so why not go in that direction first? That's what we do; we always try to use nature. The human body is a bunch of molecules and cells that are a mixture of amino acids, vitamins, minerals, cofactors, and fatty acids.

SOMERS: I believe bioidentical hormones are a game changer. Do you?

MAGAZINER: Absolutely. I think of all the things I have done in the last thirty-two years of my private practice; bioidentical hormone replacement probably makes the quickest and most dramatic change in people's lives. But once again, you have to know how to utilize it right. You have to know how to dose it, how do you assess it, how do you follow your patients appropriately. It's not a one-size-fits-all mentality, at least not for me. I individualize it for each patient. Fortunately, I learned this from

Dr. Jonathan Wright thirty-three years ago. I was with him for a year in his practice.

SOMERS: Lucky you.

MAGAZINER: Listen, he is a phenomenal doctor. He's my mentor. He taught me more than any person ever taught me in my life as far as medical treatments.

SOMERS: And he's so generous with his knowledge.

MAGAZINER: Dr. Jonathan Wright is the best in my opinion, fantastic. So, yes, we use a whole different array of different hormones. They need to be individualized, and the patients need to be monitored regularly. I have my patients fill out a questionnaire and have them rate their symptoms from one to ten. That way I can see very clearly when they come back for the follow-up visits how they're doing. I am able to see what areas have improved and what hasn't. If certain areas have not yet improved, then I need to make adjustments in one way or another. The women all concur it's one of the best things that they've ever done for themselves.

SOMERS: Well, yes, it gives them their "selves" back and in many ways better than ever. When men come in, do you have to sell them, or are they already sold?

MAGAZINER: Men are different. I usually have to explain and sell them on the concept.

SOMERS: Do men still feel hormone replacement, especially testosterone, is an attack against their "manhood"?

MAGAZINER: With a few exceptions, but men are generally not as good a patient as a woman, and they tend not to go to the doctor as much. They tend to deny their conditions and just want the simple fix. Also, they think they're invincible. So, yes, men have to be convinced that this is something to assess and to evaluate and to potentially treat them.

SOMERS: Is it because of the notion that it's only about erections?

MAGAZINER: Yes, but you just mentioned the heart and that there are many testosterone receptors in the heart compared to most other organs. So testosterone must be doing something quite important if there's that many receptors in the heart. I try to explain this to my patients.

SOMERS: What kills men?

MAGAZINER: Heart disease, heart attacks, that's it, number one. But certainly cancer, diabetes, and obesity are contributing quite a bit.

SOMERS: So it has to do with heart health and bone strength, right?

MAGAZINER: Correct. Actually, there are receptors all over the body for most of these hormones. It's not just the sexual organs; it's also the heart, the bones, the liver and kidney, and of course, the brain.

SOMERS: When you first test women, do you test for all the hormones or just the majors and minors?

MAGAZINER: I check all those at once because they all work in concert together like a well-tuned orchestra sounds. If you want a well-tuned body, you have to look at all these things. Plus I understand that sometimes I only get one or two chances to see these patients; often they live a distance away, and they've traveled for two hours, four hours, or even more. So I have to use my time with them judiciously, and the more thorough my exam, the better their health.

SOMERS: Do you do comprehensive lab work once a year or once every couple of years?

MAGAZINER: It depends. Once a year, once every two, depending.

SOMERS: Then in between they call you with symptoms, which would be an indicator to you that the ratio is not right?

MAGAZINER: Correct. I follow up with the hormone patients initially every two months but eventually every six months, and eventually, if they're doing well, it could be once a year, especially if they're all on a good track and they're doing fine.

SOMERS: Does chronic high cortisol lead to heart attack and stroke?

MAGAZINER: It's certainly one of the major factors and also leads to diabetes, and diabetes leads to stroke and heart attack as well. Once the endocrine system gets imbalanced, many different things can go awry as far as chronic illness and acute illness. As our body ages and we develop more oxidative stress, there's loss of mitochondrial function, and that's involved with the hormone dysregulation as well. So at the same time as addressing hormone imbalance, I also have to think about the sources of oxidative stress and sources of potential mitochondrial dysfunction, because that's where we make our cellular energy. It's called ATP, that's the energy center in the mitochondria. Mitochondria are so important that they comprise about ten percent of our body weight.

SOMERS: I didn't know that, but it makes sense. It's easy to build up about nine pounds of bugs [*H. pylori*, etc.] in our GI tracts, so of course mitochondria could make up ten percent of our body weight.[2] Can we rev up mitochondrial energy again?

MAGAZINER: Yes. It's hard, but you can. The number one complaint in any doctor's office is fatigue, lack of energy, and part of that is frequently due to these mitochondria dying off as we get older, so we have to try to protect them. How do you protect them? Well, one way is by trying to minimize the exposure to various environmental chemicals because they disrupt and destroy mitochondria. The plastics we're drinking out of: plastic bottles are a major problem with destroying mitochondrial function.

We have to clean up our environment and clean up our food supply from being sprayed with pesticides and herbicides. Chemicals are what we call hormone disruptors and mitochondrial disruptors. As far as getting the mitochondria [energy] to function better, we have to oxygenate our tissues. Oxygen is the most important element with regard to getting the mitochondria to work better.

SOMERS: How do we do that?

MAGAZINER: Exercise is important; there are other different options like hyperbaric oxygen. We use oxaloacetate, which is a supplement that seems to help improve mitochondrial function.

SOMERS: Where does CoQ10 enter into this?

MAGAZINER: CoQ10 is part of a very important cofactor in electron transport, helping the mitochondria work better. I measure CoQ10 levels, and we see many people are low or suboptimal, which brings up another topic, and that's the difference between suboptimal and normal ranges and optimal ranges. I feel that's another big problem with conventional medicine that is overlooked. They look at a person's lab, and they say, "Oh, you're normal," but I strive for optimal levels in my patients.

SOMERS: For their age?

MAGAZINER: Yeah, well, not even for their age. Like vitamin D normal is from 30 to 100 nanograms per milliliter, so at a range of 34 their doctors tell them, "You're fine." Well, the reality is that's not optimal vitamin D_3 to prevent diseases like cancer, which is probably a 25-hydroxyvitamin D blood level of 60 or 80 nanograms per milliliter, based on LabCorp's testing method, so 34 nanograms per milliliter is not going to cut it if you're hoping to prevent certain illnesses.

SOMERS: So in terms of supplementation, is that 5,000 IU, is it 10,000?

MAGAZINER: I get asked that all the time, I believe it's as much as you have to take to get your blood levels up to that range that I just mentioned of about 60 to 80. So it's hard to tell you exactly how much because everybody's a little bit different.

SOMERS: Once again it's individualized, as in what I need is different from what you need.

MAGAZINER: As you know, there are different kinds of estrogens in the body, and some are more troublesome than others and some are more protective. That's why you need a doctor who really understands the physiology and metabolism of these hormones. If someone's labs seem too high, you also have to look at whether they are symptomatic or not. There's too much in conventional medicine where we treat the lab work rather than using the lab work as a guide but not as a final plan for treatment. You have to look at the patient: How is your patient doing? How is he or she feeling?

SOMERS: It must be much easier to treat patients who are believers.

MAGAZINER: No question about it. I have some patients that leave me feeling so stressed, so drained after seeing them because everything I say they want to fight, but I will always try my best. Some simply aren't ready to make changes.

SOMERS: What are your feelings about eating healthy fats?

MAGAZINER: There's nothing wrong with eating healthy fats: avocados, olive oil, almonds, walnuts, salmon, those are all healthy foods. The big factor in good health is eating real food. The rest of it is junk. If we eat what nature has provided for us, most of the time that's going to be pretty good for us. Nature did not provide a McDonald's milkshake or French fries; these are loaded with various chemicals, excess omega-6 fats, and not naturally occurring fats. Things that are here on Planet Earth, that grow from trees or the soil, if they're fats, they're generally fine for us. Look at the Mediterranean countries: they eat lots of fat, and they're generally fine, because they're eating the right fats. There's a difference. You know, it's not just "Can we eat fat?," it's that we have to eat the right fats. So important.

SOMERS: Yeah, I've never seen a canola plant.

MAGAZINER: Right, exactly.

SOMERS: So what I'm getting from you is that food is medicine.

MAGAZINER: Right. That's why food should be our foundation for improving a person's life. We make decisions to eat four, five, six times a day, depending on who you are. Food can be pro-inflammatory or anti-inflammatory. Every time we eat, I tell my patients, "As you're eating or when you're getting ready to eat, ask yourself if you think this particular food will be health enhancing or perhaps health inhibiting." At least it makes you think twice before you eat. I'm not perfect and most of us aren't perfect, but it makes you think twice.

SOMERS: Do you have other doctors in your clinic?

MAGAZINER: Yes, I am the main [alpha] doctor, plus I have another doctor and also a naturopathic doctor. I also have a physician's assistant as well, so we have a total of four different medical providers in our office, and of course nurses and administrative team members.

SOMERS: When leaky gut happens, do these chemicals get to the brain and start to shrink the pituitary and hypothalamus?

MAGAZINER: Well, we do get cortical atrophy, so the brain itself, the cortex, which is the outer layer or uppermost layer of the brain, does age, and because of a lot of reasons, such as stress, free radicals, or rancid oils, the brain begins to involute and shrink. We also know that too much dietary sugar, which can also lead to insulin resistance, and exposure to various chemicals and heavy metals like lead or mercury can lead to brain dysfunction. I can't say for a fact whether the pituitary and hypothalamus themselves shrink, but I know that the cerebral cortex does as part of the aging process. We see that on PET scans.

SOMERS: Among children twelve to seventeen years of age, 5.2 percent are taking ADHD medication; among children ages twelve to seventeen with ADHD, 62 percent, according to studies, were taking medication to treat ADHD.[3] Shocking. Where will this lead?

MAGAZINER: Well, we're creating a whole culture turning to medication for any illness or condition. Once again, we should be looking for the potential causes of *why* a person isn't able to learn effectively and why they can't sit still and why they're not focusing. We do find many times that there's a metabolic reason, ranging from nutritional factors to nutrients to fatty acids to food sensitivities to even mold spores and mold toxins to various other chemical exposures. That's why I'm saying we need to be a detective as well as a good clinician. The job is to try to decipher the weaknesses and imbalances in that person's biochemistry rather than simply recommending a drug to cover up symptoms.

SOMERS: What are you doing in your arena about thyroid?

MAGAZINER: We're trying to remove, first of all, the environmental estrogens and a lot of the environmental toxins because they can all suppress thyroid function. I warn my patients about the dangers of plastics, which negatively affect thyroid function because they're endocrine disruptors. We also try to use different cofactors that build up the thyroid, like minerals such as zinc, manganese, and magnesium. We also check for iodine levels and selenium. And sometimes we use glandular substances such as thyroid glandular substances that may be beneficial as well.

The thyroid is also a hard gland to analyze or to assess properly or fully just from lab work alone. So using clinical symptoms, we have to also look at the patient once again and not just treat the lab work but treat the patient. If they have all the symptoms of low or high thyroid but have normal lab work, they may feel a heck of a lot better if we also treat them for thyroid dysfunction.

SOMERS: How significant is the inability to absorb minerals and nutrients?

MAGAZINER: There are so many reasons why a person may not be absorbing nutrients. Firstly, the nutrients in our food today are much more depleted than they were years ago, in part because the soil is becoming more devitalized because of all the insults we do to it, between herbicides, pesticides, and other chemical agents we utilize. Also, people are taking more and more medications than ever before: antacids and also acid blockers. It's crazy; they're on these things for years instead of a month or two if they have a small problem. Sometimes I see patients who have been on antacids for six years. When I ask, "Why are you still on this?," they say, "Well, my doctor told me I had acid reflux when he did an endoscopy five years ago." "It's crazy," I tell them. "You can't just rely on those things because they deplete your nutrient levels, you won't absorb your minerals." Various other medicines, antibiotics, and calcium channel blockers will have an adverse effect on nutrient absorption in regards to the vitamins and minerals. This can then lead to additional health problems that weren't present in the first place.

SOMERS: Why do we care if we absorb or not?

MAGAZINER: The body doesn't work without minerals and nutrients. A lot of people don't utilize their nutrients that well. They may be taking them for leaky gut and other factors, but they're just unable to get the minerals and nutrients into the tissues. Sometimes their transporters are adversely affected and they're not being transported to the appropriate places in their body.

SOMERS: Sort of like the car has gas, but if you put that gas into the wrong tank, like the carburetor, the car's not going to run?

MAGAZINER: Yes, a lot of it has to do with the food choices, food storage, food transportation, depleted soil. It's no longer organic, the GMOs and so many pesticides and herbicides sprayed on the foods today. All those factors are impinging our ability to absorb the nutrients effectively and optimally.

SOMERS: When someone comes in and they're highly toxic, do you do chelation?

MAGAZINER: We do a lot of chelation, but I primarily do it for heavy metals. People don't even realize that they're frequently walking around with high levels of lead, mercury, cadmium, or gadolinium, which you often get from X-ray contrast material.

SOMERS: MRIs?

MAGAZINER: Yes, MRIs where contrast is used and PET scans. I had a patient today who had high levels of gadolinium, lead, mercury, and thallium as well. He didn't realize it. Unless you test them and unless you have that level of suspicion as a physician, they won't realize that they have high levels and the damage it is creating.

SOMERS: Like a brewing storm. If you don't address it, what's the eventual outcome?

MAGAZINER: Your health will continue to decline, but you may not associate it to metals even though you have a chronic condition like autoimmune disease or chronic rheumatoid arthritis. Or your cancer may progress, because, you know, these metals will inhibit the mitochondria, damage your cells, and disrupt the hormone function of the body. So it's important to address the problem. We do a lot of intravenous chelation in my practice, which means that this substance basically grabs or binds on to different metals to help excrete them from the body.

SOMERS: And how do you feel about far-infrared sauna?

MAGAZINER: Love it. I have one in my office. It's a nice way of detoxifying, safe and very effective; it's another modality I believe should be added to a good detox and rejuvenation program.

SOMERS: The planet has been so terribly damaged; I believe what you're saying is "It's not going to go away, but here's how you can thrive and survive."

MAGAZINER: If we all make an effort and demand more chemical-free items, whether in our food, cleaning agents around the house, lawn care, or whatever, those changes will go a long way toward surviving and thriving. If we can select organic foods, the supermarkets will see there's a demand and they will continue to provide it with enthusiasm. The same with the restaurants.

It's crucial to change. We've been using toxic containers and chemicals for fifty years, and now we're seeing the ill effects: birth defects, infertility, hyperactivity, autism, dementia, autoimmune conditions, even more cancers and at younger ages. All these conditions are rising, and it's alarming.

Virtually every single one of us has traces of toxicity in our bodies, which we didn't have fifty and seventy years ago. We still need grassroots efforts by the public, who should demand to be told the real dangers of these chemical substances and continue educating ourselves.

SOMERS: Is it a pipe dream to want to get gut flora balanced so babies are born without toxins?

MAGAZINER: We do need to do better with prenatal health. It's an area that has great room for expansion in the years to come. It's not just probiotics; it's getting the mother and father to understand they need to reduce their chemical intake overall, not only during the pregnancy but before the preconception time.

SOMERS: How do they do that?

MAGAZINER: They have to clean up their bodies through detoxification and food choices, clean up the environment around them, drink clean, filtered water, avoid alcohol, and exercise regularly. A big start would be to eat only organic food starting three months before conception and go from there.

SOMERS: Do you recommend probiotics to your patients as part of your curriculum?

MAGAZINER: Yes, because there are so many elements working against us—environmental, over-the-counter drugs, prescription pharmaceuticals, poor dietary intake, and too much alcohol—that disrupt the balance in the GI tract and destroy it. There are roughly two to three times more bacteria in our GI tract than there are cells in our entire body, and we have to respect these healthy bacteria and treat them well.

SOMERS: Balance is crucial?

MAGAZINER: We have to respect balance, and unfortunately, we don't. Too many times, a person walks into a doctor's office with sniffles, a cold, congestion, and they get offered an antibiotic. Patients don't realize the true negative effects some of the medications have on their overall health, especially gut health.

In scientific studies, researchers intentionally exposed certain rats and hamsters to chemicals and then intentionally did not expose their offspring. Even after three generations, they still found traces of this stuff. So think what might be happening in humans. It takes a lifetime to study this sort of thing. But we have to start questioning, What are we really doing to ourselves?

SOMERS: I wholeheartedly agree. I wrote an entire book about the toxic effects on your health, called TOX-SICK. Clear this up for my readers: Does it make you more susceptible to cancer by taking bioidentical hormones?

MAGAZINER: When it's done responsibly and properly balanced, it actually lessens your chance of contracting cancer. I've seen it many times over in the last thirty-two years of my own private practice. But that's not to say that it's done properly by everybody; if a woman is taking too much estrone (potentially pro-carcinogenic) and not balancing it with estriol (likely cancer protective), for example, and if they're not looking at the ratios, et cetera, you might put them at risk for cancer. So replacement has to be done carefully, wisely, judiciously, and the patients need to be followed properly by a skilled and experienced clinician.

Overall, I believe with responsible replacement we have lowered the risk. Most literature has shown that, on the other hand, synthetic hormones like medroxyprogesterone have been shown that they may increase your risk of cancer. Unfortunately, the media links it all together and they just use the word *hormones*, and sadly they don't distinguish the difference, so that's where the myth of hormones causing cancer comes from.

SOMERS: What are you thinking and dreaming about for the future of this new way to age and the direction of alternative and functional medicine?

MAGAZINER: Several things. In the future it's very possible that as we begin to understand people's genetics better as time goes on—it's only in its infancy—but in the future, we might be able to tailor people's treatments better predicated in part on their genetic susceptibility toward disease. We are maybe five or ten years away from true personalized medicine. The microbiome will be a player; also, eventually we're going to have the ability to identify far greater information than where we are today as to what is going on in someone's gut, and we may be able to target certain treatments predicated on their microbiome as well as their genetics. In our office we are actively looking for what we call early warning signs of disease by identifying biomarkers; rather than waiting until you have diabetes, for example, let's focus and work on *prevention* first. The best way to treat any disease is to not get it in the first place.

SOMERS: Thank you, Allan, for your time and continued great work.

CHAPTER 2

WHAT DO YOU FEAR MOST ABOUT AGING?

You control your decisions, you control your actions, you control your outcome.
—David Kekich

When we look at aging people with all their ailments—diminishing mobility, decreasing brain function, diseases (usually one of the big three: cancer, heart disease, Alzheimer's)—we feel a sense of dread and hope that somehow this will not be our fate.

The good news is that it doesn't have to be—*YOU are in charge of your outcome.* It's all up to you. We choose our life, and it's important to know that the choices you make today, both good and bad, will directly affect your health and quality of life later on.

When we are young and invincible, some of us drink, smoke, disregard warnings about chemicals, don't value sleep; we allow stress to overcome us, all the while thinking it doesn't matter; after all, we are young, strong, vibrant.

But it all does matter, and the sooner and younger you understand this, the better your future outcome will be. Just yesterday I had a devastatingly sad conversation with a dear friend, a good person who is in the entertainment world. Being on the road is the same for most performers, and I understand this as I spent twenty-five years performing on the road until the day I heard those three words: "You have cancer." After digesting that shocking statement, I was overwhelmed by one thought: What had I done in my diet and lifestyle up to this point to play host to this monster disease? While on the road, like most performers, you can't eat on show day. You are too revved up, too excited, you have no appetite. Maybe you eat some junk food to tide you over. When the show ends, you are suddenly ravenous, but it's late and nothing is open except fast-food places selling processed foods, GMO foods, poor-quality (carcinogenic) foods, foods containing shelf-life-extending chemicals, and more. Now multiply by years of this lifestyle, and is it any wonder that cancer had invaded my body? What did I expect from years of filling myself with nonfoods and chemicals? This is most likely the same scenario as that of my entertainer friend above, and now he has incurable abdominal cancer and has been told to "get his things in order" as there is no longer any hope.

The sadness in his voice overwhelmed me, and I listened helplessly. He did not know or realize that those seemingly benign daily choices had been his death sentence. Chemicals and toxins had built up in him until his liver had given out; his high-glycemic diet had fueled tumor cell proliferation; and now he was dying. I can think of so many more friends who were "road dogs"; a great percentage of them are now either dead or have cancer or Alzheimer's disease. What's the common thread? I think we all know.

I have an exercise I do at the end of each day: I make an imaginary list in my head; on one side I place all the negative choices I made that day and on the other side the positive ones. Each night I analyze my choices to keep tabs on what I can expect as my eventual outcome. It puts me, rather than fate, into control. Just listing one day's choices can be a great indicator of what you can expect of your eventual outcome. It puts you in control.

People are always surprised when disease befalls them, but if your negative choices outweigh the good ones, what do you expect?

Imagine you owned a Maserati, one of the finest cars in the world. You would never put inferior fuel into a Maserati, yet so often we take our body, the greatest machine of all time, a true masterpiece, for granted, thoughtlessly filling it with inferior fuel (food), chemicals, and toxins. In our workaholic world we don't rest our body properly, lubricate it internally with good-quality oils, or value it—until the day comes when it gives out. Then what? You can't buy a new one, so you are stuck with all the self-inflicted damage, which in many cases is irreversible.

This is your only body, and each choice leads you toward good health and positive lifestyle habits—or away from them. It's that simple.

You can't eat sugar every day and be healthy. Sugar should be a treat, a reward. It's important to realize that sugar is cancer's favorite food, a "happy meal" of sorts. When you are hooked on sugar, how can you get off it? Here's a simple fix: There are supplements that take away cravings, like one my company makes called Dopa Renew (go to www.suzanne somers.com to order it). This supplement and others like it are nondrug. Here's how it works: Dopamine is one of our "feel-good" neurotransmitters. As we age, these neurotransmitters can decline. When they do, we often look for ways to get a "dopamine hit" by reaching for caffeine, sugar, junk food, or alcohol. But as we know, the fix is only temporary. Dopa Renew with wild green oat extract helps maintain neurotransmitter function and overall youthful cognitive support. Plus, it has been shown to assist with age-related mild temporary memory loss as well as promote cardiovascular health. Best of all, your sugar cravings diminish—for some it's sugar, or nutritionless fast food, or alcohol—leading to better health and weight loss.

Interview with

DR. JONATHAN WRIGHT

I have interviewed Dr. Wright for several of my books. He is a font of information, and he is also my friend and doctor. Whenever I have a question, from the simplest to the most complex, he always seems to have the answers. I like his kind of medicine, and in all my years with him he has never pulled out a prescription pad. He copies nature. As you will read in this interview, he knows what others don't. I remember calling him one day to ask, "What are these spots I'm getting on my arms lately?" Without hesitation he said, "Take bilberry and hawthorn supplements." Guess what? My spots went away. He knows things like this.

There was a time when you'd go to the doctor and sit for an hour or more discussing your health, but things have changed, and now, depending on your coverage, you may only get five minutes. I have a doctor friend in Canada who because of socialized medicine sees seventy patients a day. I asked him, "How can you do that?" He answered, "I say things like 'It's going around.' "

Dr. Wright is a fearless renegade, highly educated, with degrees in cultural anthropology and medicine from Harvard and the University of Michigan. Throughout the years, he has been harassed, ridiculed, and persecuted because of his rejection of the modern "allopathic-only" approach to medicine.

> Dr. Wright wrote the first prescriptions for comprehensive bio-identical hormones over forty years ago, at a time when very few people had ever heard of them.

He is a champion of natural medicines in the United States and is a sought-after teacher and lecturer to doctors and at conferences. His patients flock to him in his Tahoma Clinic in Washington State.

In forty years, I've never healed a patient; they heal themselves.

—Jonathan Wright

His modesty notwithstanding, more than thirty-five thousand patients have consulted him.

He is a sought-after speaker in Europe and a hero in Japan, and more than three thousand professionals have put their careers on hold to attend his famous seminars. Instead of aiming a chemical howitzer at health problems, which is the approach of today's standard of care, Dr. Wright attacks patients' health with the deft precision of a martial arts master. On the one hand, he utilizes treatments and breakthroughs so sophisticated that the medical establishment would rather ridicule them than embrace them for fear of looking ignorant or worse; on the other hand, so much of what he does is like the old country doctor who tells you to go home and drink plenty of fluids and get lots of rest. It's a thrill for me to speak to him and bring his knowledge to you. I like to say, "Dr. Wright is always right." We'll hear from Dr. Wright in several chapters of this book, but here he'll address some of the most common—and scariest—symptoms of aging, such as arthritis, weight gain, sleeplessness, hair loss, and skin cancer.

SOMERS: Thank you for your time, Jonathan. I have admired your work and your ethics since we first met twenty years ago at the alternative doctors' conference. As I said in your introduction, you were the first doctor to prescribe bioidentical hormones in North America forty years ago. That took a lot of courage, and you paid the price. We are going to talk about that, but let's start with the hot topic of the day: stem cells. How do you feel about stem cells?

WRIGHT: They have their place, but the problem is, they don't always address the cause. For example, we hear about stem cells for osteoarthritis, and in fact, they do help a lot of people. I will not argue with that. They also are very pricey. A patient told me that the total cost for getting stem cell treatment for a hip joint was something like $7,500 to $8,000.

Now, they did work for him, but here's the thing: the cause of the osteoarthritis is simply a lack of niacinamide, and you know how much niacinamide costs down at the health food store. It's one of the lowest-priced supplements out there. Researchers found when cartilage is deteriorating, it's because the cartilage cells are no longer supplied with sufficient energy molecules—ATP—by their mitochondria, which, as you know, are the little energy engines within all cells including cartilage cells.

SOMERS: Explain why we care about ATP.

ADENOSINE TRIPHOSPHATE (ATP)

Adenosine triphosphate (ATP) is the primary energy carrier in all living organisms on Earth. Microorganisms capture and store energy metabolized from food and light sources in the form of ATP.

When cells require energy, ATP is broken down through hydrolysis. The high-energy bond is broken, and a phosphoryl group is removed. The energy released by this process is used to drive various cellular processes. ATP is constantly formed and broken down as it participates in biological reactions and is central to the health and growth of all life. Without it, cells could not transfer energy from one location to another, making it impossible for organisms to grow and reproduce!

WRIGHT: Mitochondria make ATP, and ATP is the energy molecule, and all cells need this energy to thrive.

If cells aren't getting enough energy, they start to deteriorate. In the 1940s, Dr. William Kaufman found that sufficient niacinamide would start to take away the pain of osteoarthritis within three to four weeks, and by the end of three to four months, the very large majority of those with this issue had no more osteoarthritis pain. I read his 1949 book in 1974, and as a result I haven't had to send anyone for replacement—nobody. With niacinamide the pain subsided and they were able to walk again with no pain. The niacinamide discovery was made in the forties, but it took until about three or four years ago for researchers to finally figure out that niacinamide would reactivate the mitochondria inside the cartilage cells,[1] and get them to make more energy. By supplementing niacinamide, one can treat the cause of osteoarthritis by understanding that it is a lack of sufficient niacinamide.

SOMERS: Just this information alone is worth reading this book. Is it a derivative of niacin?

WRIGHT: They are in the same family, but it's kind of like a cousin.

SOMERS: Does one experience side effects similar to niacin, the flushing and the itching?

WRIGHT: No, thank goodness. Niacin gives the hot flash, and often a really sweaty hot flash at times. Niacinamide does not give that side effect. In fact, there are no side effects unless we take more than our livers want to process, and then our livers will tell us by giving us a low-grade nausea, kind of like getting a little seasick; if that happens, it tells you you're taking too much and to pull back. However, it takes a lot to achieve too much. Dr. William Kaufman was using very high doses back in the 1940s, and less than ten percent were getting nauseated with it. Time-release technology has rescued people from that, and now niacinamide is made in 1,500 milligrams, time released, that you only take morning and evening. If you don't get nauseous, you keep on taking it to control your joint pain and avoid joint surgery or stem cell treatment.

SOMERS: Fantastic. The body has a language.

WRIGHT: Definitely. In fact, when people first come to the clinic, I can tell from looking at them what are most likely their deficiencies. The body tells us so much with signs and symptoms.

SOMERS: I love this kind of information.

WRIGHT: Here's some interesting information: for instance, if a person has a large callus on their heels, that's a sign of vitamin A deficiency. Okay, what are we doing, treating a callus? No. We're responding to a body signal that says the whole body needs vitamin A. If a person takes enough vitamin A for a period of time, usually 50,000 units daily for an adult, which is quite safe unless you're pregnant, that callus will usually be gone in about six months.

A psychiatrist, Dr. Carl Pfeiffer, who went into nutritional medicine, taught us if we have white spots on our nails, that means we have zinc deficiency.

So if you take enough zinc the white spots go away, but you aren't just treating white spots on your nails, you're treating your zinc insufficiency. Another one: if you have too much earwax, your body needs to make more omega-3 fatty acids. So we counsel people to get the wax cleaned out and then start taking one and a half tablespoons of fish oil or cod liver oil twice a day. No kidding, that's a lot.

Just to make sure that much fish oil doesn't cause any adverse effects in the long run—as large quantities can cause something called lipid peroxidation—vitamin E should be used along with the fish oil, 400 or 500 units daily. You'll notice your earwax doesn't come back, and by the way, your dry skin will get better, too. If you're tired of taking that much fish oil, cut it back and give that some time. If your excess earwax doesn't come back, cut it back again. But your body will "talk" to you; when you cut the fish oil back enough, your excess earwax will return, and that's your body telling you that you need more fish oil than you're taking at that time. You adjust to what your body tells you. A very few of us have so much earwax that we need two tablespoonfuls a day or more to keep it under control, but that's very unusual.

SOMERS: What is generally wrong or ailing with people who come to you as a patient?

WRIGHT: I'd say a lack of realization that we're living in a very, very unnatural world. You made a terrific point of that in your book called *TOX-SICK*. Now, why is that so important? As far as we know, humans have been around for hundreds of thousands of years at least. And for most of that time humans were either created for or adapted to the natural environment of Planet Earth. When we deviate from that natural environment, our bodies don't stay healthy.

As you've pointed out in your book, there's the toxic chemicals, toxic metals, all of which get into people's bodies and systems. Our great-grandparents didn't have to go around detoxifying themselves to stay healthy, but today if we're going to stay healthy and we cannot escape the toxic pollution, we have to take extreme measures. It doesn't matter anymore if you live at the North Pole, because even there they have found that the penguins have lead and cadmium in their fat. Good grief.

So one thing we do with those who are trying for optimal health and longevity is to have tests done for levels of many common toxins and if needed suggest a detoxification method for their particular toxicities.

SOMERS: What about diet? Everyone is afraid of meat. What are your thoughts?

WRIGHT: Did you know that in the 1850s and 1860s, meat was considered healthful for us? Then that same meat, and I'm talking about mostly cattle meat, became less and less healthful.

SOMERS: Why is that?

WRIGHT: It was all organic back then compared to today. Not much in the way of chemicals, pesticides, or herbicides back then.[2] But now they've messed with nature. Also, people who raised cows discovered that if they had those cattle eating grains, they got fatter.

SOMERS: Cows are born to eat grass, but then we started feeding them corn, which goes against their natural evolution and they develop things like *E. coli* infections.

WRIGHT: Yes. The "new-style" cattle ranchers claimed that the meat tasted better and they could get it to market sooner, so we have what's called grain-fed beef. Grass-fed is nature's alternative, but it's a silly term, because nobody feeds the beef grass; they eat it themselves.

SOMERS: Cattle have been eating grass ever since there have been cattle. How does feeding cows corn and grains affect them?

WRIGHT: It gives you meat with more omega-6 fatty acids, which are pro-inflammatory, so eating grain-fed cattle is not good for us because of the overload of omega-6. Grain-fed cows cause health problems because it is another deviation from nature. When cattle first evolved, there wasn't any grain farming, so all they could eat was grass, and their bodies adapted. Meat from cows who eat what nature intended—grass—contains omega-3 fatty acids, which, as most of us know, are anti-inflammatory.

SOMERS: What about milk and dairy?

WRIGHT: The Harvard study of 28,000 male physicians showed that the more milk men drank, the more prostate cancer they got. The Harvard study of many more female nurses showed the more milk they drank, the more osteoporosis they got. So it poses the question: Did nature and creation intend for people to drink the milk of another species? Probably not. Think about this: When a little calf is born, it's not so little, is it? It can walk right away, and it has a tiny brain, whereas when a little human is born, it can't walk until it's over a year old, and it's got a big brain, so obviously, the composition of the milk for each species is the milk that belongs in that species, and if we deviate from that, some of us are going to get in trouble.

A lot of the people I see unknowingly have had milk allergies all their life, and it's been giving them trouble starting in childhood and continuing with often different symptoms into adulthood. A book by Dr. Frank Oski, who was chair of the Department of Pediatrics at Johns Hopkins University, paid attention to a letter sent to him by an Alabama pediatrician and republished the results of his research in his book that **if you've ever had a strep throat, you are a milk-allergic person.** It's as simple as that.

SOMERS: I've never heard that, but I had strep throat all throughout childhood and I bloat every time I consume dairy. Hmmm . . .

WRIGHT: I always ask when kids are having any kind of health problem, "Did you ever as a child or as a young adult have strep throat?" If the answer is yes, we always find in their allergy tests milk antibodies. Not only that, I can be working with sixty-five-year-olds who have had strep throat as a kid and find milk antibodies even if they're not drinking milk anymore.

SOMERS: Do you know how revelatory this is? I never pieced this together; I had chronic strep throat as a kid, and now I just learned from you I shouldn't have milk or cow cheese.

WRIGHT: Yes, people who have had strep throats are the ones who absolutely should never have milk or dairy. There's this old argument between Louis Pasteur and his opponent Antoine Béchamp. Pasteur says, "No, it's the germ that causes the infection." Béchamp says, "No, no, no, it's the milieu," which is French for the environment. What Béchamp was saying is that it's the environment, and he was correct. Going against nature allows the strep to proliferate. Louis Pasteur was said to have remarked on his deathbed that Béchamp was right after all. No kidding.

SOMERS: That was nice of him. So cheese is also the aggravator for the "strepers." Say no, please!

WRIGHT: Some people can get by with some cheese and it only bothers them a little, but for anybody who's ever had a strep throat, forget the stuff, folks. You'll be healthier.

SOMERS: Oh, well, thanks. An "Aha!" moment. Boo-hoo. I'll miss my Brillat [cow] cheese with truffle honey on fig crackers. I'll live.

WRIGHT: **I believe deviating from nature is what gets us into trouble. I copy nature as exactly as I can and recommend that people copy as closely as they can. Nature and creation originally intended us to live with that template if we're going to stay the healthiest.**

SOMERS: Is nutrition where your passions lie?

WRIGHT: Well, yes and no. Yes, because there is more research into the original elements that make up the human body, otherwise known as nutrients, but there is also another very important field, and that is *frequencies*. Now, Suzanne, did you know that homeopathic medicine is nothing more than frequencies? It's not laser frequencies, it's not radio frequencies. Human bodies have energies that vibrate at certain frequencies.

I am not a homeopath, but I have respect for the doctors who practice homeopathy because they are actually applying nature's natural frequencies that belong in human bodies, and certain remedies need certain frequencies for creating balance and healing.

When we're talking about good health, we have to be worried not only about the matter—the materials, atoms, and molecules—but also the frequencies at which everything vibrates. Even Albert Einstein said everything has its own frequency, every molecule has its own frequency. The reason this is so important, and thank you for allowing me to ramble on here, is that we are now living in a world of unnatural frequencies.

SOMERS: Like cell phones and electromagnetic fields?

WRIGHT: Yes, ma'am. Electromagnetic fields surround our devices, and research tells us that if a guy keeps a cell phone in his pocket too close to his testicles it may be why he can't get his wife pregnant. No kidding. It's interfering and creating the wrong frequencies.

SOMERS: I know a young boy who kept his cell phone in his pants pocket and developed a third testicle. But here's the problem: the devices aren't going away. They find more and more uses.

WRIGHT: Which is why, Suzanne, I wrote two newsletters called *Green Medicine Newsletter*, featuring an article by Dr. Arthur Firstenberg, PhD, who told us all about the hazards of cell phones. The second issue came out with research on how you can mitigate the damage from cell phones—for example, melatonin.

SOMERS: I take melatonin nightly because it promotes sleep but also for its antioxidant effects.

Switching subjects: How do we keep our hair?

MELATONIN

Melatonin is a hormone that cuts down on the damage from cell phone radiation significantly.

WRIGHT: Well, for ladies it's sometimes easier, because the older we all get, the less well we digest. It's not just our hormones that go down with age, but the stomach acid declines with age, the pancreatic enzymes decline with age.

SOMERS: Hair is determined by stomach acid?

WRIGHT: Yeah, hair maintenance definitely is.

SOMERS: Seems lack of stomach acid is the culprit in so many body issues.

WRIGHT: **Hydrochloric acid (HCl)** is one of many things that decline with age. Everyone knows estrogen and progesterone decline at menopause. Stomach acid also declines with age (and therefore causes digestive decline); this was researched and reported by Frances Vanzant, MD, and colleagues at the Mayo Clinic in 1932. Dr. Vanzant and her colleagues reviewed records of 3,746 people who had had their tummies pumped. Thankfully, we don't have to do that anymore, folks, because now there's a test called the **Heidelberg test**; it's a lot easier. The report told us that by the time we're in our sixties, we have a fifty percent chance—women 58.8 percent, men 50.1 percent—of declining stomach acid. That's a 3,746-person study from the Mayo Clinic, no less.

So something happens with time: we decline in hydrochloric acid, and the pancreas makes fewer digestive enzymes.

SOMERS: Do you mean hydrochloric acid with pepsin?

WRIGHT: Yes, it has to have pepsin, because pepsin is a protein-digesting enzyme that's activated by the hydrochloric acid.

However, less-than-optimal stomach acid for optimal digestion occurs at younger ages, too. When a premenopausal woman comes to my clinic and I notice she's losing her hair and/or her nails are going bad, I always recommend a stomach acid test. The large majority of those ladies' tests show that they are low on stomach acid.

With replacement of hydrochloric acid with pepsin, they digest their protein better because the protein is digested into amino acids, and the raw material for growing hair and nails is amino acids. Hair is protein, and amino acids become protein. I'm not going to tell you that's the only cause, but it's a major cause.

SOMERS: Now, what about guys with hair loss?

WRIGHT: That's a tough one, because there is testosterone turning into DHT, and all that. But there was one piece of research that was done in Southeast Asia. They actually had some of their students count every hair in every square centimeter in this one part of the man's head. I'm not kidding, they had to go count all the hairs in every square centimeter!

Then they had men who were losing hair take fairly high doses of tocotrienols, which are a particular form of vitamin E, and a few months later, they went back and counted every hair in every square centimeter again, not over the whole head, just on the part of the head that was counted. They found more hairs per square centimeter.

SOMERS: Well, hair loss is very vulnerable for men and women alike. Once again, I'm realizing these "things" that happen to us called aging are really about deficiencies. So by taking the tocotrienol family of vitamin E the hair grew back in men. That's great.

So our bodies are all about deficiencies and what's missing. What about autoimmune issues, fibromyalgia, lupus, MS, insufficient hydrochloric acid? Does autoimmune start in the gut?

WRIGHT: Yes, it's aggravated by the gut, but there are also other triggers for autoimmune disease. For example, we've all heard of psoriasis, which is actually an autoimmune reaction to a bacterium that causes stomach ulcers called *H. pylori* [*Helicobacter pylori*]. This was discovered by an Italian research team working to clear out *H. pylori* for people with stomach ulcers. They discovered when they got rid of the *H. pylori*, the psoriasis improved without having to use patent medicines to eliminate that bacteria. There are also other gut triggers for autoimmune disease. In his book *The Missing Diagnosis* [1983], Dr. Orian Truss describes a complete cure of lupus [an autoimmune disease] with elimination of a candida ["yeast"] infection.

SOMERS: What about rosacea? Does that originate in the gut?

WRIGHT: Oh, thank you, ma'am, I'm glad you brought that up. Killing rosacea is so easy. In 1920, researchers actually found and reported in *The Lancet* [then and now a major medical journal] the cause and cure for rosacea. If you find the cause, you can definitely treat it. Other researchers confirmed this cause and cure in other medical journals in 1925, 1927, 1928, and 1931. **Everybody with rosacea has low stomach acid**, and when you give them hydrochloric acid and pepsin to take with their meals, their rosacea goes away. In severe cases, rosacea will take a few take months to go away completely, but it will go away.

I worked with a guy from Chicago who came in with a bright red face, we checked his stomach acid with the Heidelberg capsule—that's the test we do at Tahoma Clinic—and sure enough, he was low on stomach acid. He sent us a picture from Chicago six months later, and for the first time since he was a teenager, and he was about fifty, he had no bright red face at all.

The modern so-called treatment for rosacea is to take antibiotics, the notion being it will kill the bacteria in your small intestine. Problem is, the antibiotic actually excretes the toxin that gives you rosacea. Hydrochloric acid doesn't allow those bacteria to grow. And besides that, replacing HCl improves your digestion, and that affects your whole body, so you don't just cure your rosacea, you improve your overall health, and that's what finding the cause usually does: It improves many things.

There's a wonderful book called *Death by Regulation* by Dr. Mary Ruwart. She points out the craziness as to why so many great solutions to medical problems are unavailable. Just for example, the Diamond Walnut Company, the biggest producer of walnuts, had on their website some thirty, that's over thirty, scientific studies showing that eating walnuts was good for cardiovascular health. They put the studies on their website and they were posted on the National Library of Medicine database. Then they got a warning letter from the FDA that if they didn't take down all that published research, the FDA was going to come and confiscate all their walnuts! They also did this to Michigan tart cherry growers.

So natural things rarely get approved. The only things that can get approved are patent medicines, upon which, when you have a patent, you can make megabucks.

SOMERS: Follow the money. That's why it's difficult to get TRH [thyrotropin-releasing hormone, which will be discussed later in this book]. I get mine from aging-matters.com.

Several years ago, you told me about an incredible cream for skin cancer. I've had tremendous results for three small skin cancers. For me it's a miracle, and I haven't had any dermatologist cutting things off my nose, which is great. I like my nose. It's called Curaderm. Is it easy to get?

WRIGHT: No, it's not easy to get. I wish it were.

SOMERS: Curaderm made from eggplant is for skin cancer. Explain what it does.

WRIGHT: Curaderm was researched by a brilliant PhD from Australia, Bill Cham. It was called to his attention by some cattle farmers in Australia that their cows got a certain kind of cancer on their eyeball, and when they did, the cows would rub their eyes against this particular plant and the cancer would go away. Well, Dr. Cham was intrigued, so he got some of the plants and did some research and found that they contained molecules that can only enter into cancer cells. They cannot enter into normal cells. That is the key. Therefore, they cannot hurt normal skin because they can't get into the normal cells, because cancer cells are different than normal cells.

Once cancer gets into the cells, it goes to the little bags of enzymes that are present in every cell in the body and also in cancer cells, which happen to be called lysosomes, and when they get into those lysosomes, they rupture them, and the cell digests itself to death.

SOMERS: That's fascinating. Enzymes are like little Pac-Men.

WRIGHT: No kidding. Now, there are two books; one is called *The Eggplant Cancer Cure*, and the other one is called *Inspired by Nature, Proven by Science*, and that one has all the footnotes, references, and all the studies. In *The Eggplant Cancer Cure* there's a picture of a person with a skin cancer that has eaten away the corner of their nose near the lip and the cheek, a very big, old skin cancer. So the person puts a little bit of this Curaderm cream—which, remember, can only get into cancer cells, it cannot get into normal cells—they put a little bit on there and put a Band-Aid over it and, twelve hours later, applied more and put a Band-Aid over it, and they kept doing that every twelve hours, and you can see in that book, it goes from looking like a cancer that was a big hole in the face back to looking normal, and it took twelve to fourteen weeks.

Now, here's the problem, and you can draw your own conclusions: this has cured every skin cancer for every person who's had it that I've ever worked with, and I haven't had to do a thing except tell them to go get some and use it.

SOMERS: I have had great success with it.

WRIGHT: Yes. Now, here's how good it works. It has cured over seventy-five thousand people in Australia, and guess what? Guess who complained, Suzanne? The Australasian College of Dermatologists. So what you said was exactly correct, competition here, and the dermatologists complained to the Australian version of the FDA and said, "Dr. Cham should not be allowed to sell this stuff. He hasn't been through medical school. He's not a doctor, and besides, you guys at the Australian version of the FDA haven't approved this stuff, and so it should only be available by prescription." And guess what, the Australian version of the FDA said, "Oh, yes, that should only be available on prescription."

SOMERS: That's why I have to get it circuitously? I mean, it's made from eggplant!

WRIGHT: Dr. Cham and his wife moved out of Australia, but to order one can go to the website www.curaderm.net.

There happens to be a very small loophole in our not-so-free health-wise country that says you can import something for your own use, but you better not tell anybody what to do with it and sell it to them, because then they're going to get you. But you can import it for your own use. By doing this, they are able to keep the use of it down to a minimum.

CHAPTER 3

STRESS:

The Real Killer—and the Part You Play in It

CHOICES!
YOU ARE IN CONTROL!

Do you realize that each of us determines our own longevity? Sixty-five to 75 percent of the length of our lives is determined by the lifestyle choices we make. Our genes account for less than 35 percent. This is backed up by hard science.

Mayo Clinic research shows that people who are stressed have telomeres that are almost 50 percent shorter than those of non-stressed people. This equates to a nine- to seventeen-year difference in biological age. (I will explain telomeres in detail later on.)

The Mayo Clinic research also shows that **people with a positive outlook live 19 percent longer!** Live longer by thinking positively; what a concept! One of my favorite quotes, by John Assaraf in *The Secret*, is:

Worry is a prayer for what you don't want.

I use his quote daily as one of my tools to dismiss negatives the moment a worrisome thought comes into my mind, which is usually a projection.

Think about this: Did you know that the majority of all doctor visits are related to stress-induced conditions and a significant percentage of all diseases is caused or complicated by stress?

One of several things you can do to control your stress is to eliminate artificial chemicals. This is a big one. We are under tremendous environmental assault. It's hard enough to manage stress without your stress management system being turned on by artificial chemicals.

It sounds simple, but diet, exercise, sleep, and rest are crucial for managing stress.

Optimal health that manages and controls stress levels allows you to focus. *Focus* is what separates peak performers from average performers, which is why so many high-profile leaders practice meditation. I have found the greatest stress reliever I do regularly is my every-other-day yoga sessions. Having focus and an intentional practice is more effective than passive relaxation. It all works: yoga, meditation, prayer, self-hypnosis, deep breathing, exercising, creative visualization, all have calming effects and bring great pleasure. Stress makes you fatigued, and fatigue reduces your immune functions and healing abilities. **If you are constantly exposed to stress, it will accelerate aging.** (Now you're listening.)

For me, the key to conquering stress is self-examination: continual, honest self-examination. I believe an honest review of the harmony and disharmony in my life enables me to face who I really am, the one that's hard to look at sometimes.

It's said that the two big questions in life are "Who am I?" and "What do I want?" Most people die never being able to answer either of these.

Therapy is a wonderful tool for self-examination and stress reduction. It's your opportunity with a neutral arbitrator in the privacy of your personal session to question yourself: Why do I do and think the things I do, good or bad? A good therapist can help you align your thoughts so you can come to your own conclusions. I like to do phone therapy. Fewer distractions.

My issue in life has been perfectionism. Perfectionism is stressful, and it's taken me a long time to accept myself as the imperfect person that I am. When your goal is perfection, you will always fail, and that causes stress because the underlying message is "I'm not enough." I've finally learned through therapy that no one is perfect. What a relief! That only took me most of a lifetime, but I did it, and today I feel relaxed about most all things in my life. Aging has many wonderful attributes: "knowing," wisdom, perspective, letting yourself off the hook. We all do the best we can with the information we have. The decisions you made earlier in life are probably not the same decisions you would make today unless you've done no work on correcting yourself, but that's rare. At some point we all start to question who we are and the cumulative effects of our choices. I have finally learned: I am enough.

Acceptance reduces stress.

> *For every minute you are angry, you lose sixty seconds of happiness.*
>
> —Ralph Waldo Emerson

Science has proven that we are "wired" for direct connections among our thoughts, our emotions, and our health. Think about that. You are in control of all of it by what you think. Thoughts create. That is why prayer is so powerful.

Your genes and DNA do not control all your biology. **DNA expression can be controlled by signals from outside your cells,** including positive and negative thoughts. You can modify the way your genes are expressed without changing their blueprint by modifying their environment through changes in your diet, emotions, toxins, and stress. This change in gene expression signaling can then be passed on to future generations. This is called **epigenetics.**

Everything you eat, drink, breathe, think, and expose yourself to affects your genes and triggers them to act in certain ways, good or bad. We have now learned that each of us is in control of our health and happiness through our thoughts and our choices.

Genes cannot turn themselves on or off. Only we can do it with our thoughts. We have within us powerful tools to modify our gene expression—the ability to control our programming for health and happiness by our life choices and our thoughts—yet we continually ignore taking preventive measures, as if we don't want to accept the idea that we are damaging ourselves by the negative choices we are making for ourselves.

I practice a meditation every morning. I've been doing it for the last fifteen years, and it has changed my life. Here it is: In 2013, a team of researchers from Greece, Italy, and Spain estimated that the human body contains approximately 37 trillion cells. (Wonder who did the counting?) I know that all cells communicate with one another. It's our messaging system, so every morning I mentally isolate just one of my

37 trillion cells, and I feed it with gratitude: I love my life, I love my husband, I love my family, I love my work, I love the food I get to eat, I love that I get to live in America, I love my good health. I then release that one cell, knowing that it has no choice but to blab it to all the rest of the 37 trillion cells, and in a nanosecond I feel ecstatically happy. I have programmed gratitude.

Conversely, imagine if I woke up each morning and programmed hate and anger, how differently I would feel throughout the day. Try this simple exercise. It takes only minutes to do, and the effects last all day.

When cells are ailing, first look to their environment for the cause, not to the cells themselves. In a healthy environment, cells thrive; in a suboptimal environment, they falter. Here's where your choices come in. If you eat processed food, expose yourself to chemicals, and so on, you're going to pay a price. We are talking about cumulative effects. A lifetime of exposure will take some major detoxifying to undo, but it's possible and is happening at alternative and antiaging doctors' offices all over the country. People sit in clinics with IVs of glutathione (our amazing and versatile antioxidant) or mineral drips for people whose stomach and GI tracts are so imbalanced that they can no longer absorb minerals. The body can't run without minerals and nutrients; it's like trying to run a car without gas.

Antiaging doctors determine your vitamin deficiencies through lab work and compose a recipe of sorts individualized for you to "fill the tank." They also determine your hormonal decline through lab work, and they can measure your toxic burden through labs. Your toxic burden includes how much lead you have accumulated in your bones and brain and what your chemical load from all the nonorganic skin care and poison food you have been using and eating is, coupled with the polluted air you've been breathing. (HEPA filters for the air in your home are now a necessity.)

What I'm saying is that regardless of what you didn't know or understand earlier on, you can turn your life around. When Alan's and my bodies were filled with black mold after our home burned down and we had to move to another home, it took us five years of detoxification to clear it out. It was a real commitment and hard work. The needles hurt some days, but we stayed with the treatment because we believed in it, and it worked. Today we are both in peak health again.

It's very clear that there is a flow of information among cells, and we can regulate a lot of this with our minds.

When you think a grateful thought, there's no room in your mind for anything else.

Genomics is the ability to read the information encoded in our DNA. The good news is that now through science we can read it, and after reading it, we can reprogram it. For instance, scientific advances have given us the ability to leverage biological processes related to RNA to inhibit selected genes; the process of genomics can actually turn off the bad genes by blocking the messenger RNA that is expressing that gene. This technology is currently being studied in clinical trials for many conditions. RNA is that powerful. In fact, in one study when the fat insulin receptor was turned off in mice, the mice ate like horses, stayed slim, didn't get heart disease, and lived 20 percent longer.[1]

So, to sum up, stress makes us sick, shortens our life spans, and then kills us. Whatever measures you can take to reprogram your thoughts through meditation or yoga or whatever form of destressing you choose will go a long way to reverse aging and keep you healthier. How about going for optimal health? That's my goal.

> It is in your moments of decision that your destiny is shaped.
>
> —Tony Robbins

The famed gerontologist Dr. Aubrey de Grey asked, "How long does a house last?" There are houses on the planet that are more than a thousand years old. Along the way they need shoring up, repairing, parts replaced, but with each improvement the house gets a considerable number of added years of life.

That's the way to think of your body. Envision your end point; what does it look like? I know that I want to be here as long as my brain is sharp and my bones are strong. What do you want and envision?

We are all very lucky to be alive right now because so much is happening to address aging, making the present aging process healthy, full of energy, and vital. Read the interview with Bill Faloon in chapter 16 to learn more about the latest age reversal experiments and protocols. There are now validated ways to repair broken DNA and help clean out the debris in our cells.

Think about it: You know how much better the pipes in your house work when they are cleared of debris? Same thing with our cells: a lifetime of debris accumulates, and our cells start to die and malfunction from the weight of it. Then the debris needs to be cleared out.

There's a lot to consider at this stage of life. Ask yourself some questions such as: What will be your end point? What does it look like? Are you healthy and robust, of sound mind, or decrepit and frail? Do you envision getting one of the big three—cancer, heart disease, Alzheimer's disease—or all three?

Believe it or not, most people do envision this terrible scenario as their end because at present it's all we see before us; therefore, it's all we know. Because of the terrible scenario we witness daily with our friends and loved ones, many people have already decided that the effort required to take precautions regarding food and lifestyle choices is hard work and a waste of time. Their thinking is "We're all going to end up sick in the end anyway." This kind of thinking is dangerous because you are programming your outcome.

Cancer is more prone to form in cells that are damaged and stressed. Cancer results from the accumulation of mutations in genes that regulate cellular proliferation. These gene mutations can be caused by stress, toxins, poor diet, nutrient deficiency, and lack of exercise. All of these factors weaken our ability to prevent normal cells from turning malignant. But a good diet lowers your risk of death from all causes. Did you know that the largest amount of chemicals to which your internal organs are exposed comes from your food? It's said that 30 to 50 percent of your food each day should be raw; simple changes such as vegetable juicing and having a salad for lunch can do this.

Very bad diets with no fresh organic fruits and vegetables, filled with fried high-calorie food, low-fiber food, and grilled meats may do more damage to you than even smoking. Think about that. Also, you may have noticed that as you age, you become less tolerant to grains, dairy products, and legumes.

That's a drag.

Our skin, lungs, liver, and kidneys are designed to remove toxins, but today they are stretched beyond their limits. Sadly, our livers are "groaning." This is not good, because the liver is our major detox organ. When it doesn't work and we are trying to wade through all the environmental pollution, we are going to have a difficult (but not impossible) time staying healthy.

So here's the deal: periodic detoxing is now essential. The doctors interviewed in this book introduce you to detox protocols among many other cutting-edge medical advances. Many other doctors versed in this "new way" can be found at www.foreverhealth.com, a free service that can direct you to a qualified doctor near you.

Here's the bad news: over the course of your lifetime, you have a one-in-three chance of developing cancer as a woman and a 40 percent chance of developing cancer as a man [2] if you follow the crowd and don't take preventive measures. Furthermore, 25 percent of all women die of heart disease, and 3 percent die of breast cancer. [3]

America is backward and upside down; we in this country consume a huge percentage of all the world's prescription drugs, yet the average health status and longevity in the United States are pathetically low compared to those of other modern societies. The other 95 percent of the world consumes the remaining 5 percent of the pharmaceuticals.

A study published in 2018 showed that the United States ranked a pathetic forty-third among 195 nations in life expectancy, with an average life span of 78.7 years. Furthermore, the study projected a significant increase in deaths from diabetes, chronic obstructive pulmonary disease (COPD), chronic kidney disease, and lung cancer, as well as worsening health outcomes linked to obesity. [4]

> For all our advances, our beautiful way of life, our hedonism and bounty are killing us. It *was* too good to be true. But—and I will say this over and over again—it's never too late to turn the ship around.

I have sprung back from childhood abuse, violence, traumatic teen years with a teenage pregnancy, shame and defeat, breast cancer, my home being burned to the ground, being fired from my greatest job unfairly, and black mold. It's taken a lot of work to arrive at where I am today. I feel proud and good about myself. I wake up happy, healthy, and grateful. I did it. You can do it, too.

In everything I read, with every interview I do with doctors, scientists, and professionals, I hear the same thing: science has proven that we are hardwired for direct connections among our thoughts, our emotions, and our health. DNA gene expression is controlled in part by signals from outside your cells: your thoughts and everything you eat, drink, and think control the expression of your genes.

Think about this: your thoughts, your lifestyle choices, and your environmental factors control whether beneficial "pro-youth" genes are turned on or off.

How long do you want to live? Ask yourself. Give yourself an answer. Your cells will receive the information. Take control. What is your real age now, meaning how young or old do you feel, not your chronological age? Do you feel fifty but look sixty? Your answer will reflect the attention you pay to diet, supplements, skin elasticity, respiratory function, reaction time, immune profile, and neurological scores.

How long can you stay sexual? Hormone replacement, along with all your other good and positive choices, can allow you to remain sexual forever. What a nice thought.

It's all up to you.

Interview with

DR. JEFFREY R. GLADDEN

Dr. Jeffrey R. Gladden is the founder and medical director of Apex Health, Human Performance & Longevity Optimization.

Dr. Gladden's transition is interesting. Trained as an interventional cardiologist, he realized early on that the heart is a part of the body system and wanted to create a new dynamic and approach to treating it as part of the whole body system.

He began his career as an interventional cardiologist, and in his more than twenty-five years of practice, he has treated thousands of patients for cardiovascular disease. His interventional passion has shifted, however. Instead of intervening late in the course of heart disease, when stents and bypasses are the primary options, he has shifted his focus to heart attack and stroke prevention. His true passion is integrating the prevention of cardiovascular disease with the optimization of cardiovascular performance. Applying his interventional mind-set to age management and integrative medicine, he created Apex HHPLO. Apex is a multifaceted, all-encompassing, comprehensive, integrative approach that has led to both the effective arrest and, in many cases, reversal of heart disease while enabling people to turn back the clock and enjoy levels of performance and participation they never thought possible.

Dr. Gladden's vision of Apex is based on his passion for integrative medicine, age management medicine, and health and human performance optimization in every area of life. He is actively dedicated to every Apex client's success. More information is available at www.apexhhplo.com.

In his free time, Dr. Gladden enjoys mountain biking, running, heli and snowcat snowboarding, bodysurfing, stand-up paddleboarding, playing the guitar, writing songs, and living an active Apex lifestyle. He continues to explore and test the reach of his own global performance while avidly working to reverse the decline that is traditionally associated with chronological aging. His goal is to help himself and others create optimized relationships and cultivate spiritual wisdom, while enjoying vocational and avocational pursuits in addition to vibrant health.

He also cofounded Living Beyond 120 (www.livingbeyond120.com) with his partner Mark Young in 2017. It is a company devoted to democratizing information about optimizing health and performance in every area of life. Living Beyond 120 produces a podcast of the same title cohosted by Mark and Dr. Gladden.

So much of what they discuss is stress management and the power of one's thoughts to go forward with optimal health or conversely away from it. Once again, it's all about the fact that our personal choices control our degree of happiness—or unhappiness—and our outcome.

SOMERS: Thanks for your time, Dr. Gladden. What is it that draws people to your Apex program?

GLADDEN: Thanks for the opportunity to speak with you, Suzanne. What draws people to Apex is that we are asking a completely different question about their health than is traditionally being asked. We are asking "How good can you be?" The questions asked in traditional health care, or "sick care," as I refer to it, are "Are you sick?," "Are you having symptoms?," "Is there something wrong?" During my life experiences, I've discovered that questions are much more powerful than answers; asking the right questions is the key to growth and discovery. Something I learned from Lee Brower at the Strategic Coach is that questions empower our minds to find new answers; statements do not. At Apex our empowering question is "How good can you be?," meaning how healthy, how fit, how strong, how mentally sharp, how relationally connected, and how spiritually centered can we be, and for how many years and decades can we carry those levels forward? Our questions open up entirely new pathways of healing, health, and performance optimization.

We start each prospective client interview with a series of questions to understand their mind-set. Many people need what Apex has to offer; however, we chose to only work with people who share our mind-set and are asking the same questions about health and life that we are. To that end they complete a Mindset Scorecard, where we ask questions to understand their specific aspirations for their health, performance, and longevity. We then have them identify perceived roadblocks or hurdles based on their health history, family health history, work stress, relationship stress, et cetera.

We then go on to ask three multipart questions:

• Go back and remember the age at which you were at your peak for health and fitness. How fit were you?

• At what age were your mental capabilities, creative energy, problem-solving ability, and intellectual capability at their peak? When was that? How sharp were you?

• At what age were you at your peak of spiritual insight, relational insight, and wisdom? How good was that? What characterized it?

It's interesting to get the answers back and plot the peaks against the ages at which they occurred or are occurring. We typically find a large disconnect between the ages of peak health and athletic performance and the other peaks. As we age, we get better and better, while our health and performance levels get worse and worse.

SOMERS: Very interesting to ask about their mind-set. Never had a doc ask me that other than my therapist.

GLADDEN: Mind-set is interesting, Suzanne, because, as you know, it is so powerful in determining our health, happiness, and levels of performance. Circling back to our prior multipart questions, we hear many times that people are their wisest now, they are most spiritually centered now, and they have the most relational insight now. Intellectually, they are capable of doing things as well as or better than ever, or they are within a few years of their peak mental powers. When we come to health, fitness, and athletic performance, this is not the case. Typically, peak health was years if not decades ago, and peak fitness and athletic performance occurred in their twenties or thirties. Occasionally, peak health and athletic performance might be later. For example, if at age fifty someone has a "wake-up call" and starts mixing and matching P90X, yoga, CrossFit, spin class, et cetera, et cetera, they report they got into the "best shape of their life." However, even here I still find a chronological disconnect between their health and fitness peak and the other peaks. I mean, look at what you're doing now; you're probably at the peak of your powers in terms of your ability to integrate and synthesize information, and yet you might not say that you are at your peak for athletic ability or athletic performance. In my opinion the beauty of what you do makes new possibilities come alive for people, positively changing their mind-sets about their health and leading them to ask new, empowering questions.

When Apex is asking the question "How good can you be?," it's actually based on the possibility of changing the trajectory of aging. Working with us, we see people turn back their functional clock five, ten, fifteen, even twenty-plus years all the time.

SOMERS: I have found that after fifty, the wisdom starts to pour. You don't sweat the small stuff, the angst calms down, and you no longer have to be perfect.

GLADDEN: Yes, I would agree if we pay attention, cumulative experience provides the building blocks of wisdom. With time I've found that perspective, insight, wisdom, gratitude, love, and relationship have all become much more important, fulfilling, centering, and healing than anything else in my life.

SOMERS: So age is just a number but the important question is "How young is your energy?"

GLADDEN: Agreed! I am saying age is just a number and that this statement has never been more true than it is today. Chronology is inevitable, but how we age is becoming truly optional. Back to mind-set for a minute. One of the most important determinants of age is the question, How youthful is your mind-set? Culture, society, family, the medical profession, the professional world, and the government have all institutionalized and normalized the aging process as we know it. The mantra is that aging and its associated decline are inevitable. Given what we now know, the actionable knowledge we have, and the results we have experienced for ourselves and our Apex clients, I believe that aging as we did in prior generations is not inevitable and is actually optional. But we will never age differently if our mind-set reinforces the ubiquitous paradigm of aging we all grew up with.

You can't become something that you haven't envisioned becoming.

If you envision yourself as young, that's a good first step. But then you have to ask the right questions and discover the appropriate tools to optimize your physiology, relationships, and spirituality. Having an optimization mind-set fueled by an empowering question such as "How good can you be?" allows you to have a revolutionary experience of life where wisdom is growing, spiritual insight is growing, intellectual capabilities and creativity are all growing, and your health and athletic performance are improving as well!

SOMERS: Revolutionary in its simplicity! We've made it complex by turning our health over to doctors, expecting a pill for every ailment. I've had a number of doctors in this book talk about "pharmaceuticalization" as the end of humanity at best. People are so pilled up that wisdom is dwindling, which is tragic because with that paradigm, by the time you are old enough to acquire wisdom, you can't think anymore.

You mentioned the tools; I would imagine you mean your regimen. If I am a patient of yours, I come to you hopefully somewhat educated in this new way, so you don't have to start in kindergarten, right?

GLADDEN: First, you wouldn't be a patient. The word *patient* is for people in the sick care system asking sick care questions of sick care physicians. You would actually be a "client" or a "health partner," and we would leverage your optimization mind-set to refocus your questions and provide you with new answers.

SOMERS: Okay. If a client has been listening to your podcast *Living Beyond 120* and gets turned on with the possibilities, what are the tools you provide to achieve this kind of health?

GLADDEN: Central to the process is understanding what food to eat, what nutrients to take, and what exercises to do. With exercise it is critical to know at what intensity and duration one should partake based on your body's recovery and ability to take on strain. Being precise about each of these elements makes us stronger, healthier, and less prone to injury. Couple those themes with a deep understanding of hormonal decline, telomere biology, cognitive function optimization, gut function optimization, cardiovascular function optimization, cancer risk mitigation, dementia and neurodegenerative disease risk mitigation, et cetera, and we are in a position to develop a blueprint for action that leverages your assets and minimizes your liabilities, restores health and minimizes risk, and optimizes performance levels.

In our genetic testing we focus on what is actionable. We do this by focusing a great deal of attention on the area known as **nutrigenomics**, the field devoted to understanding how our DNA expression is influenced by what we do, what we eat, and what supplements we might take.

We were all taught in high school biology that our genes are a blueprint and that as such they are our destiny. Yet in actual fact, apart from someone who is born with a true genetic disorder such as cystic fibrosis or Down syndrome, our genes are not necessarily our destiny. It is more accurate to think of our genes as a set of proclivities or tendencies that actually are expressed in response to the environment in which they reside. Understanding environmental influences on gene expression is the study of **epigenetics**.

Once you understand your own genetics and the environment in which they are optimally expressed, you can start to take action to create a health-promoting environment and optimize your own genetic expression. To me that is revolutionary.

SOMERS: How powerful are thoughts relative to epigenetics?

GLADDEN: Thoughts are massively important to our genetic expression. We can will ourselves to die. My grandmother did this at ninety-six after my grandfather died. After he passed, she lost the will to live and essentially willed herself to die. She was gone six weeks later.

Thoughts and emotions can lead to either stress and anger or peace and love, and both are important epigenetic influences. When we carry stress, anger, and resentment, we are literally shortening our lives. The opposite is true when we are at peace and have a life full of loving relationships with ourselves and others.

In addition, there are other important contributors to the environment that affect our genetic expression. Nutrition, micronutrient levels, exercise, toxins, hormone levels, et cetera all play a large role. To your point, however:

Our thoughts and beliefs ultimately drive everything because they drive the questions we are asking.

If I might add, one of the big problems in our sick care system is that very smart people get married to their answers. As doctors we go to medical school, graduate from great universities, go on to do our training at great training programs, and over time we become recognized experts in our fields. In the process we get married to what we've been taught and the answers we were trained to use. We believe that what we were taught gives us the best set of answers for any illness.

We have our sick care questions and our insurance-reimbursed answers, and we become married to those answers. Our sick care system is in essence orchestrated by the payer system of insurance. That insurance system only reimburses doctors and hospitals for treating patients with answers that align with the insurance companies' policies of reimbursement. These policies are conveniently lifted selectively from our medical training programs and literature. The entire system becomes insular and circular and close minded. It therefore becomes impossible to implement new diagnostic and treatment technologies at the pace they are being discovered, tested, and validated.

SOMERS: What do you mean by "married to their answers"?

GLADDEN: As human beings we get married to our answers when we stop asking deeper questions; for instance, we might get married to the idea. For example, one idea we were married to in the past is that the earth is flat. When we are married to the answer, it stops us looking for better answers. Note the difference in energy created in your mind between saying "The earth is flat" and asking "Is the earth flat?" Statements we are married to make our brains take on a defensive posture to defend the answers we already have. From that position: (1) We look for evidence to support our conclusion. Lo and behold, we find some; therefore our answer is obviously true and obviously the only truth. (2) From our defensive posture we spend our psychic energy denigrating alternative answers and leave a trail of martyrs and heretics in our wake.

I met with a thirty-seven-year-old in my office yesterday morning who went to his doctor for an annual physical exam. He was told, "Everything looks great." His doctor said, "You are healthy, your lab work looks great." But the patient said, "My back is killing me, I'm in so much pain all the time, and it gets stiff whenever I don't move for a little while. My knees are bothering me, too." His doctor did not have an answer for him and therefore was relatively dismissive: "Well, let's give it another six weeks and see how it goes. Maybe we can put you on an anti-inflammatory pill if it doesn't improve, but I have to tell you, although you are not old, you are not young anymore, either."

At thirty-seven, this patient was being groomed to accept aging and decline as the norm. This is the present paradigm in medicine of normalizing the aging process: an entire "health care" system with no investment or interest in you being young and healthy. We've normalized the fact that people are going to age and develop disease and that we are going to treat it with our sick care answers. It's a classic case of us getting married to our worldview and married to our answers. The difference at Apex is that we are not married to our answers, and we have a lot of answers, but we are only married to our questions.

SOMERS: I often say a lot of doctors are "down on what they're not up on." It takes courage for a doctor such as yourself and the others in this book who have all had that same epiphany where there has to be another way because the conditions of today are so different than ever before. We talked on your *Living Beyond 120* podcast about this: we are experiencing the greatest environmental assault in the history of humanity. How much of what you are treating on a daily basis is environmental?

GLADDEN: The environmental toxins include excess sunlight, excess artificial light, toxins in our air and water, high-calorie, poor-nutrient-quality food, the exercise that we do or don't do, the sleep that we get or don't get, the electromagnetic radiation that we are exposed to, et cetera, et cetera—including all these elements as part of the environment, I think probably eighty-five percent of what we see has an environmental link. There are biological mechanisms triggered by these environmental challenges: telomeres are shortening, hormone levels are declining, inflammation and oxidative stress are increased, et cetera. Like you, I think the environment counts for a great deal of our health-related issues.

SOMERS: If the environment counts for a great deal of it, I would imagine food choices, the kind of food that's not contaminated with pesticides, et cetera, has got to be paramount.

GLADDEN: Agreed! Food choices are paramount. I rarely find a person who isn't trying to eat better, but the problem is, nobody actually knows what that means for them. The problem with most diet plans is they start by talking about the food. At Apex we start with the person and then work back to the food and foods that work best for them.

SOMERS: As a heart doctor, I'm sure you tell everybody, "No fat"?

GLADDEN: Well, that was the party line for many years, but now we've learned that no-fat diets are high-sugar diets and high-sugar diets lead to more obesity, diabetes, and heart disease, not less.

SOMERS: I was being facetious. I know you know good fats are good.

GLADDEN: You got me going there, Suzanne! Healthy fats are certainly part of what we would recommend, but we don't recommend things on a generic basis. Kale and fish oil may be terrific, but the question needs to be, Is it right for you?

Until we actually do our genetics, understand our nutrigenomics, our immune system–mediated food sensitivities, our gut biome, gut integrity, and gut function, and look at the food-mediated immune systems and brain interaction, I think it's impossible for us to know what to eat for optimal health. Until you put all these pieces together and connect the dots, you can't really start to recommend with any real certainty what food is good for an individual.

People are trying to do the right thing, but they don't know whether they should be putting butter in their coffee, whether they should be vegan or paleo, keto, low carb, high fat, low fat?

God bless us, we just don't know. Until you actually do the work to unravel the knot and understand how you're built and the current status of your body, you can never get the food piece right. And to your point, yes, eating organic foods is very important, but it's also very hard to get clean food, even organic food, unless you are growing it yourself, controlling the water, air, and soil. It's almost virtually impossible to get clean food these days.

That being said, to the extent that we can eat food that is clean, it is incredibly helpful, but if you are eating the wrong "good" foods, you are just inflaming your system and causing more problems than you're solving.

SOMERS: What are the wrong foods? Are we talking dairy?

GLADDEN: Categorically, we are not talking about anything. We are asking whether our body is reacting poorly and generating inflammation from certain foods. For some people, dairy works great; for other people, it's very inflammatory. Some people are built genetically to have MCT oil or put butter in their coffee; for others of us, it is harmful.

SOMERS: We are unique individuals.

GLADDEN: That's right. The best solution is a custom solution, not a one-size-fits-all recommendation.

SOMERS: Relative to heart issues, how important is alignment? I'm thinking specifically of the jaw. I've come to find the jaw an interesting player. I do know that the vagus and trigeminal nerves flow right behind the ear and people get hit in the head, neck, or jaw or fall as kids or as football players in high school, and then twenty, thirty, forty years later, this misalignment rears its ugly head and causes vertigo and multiple other problems.

GLADDEN: Misalignment causes stress in the body, whether it's the cervical spine, the neck, the thoracic or lumbar spine, the jaw, or the shoulders. All of these things can become misaligned, and that stresses the body. The way I think about alignment is that the entire body, not just what's between our ears, is our brain. The reason I think of it this way is because our nerves travel through and to every structure in our bodies. Everything is actually neuro-something: neuromuscular, neuroskeletal, neurofascial, neurocardiac, et cetera, et cetera. When trauma occurs in the jaw, back, knee, shoulder, et cetera, it is now structurally out of alignment. The brain also becomes out of alignment. The brain realigns itself to accommodate and protect the injured area. We put so much attention on structural misalignment as causes of pain, and rightly so; we want to relieve pain. The question, however, is how do we realign the structure and the brain to enable healing and make the injured area less prone to injury in the future? Adequately answering these questions enables a full return of function, but it can't be done without retraining or reprogramming the brain to work in an optimal way with respect to that area of the body. Our traditional approach typically employs an external tool to realign the injured area, and then time is permitted to allow the body to heal. But I believe that is not enough. While the body part was injured and out of alignment, the brain reprogrammed itself and compensatory protective mechanisms were hardwired into our neurons. Those compensatory mechanisms prevent both a full return to function and also the development of a better neurostructural unit that will take undue stress off of other body parts and decrease the risk of injury in the future.

For example, let's say your jaw is "out." Being "out" causes pain at the jaw but also elsewhere as the brain realigns the chewing mechanism to accommodate the jaw being out of alignment. Consequently, headaches ensue, nausea may occur, et cetera, et cetera. Putting the jaw back into alignment does not necessarily resolve the other symptoms because the brain has not been realigned. Putting the jaw back also doesn't make it less prone to going out in the future; in many instances it will be more prone to go out again. Until the brain is reprogrammed—i.e., the neuromuscular, neuroskeletal systems are realigned and strengthened—the jaw can continue to be a source of other problems, say headaches, and will be prone to go out again. Until the area is fully healed, it places a lot of stress on the body. The body only has a few ways to respond to stress. And while there are an infinite number of insults, the body has a limited number of responses.

Increased stress triggers the sympathetic nervous system, which is our fight-or-flight response. Stress also turns down the parasympathetic nervous system tone. This imbalance within the autonomic nervous system drives a lot of stress-related illnesses.

When vagal tone, parasympathetic tone, is turned down, GI health is compromised. Once GI health and integrity are compromised, structural misalignment elsewhere occurs or there is excess psychological stress. Then heart rate variability is compromised, and the heart becomes more prone to arrhythmias and to developing heart disease. There is a cascade of misalignments and imbalances in nervous system tone that results in these kinds of chronic insults becoming hardwired into our brains that create more stress. The same is also true for psychological issues such as PTSD.

Misalignment causes chronic stress. Concussions or traumatic brain injuries, even in the remote past, cause misalignment, and it may be twenty years or later before symptoms occur.

One underlying root cause of every disorder is compensatory brain reprogramming that occurs with the injury; another root cause is inflammation. What's actually happening at the cellular level in these situations of prolonged inflammation is excessive oxidative stress. When there's an imbalance of oxidative stress relative to the cells' ability to handle that oxidative stress, bad things happen, chronic conditions develop, and all elements of aging are accelerated.

For example, if we are genetically predisposed to develop Parkinson's and we are exposed to an environmental toxin that creates higher levels of oxidative stress in the substantia nigra, we develop Parkinson's disease. It's the excess oxidative stress layered into a system that has a genetic predisposition toward developing Parkinson's disease that results in the disorder. It's not that everybody with Parkinson's has a misaligned jaw. It's more about looking at root causes like genetic predispositions, misalignments perhaps of the jaw, and the subsequent misalignment of the brain while simultaneously managing the inflammation and resultant excess oxidative stress that really cause the damage at the cellular level.

We have found so many applications for our idea that **the entire body is the brain**. What really excites us is the work we are doing to reprogram the brain in the face of injury to enable not only complete healing but also increased resilience to future injury.

SOMERS: What are those techniques?

GLADDEN: We are using something called transcranial direct stimulation in the form of Halo Sport headphones. They look like headphones with little transducers that basically run from ear to ear over the scalp. The headphones run across the top of the head, and below them is where the motor cortex resides. Using transcranial direct stimulation, we can actually run a very light electrical current into that motor cortex and you can actually increase its neuroplasticity to the point where it can actually learn, unlearn, and relearn things faster.

Let's say we injure our knee, and now the next thing we know, because of the way our brain compensated for this with a change of gait, our left hip starts to hurt. As we discussed above, it's not enough to get our knee "fixed," because the brain will have reprogrammed itself to protect the knee and in so doing places more stress elsewhere. We have to heal the joint, then realign the functional brain/neurojoint, neuromuscular, neuromotor unit to optimize and strengthen that alignment in order to minimize injury in the future both at the knee and the hip. It's fascinating stuff.

SOMERS: Is that a microcurrent?

GLADDEN: Yes, transcranial direct stimulation, TCDS, is a microcurrent.

SOMERS: Does someone need to come every week, every day to use the machine?

GLADDEN: Actually, you can buy these on the internet from a company called Halo Neuro. FYI: I have no relationship with Halo Neuro. The technology works. Musicians are using the headphones to learn music faster and perfect their craft faster. I play the guitar, and when I put the headphones on, my musician friends say, "Wow, you are a much better guitarist!" I can play the guitar, but when I wear the headphones and the TCDS increases the neuroplasticity of my motor cortex, I'm seriously a better guitarist both technically and creatively.

SOMERS: Does it put you more in a zone?

GLADDEN: Much more in a zone. I refer to "the zone" as a "flow state." When I go mountain biking and I use the headphones to neuroprime before I get to the trail, I immediately go into a flow state where I'm one with the trail, one with the bike. I mean, my riding is just spot-on. It's really fantastic.

SOMERS: It's high vibration?

GLADDEN: In a way. But these transcranial direct stimulations are interesting because you can stimulate the brain for twenty minutes, and while you are doing that, you can do other things, like warm up or just sit there. I tend to neural prime on my way to the mountain bike trail in the car, and when I get there, I take them off, put on my bike helmet, and take off, and the effect lasts for another hour or so.

We've got a major-league pitcher we're working with who has had Tommy John surgery, a common elbow surgery used for stress-induced ligament injury, a couple of times and was trying to get back to the majors. We were able to decrease his pain by decreasing his inflammation and excess oxidative stress, and then we were able to realign his neuromuscular, neuroskeletal system to improve his throwing while decreasing the stress on his elbow. When he was rehabbing his arm, he pitched wearing a special sleeve that measured strain on his elbow. Using the

Halo Sport headphones, we were able to decrease the strain on his elbow by twenty percent and have him pitching pain free. Think about that from the standpoint of career extension.

Central to effectively utilizing these techniques is understanding that **brain reprogramming** is required for complete healing and improved resilience. Back to your comment about the power of thought, realignment of the brain dovetails nicely with the idea of the overall power of the brain to heal.

I've come to believe that health itself is ninety-eight percent behavioral; it's the choices we've made, things we do, how we exercise, and how we think about things.

What we do at Apex is essentially reprogramming of the brain, not in a big-brother kind of way, but we give people the tools, the ability and coaching, to help them retrain their brains, allowing a much more expansive view of what's possible and the tools to implement, with personalized precision, what needs to be done. Our clients say they feel and perform better than they ever have in their adult lives.

SOMERS: It shows that we are each in control. It does go back to our thoughts. When I think of the success I've had in my career, I think back to my childhood thoughts. I didn't realize I was doing it, but I saw it my whole life, I always saw it, like this star up there, and I just never took my eye off of it. When it worked out, it didn't surprise me because it was always my vision. I guess happiness, health, how long you want to live, how healthy you will be in these extra years are up to each of us to imagine and then do the right things to manifest that vision. It's all up to each of us.

GLADDEN: That's a beautiful image of you as a young person, Suzanne, seeing your future direction. And you're right, but our traditional medical system is not acknowledging that thoughts and vision are the primary drivers in creating health and disease. Let me just comment on a vision of what antiaging looks like. We didn't see this kind of antiaging mind-set in our parents and our grandparents or our family and friends.

My intention is to use Apex questions and answers to recapture and stay between twenty-seven and thirty-five; then, if I live to be 120 years or beyond, I want to leverage the available and emerging technology to keep my health age in that twenty-seven-to-thirty-five-year age range.

SOMERS: I think EMFs are the next wave of trouble for brain, heart, and the nervous system. Do you have any feelings about EMFs [electromagnetic fields]?

GLADDEN: I think EMFs have a huge impact and can be healing or destructive. Just as we were talking about transcranial direct stimulation being integral to healing by improved neuromotor function, there are other devices out there that can also help. One is called Alpha-Stim, and another is a Fisher Wallace device. In both instances you can apply these to your head and run microcurrents through your brain to actually lower anxiety, treat depression, improve your ability to meditate, and even improve cognitive clarity for people.

The whole body is energy, and how it interfaces with other energy sources, whether it's food, electrical, or sunlight, is key to health. So a body made of energy depends on the frequencies of what's coming in and how it's interfacing to help optimize cellular function.

We are looking at something now using pulsed electromagnetic frequencies to actually enhance ATP production.

SOMERS: Is that Ondamed?

GLADDEN: Yes, very similar to Ondamed. Fascinating, right? We are looking at it from the standpoint of rehabilitating mitochondrial function, which is another reason that people get old: they can't make ATP, they can't repair themselves, they don't have any energy.

SOMERS: I always say the difference between a young person and an old person is energy. Ironically, it doesn't really have to do with age. I know a lot of forty-year-olds who are a lot older than me.

GLADDEN: Lack of energy is part of the excess oxidative stress and decline of energy that occurs. We are looking at numerous strategies inside of Apex to rejuvenate mitochondrial function and ATP production. We are looking at and still experimenting with pulsed electromagnetic frequency. Electrical current can be good, or it could be bad; it just depends on what kind and what you're doing with it.

SOMERS: I read a book on EMFs by Elizabeth Plourde, PhD. There are some people so sensitive to EMFs that they have to create tinfoil barriers in between their windows and, let's say, the EMF fake tree that's at the hotel down the street because EMFs can go through walls, windows, and more. Shocking. What is this going to do to all of us down the line? What are the negative effects? I think we know.

GLADDEN: We can't avoid toxins completely even if you are going to live in a bubble. It's very hard to avoid Wi-Fi, radio waves, and environmental assaults. This has been going on ever since radio came around, so I don't know if it's realistic to say we are ever going to change that, but I think making ourselves resilient and more robust is a strategy that can work.

SOMERS: Thank you for this time. I have really enjoyed talking with you and learning about your business model for "clients."

GLADDEN: Likewise, a pleasure. I admire your passion for what you're doing and the way you're bringing the information of what's possible to people at large. I know you have a huge audience, and it's fantastic what you're doing.

CHAPTER 4

SUPPLEMENTATION

Aging is an extraordinary process where you become the person you always should have been.
—David Bowie

To take or not to take? Are supplements just "expensive urine"? That is often the argument for not taking them. If you truly believe the planet is not a toxic soup and is not depleting each of us of the "fuel" that keeps our body engine running, you probably shouldn't supplement.

But I firmly believe, as do the doctors in this book, that because of the enormous stress people experience in today's world and the fact that our soil has been depleted of essential nutrients and minerals—then add in genetically engineered food being so abundant—it is now crucial to supplement our bodies with vitamins, nutrients, and minerals. It's no longer a joke. It's not "expensive urine," it's now essential, and yes, it is a pain in the butt to take so many pills daily, but be grateful that you can. Without supplementation, it's very difficult to get the nutrients necessary to have a well-running body.

There are days I don't want to take my large handful of supplements; it's gaggy (my word), but I do it. I know it's that important for life quality.

I have my supplemental protocol determined by blood testing that indicates my deficiencies. I supplement to "fill the tank" with that which is missing. I want to live a long, healthy life with my incredible husband, and I want us both to have great brains, well-working livers, calm, healthy gastrointestinal tracts, and strong bones; can't achieve that eating Cheetos.

In the following pages I am going to list some of the more important supplements, giving insight into what they do. Recent research has proven that these supplements do truly make a difference. I highly suggest that you choose one of your favorite doctors from this book, look at the tests offered by Life Extension listed at the back of the book, or go to www.foreverhealth.com to find a qualified doctor near you to give you the proper tests to determine your deficiencies, be they hormonal, mineral, or nutrient.

That's what the "new aging" is about: putting back what you've lost in the normal aging process or due to environmental toxicity.

This step really matters. This is your starting point, and it is affordable. When your deficiencies are counteracted, when your toxic burden is greatly lowered, your quality of life and good health will remain—or return if it has been degraded.

NUTRIENTS

Nutrients are fertilizer for your brain and body.

Vitamins and minerals are essential nutrients. Without them, you would structurally fall apart and your cells would lose life-sustaining functionality.

Ever wonder why your body is sluggish and not operating at optimum? What are you feeding yourself? Are you cognizant of the proper balance of nutrients that would keep you operating in tip-top health and energy?

The difference between an old person and a young person is energy. How is yours?

If you're not thrilled with your daily performance, it's time to take supplementation seriously. To brush it off as nothing more than "expensive urine" is doing yourself a big disservice.

> *Your life is sustained by millions of enzymatic reactions that occur inside your cells every second. Vitamins and minerals are required to keep vital enzymes inside your cells working.*

Here's just one example: magnesium is a cofactor for over three hundred enzymes responsible for DNA/RNA synthesis, protein synthesis, cell growth, cell energy production, and on and on. Without magnesium, these life-sustaining enzymes would not be able to do their job.

VITAMIN B$_{12}$

I remember many years ago I was working with Dr. Diana Schwarzbein, my brilliant first endocrinologist. I apologetically called her on a Christmas morning, tearfully saying I didn't know what was wrong, I was so depressed and couldn't figure out why. I told her sleeping was impossible; that I had been awake all night long and it had been going on for weeks. I told her that Christmas was normally the happiest day of the year for me, yet I was depressed, that I love Christmas and I love my family and I love my life, so what was wrong? There was a long pause on the other end of the phone, and then she said without emotion, "What did you expect? You keep burning up your biochemicals and not giving yourself sufficient time to build them back up. You work to the point of stress, and then you fall apart. You think you take good care of yourself, but here you are: your adrenals have now flatlined, and that's where your depression is coming from. And let me tell you something else," she continued, "the next call you make to me is that you have had a heart attack." I asked through tears, "So what do I do?" She said, "Sleep, sleep, and more sleep and daily vitamin B$_{12}$ injections." Repair!

I realized I had been burning the candle at both ends for quite some time. But I was young! I could take it, couldn't I?

Her words resonated with me. Something was clearly wrong, so I took her advice.

Besides causing flatlined adrenals and "dog-tired" fatigue (a big reason we don't sleep, as well as why we gain unexplained weight), vitamin B deficiency can ultimately be devastating to your brain.

The conditions most associated with vitamin B$_{12}$ deficiency include toxic brain syndrome, paranoia, violence, heart attack, and depression. There's a well-documented association between B$_{12}$ deficiency and dementia. Nice, huh?

There's an interesting article entitled "Subtle Vitamin-B$_{12}$ Deficiency in Psychiatry: A Largely Unnoticed but Devastating Relationship?" It was published in 1991 and provided an interesting hypothesis that some cases of so-called Alzheimer's dementia may actually be caused by B_{12} deficiency.

Since then, hundreds of studies have identified nutrient deficiencies and unhealthy lifestyle choices that contribute to higher dementia risk. (Later in this book we will also see the relationship between decreased estrogen, in particular estradiol levels and Alzheimer's.)

B_{12} deficiency can cause depression and even in certain cases bipolar-1 disorder (manic depressive illness) and more commonly bipolar-2 disorder.

Factoring in the nutritional deficiencies of so many people today, you begin to understand the crazy shoot-'em-ups and senseless killings being committed. That's how important it is to keep your vitamin B_{12} and other nutrient levels in perfect balance. You're not going to find healthy nutrition and adequate B vitamins in processed food.

Throughout this book, you're going to see that we, as humans, are one giant system, all of its parts interacting at all times with all of the others that make up this wondrous creation called our body.

> *Don't dig your grave with your own knife and fork.*
> —Proverb

The fuel and fertilizers for optimal health are the nutrients, minerals, and vitamins we need to take to achieve optimal health. Eating real food, organic food, is the best thing you can do for your body. After that it's crucial to understand that unfortunately the soil and the water so often used in growing our food have been depleted of vital nutrients. That's where supplementation comes in: fill the tank, put back what is missing in your food, and replace low or missing nutrients and minerals.

For me to get back to good health after the episode described above with Dr. Schwarzbein required me to take vitamin B complex shots daily for a year. It was quite a commitment and slightly painful, but I chose to look at it as an opportunity. Had I not been working with such a cutting-edge doctor who understood what was going on with me, I might have been put on the pharmaceutical protocol, a life of what I call "Band-Aid medicine," meaning never healing, just keeping the condition at bay, until it no longer worked, then switching to a stronger version, and on and on. And what, I ask you, does filling your body with all these dangerous chemicals over a lifetime do to you? Certainly, for starters, it can't be helpful to the brain.

Luckily for me, my doctor understood my situation. She did not put me on antidepressants or sleeping pills plus all the various other drugs given to patients with similar conditions, and for that I am so grateful. When a doctor doesn't understand physiology, drugs are all he or she has in his or her arsenal. I was able to return to optimal health and at the same time build up my vitamin B_{12}, the lack of which was the major reason I had a high homocysteine level, which was what was causing my condition.

Why do I care? Because a high homocysteine level can lead to heart attack, and in fact, heart attack is what has historically killed my family members. Maybe throughout the generations my people were all low in B vitamins and suffered from lowered homocysteine levels.

Fatigue is another symptom of vitamin B deficiency, but the medical community has been slow to recognize the condition.

The cyanocobalamin form of vitamin B_{12} has been used for many decades. A more effective approach is to supplement with the biologically active form of B_{12} called *methylcobalamin*. Oral doses of 1,000 to 5,000 micrograms of B_{12} daily have been used in cases of anemia to maintain patients' vitamin B_{12} levels.

Symptoms of vitamin B_{12} deficiency include anemia, a pale, smooth tongue, brown spots over the joints, paranoia, bursitis, poor memory, dementia, psychosis, depression, restlessness, diarrhea, schizophrenia, dizziness, a sore tongue, irritability, temper outbursts, mood swings, tingling, nausea, violence, negative thinking, and weakness. When taking B_{12}, be sure to take folic acid along with it, as both are needed for **methylation**.* A deficiency of either can produce anemia, so always correct both if you are deficient.

---

* Methylation is a vital metabolic process that happens in every cell and every organ of our body. Life would not exist without it. It takes place more than a billion times per second.

If your blood test for homocysteine is high, always use the methyl forms of B_6, B_{12}, and folic acid (5-MTHF).

GLUTATHIONE

It's important to understand the crucial role of glutathione in keeping you healthy and living longer. You must understand that the longer we live, the higher our toxic burden. As I say over and over, we are under the greatest environmental assault in the history of humanity. Dr. Walter Pierpaoli, featured later in this book, feels it's possible that the younger generation is not going to live as long as we are because of their exposure to massive amounts of toxins and chemicals. Imagine. Our livers are "groaning," unable to perform at peak because they are so overloaded with toxins never meant to be metabolized in the human body. The liver makes glutathione, but our reserves run out earlier and earlier in today's world. It's important to understand that glutathione is a critical and versatile antioxidant.

In the polluted and toxic world in which we live, you want optimal liver function. Your liver is where most detoxification occurs in your body. Your liver utilizes glutathione to fight off free radicals, mercury, chemicals, and more.

Glutathione also plays a major role in numerous metabolic and biochemical reactions, such as DNA synthesis and repairs, protein synthesis, prostaglandin synthesis, amino acid transport, and enzyme activation. According to Prescribers' Digital Reference, "Most systems in the body can be affected by the state of the glutathione system, especially the immune system, the nervous system, the gastrointestinal system and the lungs."

Glutathione is also necessary for optimal conversion of T_4 to T_3 thyroid hormones.[1] In addition, it's necessary for transferring electrons from the cell membrane to the mitochondria, your energy center.

Recent studies have shown that daily consumption of glutathione can increase blood and RBC levels.

What many people do today to boost their plasma and liver glutathione concentrations is supplement with S-adenosylmethionine

(SAM-E), n-acetylcysteine (NAC), and/or whey protein. These nutrients increase the glutathione content within cells. Also, you can get IV glutathione treatments from your antiaging doctor.

Lipoic acid has also been shown to restore intercellular glutathione, as does melatonin, which stimulates a related enzyme, glutathione peroxidase, and silymarin, an extract of the seeds of the milk thistle plant. By the way, milk thistle and nutrients such as NAC and SAM-E can help mitigate the effects of alcohol consumption. It makes sense, because this is another example of antioxidants at work. In the simplest terms, glutathione-boosting nutrients help restore some of what the alcohol depletes.

Enlightened individuals today take formulas providing vitamins C and B$_1$, glutathione-boosting nutrients such as NAC, and NAD+ precursor supplements before and/or after ingesting alcohol.

According to Wikipedia, "Low glutathione is commonly observed in wasting and negative nitrogen balance, as seen in cancer, HIV/AIDS, sepsis, trauma, burns, and athletic overtraining." Glutathione supplementation can oppose this process and in AIDS, for example, result in improved survival rates.

MAGNESIUM

Magnesium plays a critical role in the functioning of more than three hundred enzymes, many of which play an important role in energy production. Magnesium is a mineral found in many different types of foods; it plays an essential role in human DNA production and repair and in maintaining healthy bones, nerves, and muscles. Most Americans are magnesium deficient.

People who eat a diet high in pesticides, chemicals, and processed foods should take note that magnesium supplementation is a matter of life and death. It's that important. There's a magnesium research organization run by Paul Mason, who has dedicated his life to educating people that if they would consume more magnesium, the number of heart attacks would go down. He's found more than eighty scientific studies showing that small amounts of magnesium lowered the risk of heart disease. The Life Extension group, founded by Bill Faloon, recommends taking 400 to 800 milligrams of magnesium daily.

There are many serious problems caused by magnesium deficiency. Low magnesium can magnify free radical damage and precipitate the production of free radicals. Free radicals are the "bad guys." Antioxidants, in the simplest terms, "eat" the "bad guys," i.e., free radicals.

The following symptoms could indicate that you have a magnesium deficiency.

- **Low energy.**

- **Muscle twitching or cramping.** Magnesium plays an important role in muscle relaxation.

- **Frequent headaches.** Magnesium deficiency lowers serotonin levels, causes blood vessels to twitch, and affects neurotransmitter function, all related to headaches. It is said that migraine sufferers most often have a magnesium deficiency.

- **Difficulty sleeping.** According to Dr. Ronald Hoffman, the founder of the Hoffman Center in New York City and host of the radio show *Intelligent Medicine*, "If there isn't enough magnesium available for the body to replenish itself, sleeping becomes difficult."

- **Irregular heartbeat.** With low magnesium levels, the heart has difficulty staying in its regular rhythm.

- **Sensitivity to noise.** Dr. Hoffman says, "Without enough magnesium the body can't stabilize its nervous system. This often results in hyperreflexia, an enhanced startle reflex."

- **Seizures.** Startle epilepsy and the above symptoms can result when the nervous system is severely compromised as a result of a magnesium deficiency.

- **Low bone density.** Magnesium is essential for bone formation. The majority of the body's magnesium is stored in the bones.

- **Constipation.** Bowel movements slow down without enough magnesium. A great way to take in magnesium is to take a relaxing twenty-minute Epsom salts bath before bedtime. After doing so, you may find you sleep seven to eight hours without drugs.

- **High blood pressure.** Magnesium deficiency can cause blood pressure to be too high.

- **Type 2 diabetes.** Magnesium may help support healthy blood sugar metabolism.[2]

- **Depression, anxiety, confusion.** Low levels of magnesium in the brain can affect neurological functions and even cause agoraphobia.

Magnesium is a vital mineral, essential to body functioning. Three other vital minerals are calcium, potassium. and sodium. It's a simple fix: go to your favorite supplier to order them (I get my minerals from Life Extension at www.lifeextension.com/goodhealth), and begin taking magnesium immediately and for life. Yes, for life. If you want to age the new way, you have to give your body the essentials it once had in order for it to function at optimum. The benefits to your sleep and heart health alone should be enough of an impetus to do so.

CURCUMIN

Curcumin is a powerful antioxidant. It has a broad-spectrum effect, and it is thought that it may help prevent Alzheimer's disease, cancer, atherosclerosis, and chronic inflammatory disorders. It seems to have a beneficial effect on just about every medical condition, and it costs very little.

MULTIVITAMIN

If you are going to take only one supplement for the rest of your life, make sure it's a multivitamin with meaningful potencies. A formula called Two-Per-Day provides higher potencies of vitamins, minerals, and plant extracts than are found in other supplements. It's formulated by the Life Extension group and regularly updated to reflect new scientific advances.

ZINC

According again to Dr. Jonathan Wright: zinc is best absorbed in the zinc picolinate form at a minimum of 30 milligrams daily, along with a bit of copper. Nature's Life is the only company selling zinc picolinate combined with copper.

For men, zinc is also a prostate protector; the recommended dose is 60 milligrams zinc (with copper) daily. Without enough zinc, the thymus gland in both genders shrivels and dies. This is important because healthy immune function is highly reliant on the thymus gland.

PREBIOTICS AND PROBIOTICS

There are many supplements that are crucial to survival, including those listed above, but because of the overuse of antibiotics, the toxicity from the environment, and the daily stress levels we all encounter, the gut balance takes the biggest hit. Having sufficient flora in the GI tract is essential for good health. Let's look at gut flora simply: there are the "good guys" and the "bad guys," and they are equally important and need to be in perfect balance.

Are you bloated? Constipated? Do you suffer from unexplained weight gain, brain fog, attention deficit, autoimmune disorders? Is your immune system degraded? Imbalanced gut flora is at the root of all these conditions.

Probiotics help balance the ratio of good-to-bad bacteria in your intestines by providing beneficial strains. The objective is to overwhelm "bad" bacteria with beneficial bacterial strains.

For support, you can take a prebiotic fiber supplement containing 70 percent xylooligosaccharides to promote the optimal growth of the beneficial bacteria you are introducing to your GI tract in the probiotic.

This is my opinion, but if I had to choose only one supplement to take for the rest of my life, it would be probiotics. Most cutting-edge doctors suggest starting with a good probiotic; if you don't see results in three weeks, consider adding a low-cost prebiotic supplement (available at www.suzannesomers.com) to better nourish your beneficial bacteria.

MINERALS

Minerals play an important role in good health, and some can act as an "on-off" switch in the body. This is particularly true of calcium and magnesium. For example, to contract a muscle, calcium is necessary. Calcium turns things on, and magnesium turns things off. If you run out of either of them, you get stuck in either the "on" or the "off" position. **It's important to take vitamin K along with calcium.** Here's why: Calcium is an essential mineral, but it tends to want to go to the soft tissues (arteries), where it can cause harmful calcium deposits on the heart valves (aortic stenosis) and in the arteries (arteriosclerosis). Vitamin K acts like a traffic cop, rerouting the calcium to go to the bones, where it is needed, and keeping it out of the arteries. Vitamin K is described as being good for the heart because of this protective measure.

Anything you put into your body that can't be used to make a new cell must be eliminated from the body at some cost to the system. That includes chemicals used as pharmaceuticals or food preservatives; environmental toxins; materials used in dental fillings that leach chemicals, such as mercury; and chemicals and other things we put onto our skin, such as soap and cosmetics. You should also be aware of the dirty air we breathe. At home, use HEPA filters to clean your air. Finally, switch out all chemical home cleaning products to natural nontoxic ones (you can order good ones at www.suzannesomers.com).

The basic diet for good health is one that is free of chemicals and has not been processed in order to increase foods' shelf life.

As I said in my original Somersize books, shop the periphery of the grocery store, where all the fresh foods are located. Common sense says to stop smoking, stop eating artificial sweeteners and MSG, stop eating soy products (soybeans are now mostly genetically modified (GMO), and according to the movie documentarian Michael Pollan of *Genetic Roulette*, GMO food creates a kind of "insecticide factory" in your intestines).

I say eat organic if you can afford it in order to avoid the negative effects of pesticides and the herbicide glyphosate. If you want to see what some people are saying about GMOs, you'll get a wake-up if you google *Genetic Roulette*. The producer is not a doctor but a passionate documentarian who does his homework. It's important to stop eating "plastic" fats (as I've described earlier) and partially hydrogenated oils. Also, get house filters for your tap water so you can eliminate chlorine, fluoride, and other compounds from it.

This is what you have to do to survive in today's polluted environment. It sounds harsh, but it's a waste of time to get upset or depressed over the damage that's happened to our planet. I always try to find hope, and here it is: you can control the environment in your own home by what you clean it with, the food you buy, what you put onto your skin, and keeping the air in your home free of toxicity through the use of HEPA filters. We spend most of our time in our homes, so this will be a huge step toward protecting against this great environmental assault.

HUMIC AND FULVIC ACIDS

Huh? you say. What are humic and fulvic acids? I learned about the benefits of humic acid and fulvic acid after our home burned down and Alan and I moved into a leased home that unbeknownst to us was saturated with the worst kind of black mold. You couldn't see it or smell it, but the mold was there like the little shop of horrors, crawling throughout the drywall and into the air-conditioning and heating ducts. After a couple of years there, we both started feeling low-grade sick all the time. My intestines were bloated and painful, I gained weight, and Alan developed facial tics and vulnerable facial spasms plus red, swollen, watery eyes. He's a healthy guy; he had never had that before. I've since found out that toxicity often finds its home in people's eyes. Next time you are out, notice how many people, especially older people, have watery, bloodshot, sick-looking eyes. Could it be toxic buildup?

For me, my symptoms were bloating and absorption problems. I wasn't absorbing minerals due to the mold in my intestines. One capful a day of humic/fulvic worked for me, allowing my body to once again absorb my vital-to-life minerals.

All toxicity, be it due to mold, chemicals, multiple chemical sensitivities, or fungus, needs to be eliminated through detoxification; there is no effective drug-based answer for these new conditions of today. This is where the antiaging and alternative doctors excel. They are equipped to deal with and understand your toxic burden and can alleviate it in a myriad of ways. IV drips are commonly used, as is far-infrared sauna, which helps you sweat out the toxins. Make sure to wipe down in the sauna regularly so as not to reabsorb the toxins you just excreted. Also, take extra magnesium when you detoxify.

But there is a miracle in a bottle that comes from nature, called humic and fulvic acids.

When a leaf on a tree is alive, it contains oxygen, which suppresses the growth of the fungal spores that are always present on the leaf. When the leaf falls off the tree, it loses its oxygen, and this loss of oxygen causes cell wall–deficient organisms to become fungi and causes the fungal spores on the leaf to "wake up" so the fungi can do what they were designed to do: begin the process of turning the leaf into "dirt." The dirt contains a mixture of organic acids collectively called **humic acid**. A series of complex acids in the humic acid is called **fulvic acid**. It contains *all* the well-known vitamins, minerals, and amino acids.

Now imagine that a seed blows into this dirt. Add water, and the fulvic acid opens the cell membrane of the seed, allowing the humic acid to enter. With this nutrition and water and all the inherent minerals, vitamins, and amino acids, the seed will grow into a plant full of nutrition that we will then ingest when we eat it.

That is, in a perfect world.

But sadly, farmers use pesticides and horrible substances such as glyphosate to kill weeds. These chemicals then get into our GI tracts. Ever wonder why almost everyone seems to have gut problems? Our food has been degraded, and natural growing processes have been torpedoed. Our GI tracts are filled with toxins that are eating little holes in them, causing leaks (leaky gut) that allow the toxins to travel throughout our bloodstreams, causing havoc with our other organs and glands. Meanwhile, eating foods without sufficient nutrition makes it difficult for us to extract enough good things from the food we go out of our way to put into our bodies.

Here's why I am explaining this: Today's crops contain only a fraction as much (80 percent less) of the humic substances (especially fulvic acid) as they did a century ago, according to the US Department of Agriculture. This deficit of natural humic and fulvic acids results in people obtaining less of the vitamins, minerals, amino acids, phytochemicals, and other beneficial plant nutrients.

The reduction in specific nutrients per unit of farmed plant foods today as compared to a hundred years ago is largely explained by industrial farming methods that provide far greater yields per acre but less nutrition per unit of food.

Fruits and vegetables are still healthy food categories, especially when organically grown. What few people realize is that the nutrients that were once abundant in plant foods are now often depleted, which is why supplementation is so important.

Depletion of fulvic acid and humic acid is regrettable because these compounds help protect against the loss of mitochondrial function, which works synergistically with **coenzyme Q10 (CoQ10)** to slow cellular aging.

Fulvic acid stimulates mitochondrial energy transfer, while humic acid speeds the transfer of energy-producing electrons in the mitochondria.

An easy way to supplement with fulvic acid and humic acid is to take 100 to 400 milligrams per day of shilajit, which can be found today in more advanced CoQ10 formulas. There is exciting evidence that one of the principal substances in shilajit, fulvic acid, inhibits the buildup of toxic tau proteins and untangles filaments of tau proteins in the brain. This has the potential to protect against the underlying pathology involved in dementia.

I've spoken with researchers about how adding fulvic-activated minerals to our bodies neutralizes the acidity that contributes to health problems. The claim is that fulvic acid assists in excreting acidic waste and toxins from our bodies that can otherwise build up in our cells and tissues.[3]

As we age, our bodies have difficulty absorbing vitamins and minerals. I take a capsule or two a day of humic and fulvic acid to help my body absorb minerals. I also use humic/fulvic acid fertilizer in my organic garden to help my food absorb valuable nutrients. You can order it from HUmineral at www.humineral.com or call 888-765-0087.

CHAPTER 5

YOGA:

An Exercise for the Rest of Your Life

We all know we *should* exercise and reduce stress for the rest of our lives, but aging unfortunately brings a lack of energy and drive. The desire for the "perfect" body diminishes somewhat, and we start saying things such as "I look pretty good for my age."

How about having a beautiful and healthy body forever?

Let me introduce you to yoga, the exercise I will do until I die. It's ageless. I love it; it's as intensive as I want, as cardio as I want, and, like my cat in the morning, it gets me to stretch gently to wake things up. We start slowly, moving, stretching, getting the blood moving.

If you eat right, stick to real food, consume little sugar and grain, and follow the examples of what you have learned so far from the doctors in this book, you can sail through life with a beautiful body, little to no cellulite, and very little wrinkling. **It's all about how much you put into it.**

The nice thing about yoga is you can go to a class, you can have a teacher come to your home, as I am privileged to do, or you can follow classes online.

Because it is so accessible in so many ways, you can do it whenever and wherever you are. You won't have to find a gym and go to some awkward place where everyone looks like Arnold Schwarzenegger.

Chapter 3 focuses on "Stress: the Real Killer" and that its effects are not so silent, emphasizing the importance of calming the mind with meditation. Yoga gives you that calm while providing you with all the benefits of exercise that is not violent. You progress according to your abilities, never more rapidly. There is no competition or pushing beyond what your body can do; rather, you go with the flow of what your body wants to do on any given day.

Interview with

JULIE CARMEN

I have been practicing yoga with Julie Carmen, my friend and yoga instructor, for nineteen years. She is also a yoga therapist in Malibu, California. A yoga therapist is different from a yoga teacher. She is a licensed marriage and family therapist, a certified yoga therapist, and the director of Yoga Therapy for Mental Health at Loyola Marymount University Extension. She is also the founder and director of Yoga Therapy for Mental Health at Venice Family Clinic, a supervised clinical practicum.

SOMERS: Thanks, Julie. You and I spoke last week, and you said something so interesting: "the wisdom of yoga." Can you explain what you mean by that?

CARMEN: Yes, what I mentioned was a phrase that is *prajnaparadha*—that's P-R-A-J-N-A, which means "wisdom," paradha, P-A-R-A-D-H-A, which means "to go against wisdom" or "crimes against wisdom."

SOMERS: So what does that mean?

CARMEN: Well, for instance, I had a cup of coffee before having a cavity filled this morning, which was not my most evolved choice. It made a stressful experience more stressful. All of us do this, especially when stressed: we eat things that taste delicious but cause indigestion or worse. Or we have heart issues but don't practice cardio to strengthen the heart. These simple things or choices are crimes against our own innate wisdom.

SOMERS: You mean that we know inherently it's wrong but we choose to do it anyway?

CARMEN: Yes, and then we experience the consequences.

Yoga works with lifestyle choices; I call it "mind/body hygiene." That phrase comes from as far back as when dental hygiene was first being taught; if plaque creates decay, we know if we floss, we can remove the plaque.

In yoga we practice mind/body hygiene, meaning looking at our thoughts, our posture, how we move, breathe, and communicate. Then we modify our lifestyle practices. We interrupt sabotaging self-talk and replace those thoughts with phrases that help us stay present, such as "I am breathing in. I am breathing out."

I teach how to stay on top of our lifestyle practices and our mind/body hygiene so we don't create dis-ease through negligence and old habits.

SOMERS: Deep breathing is such an important part of our practice. I can feel that I'm using more of my lungs when I exhale fully and allow the new air to come in slowly. Why would we care about vagus nerve activity?

CARMEN: Yoga breathing and a yogic mind-set of grace under pressure is known to increase vagal tone, which reduces stress and inflammation. When someone has had a traumatic event in their lives, psychological or physical, their window of tolerance or of frustration becomes narrower, uncomfortable at best. In yoga we practice expanding our window of tolerance, and eventually the breath starts slowing and becoming deeper. Then the heart rate becomes less agitated.

SOMERS: That explanation makes me understand the wisdom of yoga and its ability to destress. What's micro–yoga practice?

CARMEN: I ask students to find one posture or sequence they love, that they know will work, and just do it throughout the day. That way we are not chasing stress but we are ahead of it. If we spend more of the day within that *window of tolerance*, we won't have to wind down quite as much at night.

SOMERS: Sort of reminds me of when I was in kindergarten, we had to put our heads on the desk and take a little nap. It was probably a way of getting the kids to calm down after lunch and recess.

CARMEN: Yes, and to be less reactive and more self-reflective and maybe to breathe a little bit.

SOMERS: Is yoga ageless? I mean, can you do it from your youngest years to the end of life?

CARMEN: Absolutely. There are certain parts of yoga that are more appropriate for different age groups. With children we like to imitate the animals. That's why a lot of the postures the children do are named after animals, but subliminally it teaches them meditative practice. Most children are too active to be able to sit still and gaze at a single point of focus and observe their breath.

Contrary, most older people misunderstand and think yoga is a teacher in a gym having them jump through the hoops doing different advanced asanas.

SOMERS: Well, yoga can appear intimidating if you have never done it.

CARMEN: Right—all these pretzel poses or lotus poses, and people think they can't do that so they can't do yoga. There are many accessible types of yoga: chair yoga, yoga for Parkinson's, yoga for cancer survivors, yoga for multiple sclerosis, yoga for arthritis, and prime-of-life yoga.

As a yoga therapist we are required to have a minimum of a thousand hours' training. The three thousand certified yoga therapists in the United States are often dual credentialed, where in addition we have a license as either a psychotherapist, like myself, occupational therapist, or physical therapist. Some MDs are also certified yoga therapists. On the other hand, a yoga teacher may only have two to three hundred hours of training.

Many people are under the impression that yoga is to lose weight and that yoga is simply doing a limited set of physical postures because that is what is taught in many yoga classes. But it's much deeper than that. A yoga therapist adjusts every practice individually to the person in front of them. They watch the breath, they sometimes take the pulse, and they do an intake assessment. They take into account stage of life, energy, and any current or past trauma.

So to answer your question about how long we can do yoga, there are people who are a hundred years old and still doing yoga.

SOMERS: That will be me. I started with you having never done yoga in my life, not quite knowing what it was, but something about it appealed to me and you are such a good teacher. I have found the added component of you as a psychotherapist to be beneficial also, as our talks often have wandered off and you put on your other hat. Over the years I have found your psychological "take" equally as beneficial as the yoga itself. Long ago I would have thought that seventy-three years would be too old to be doing yoga, but I find the contrary. Instead, I feel strong inside. That's one of the main things I like about it, the inner strength. I am also doing it for my body. I enjoy looking good, and yoga is having that effect. But I also love the inner strength, the core work. How important is a strong core?

CARMEN: I like doing core work myself and with all students so they don't get injured. There is a misconception that yoga is only about stretching and stabilizing. But the real key is the integration between what's going on in your mind.

Yoga is now, and what's going on with the breath connects you to your core.

There is a phrase that translates to mean "Keeping my heart rate and breath steady even as I increase the intensity of my physical practice." In Sanskrit we call that *sthira sukham asanam*, which translates to mean "steadiness and effortlessness."

Keeping the mind-set—

So let's say we are holding plank either on the forearms or on the palms, and you are breathing and drawing the belly toward the spine, and you are starting to feel "I can't wait till this is over." Then you are challenging that sattvic state; you have a choice to expand your window of tolerance by consciously maintaining emotional equilibrium.

SOMERS: I promise never to complain about plank again. Haha.

What if you are overweight? Is yoga for you?

CARMEN: Absolutely. I would start gently; you don't want to sprain the joints. Improper alignment puts pressure on the joints. Strain on the joints, plus excess weight or previous injuries that may have thrown the skeleton out of alignment, has to be taken into consideration. I'd suggest learning from a physical therapist or yoga therapist how to properly forward bend or twist. Some injuries get worse from forward bending and twisting. I would suggest neutral breath-centric postures that are stabilizing for the joints.

SOMERS: In order to strengthen?

CARMEN: Yes, to strengthen, keep limber, and to keep the mind forming new positive connections. Yoga helps us control body sensations like craving foods we may not want. Yoga also helps us watch and regulate our emotions, so that if we are feeling deprived, like "Oh, I was on the bike for twenty minutes, I deserve a piece of chocolate cake," that's negative self-talk that's self-sabotaging if one is trying to lose weight or prevent diabetes.

In yoga we learn to "watch our thoughts" in a self-reflective way, as though we are in cognitive behavioral therapy.

Svadyaya is that self-study in yoga language where we might say to ourselves, "Boy, I just noticed a thought that's working against my goal." And that brings us back to the *prajnaparadha*, which is crimes against wisdom.

If our wisdom tells us that we would have a better quality of life if we dropped twenty, forty, or a hundred pounds, then we have to figure out what lifestyle practices we can adjust and what positive new ones we can adopt. It's always easier to increase positive lifestyle practices than let go of things that are habitual.

This all brings us back to the mind/body hygiene. We want to not only use dental floss with our teeth, but we also want to "dental floss" our brains from self-sabotaging thoughts.

For instance, food is not a way to manage stress, as in "I had a hard day, so I want a beer." Instead, what are the healthy coping skills that will work toward my end goal, which is longevity with great quality of life?

SOMERS: And there you have it. Once again, we are all in control by the choices we make and the thoughts we think. That's the point of this book. We each have the power to make our lives what we want.

BIOIDENTICAL HORMONES:
The Game Changer

CHAPTER 6

NO ONE SIZE FITS ALL

I'm out of estrogen, and I have a gun!
—Anonymous

The above quote makes me laugh. Anyone who has experienced PMS or severe hormonal decline can relate to it. Haha.

Bioidentical hormones, which are biologically identical to the human hormone, an exact replica of what you still make or once made, *are* a game changer for both aging men and women.

I began taking bioidentical hormone replacement therapy (BHRT) twenty-five years ago, a decision that changed the course of my life. As a result, I don't have any of the negative symptoms of aging, I sleep eight hours without drugs, my weight is good, my libido is good, my skin is not very wrinkled for my chronological age. (As you'll see from the interview in chapter 9, Dr. Thierry Hertoghe believes that what we expect and accept as normal aging is really a result of deficiencies—yes, wrinkles, too! It's quite exciting to read how far he has come in the understanding of hormones.) Due to my bioidentical hormone replacement, I don't get rashes and breakouts, my hair is thick and shiny, my nails are strong, I have no bone loss, and my mind is sharper than ever. There are limits to how long we can depend on healthy lifestyle choices to keep us youthful, but overall, my mind is working better than ever, and, best of all, I am able to access my wisdom and perspective, the two things no young person can buy or have. If we get to this age not all pilled up, the gift that awaits us is the "knowing" that comes with having lived long enough to "get it."

At seventy-three, my mind is working great. I remember everything; I am proud of that. I deliberately take lots of brain supplements that include mind-enhancing nutrients. In the interview with Dr. Jonathan Wright in chapter 11, he explains ReMIND supplementation for the brain. I take six a day. I also take over-the-counter lithium, 20 milligrams daily, and two capsules of turmeric, along with what I use liberally in cooking. Older people joke about "senior moments," but make no mistake, the memory lapses common to seniors are no joke; rather, they are an indicator that the brain has ceased to "fire" at optimum.

As you get older, the situation will become exacerbated. The marvelous and crucial natural hormones are your ticket to happiness and quality of life. Through BHRT, I can better access my well-earned wisdom and perspective; my stress levels are very low because I can calmly assess each situation for what it is without experiencing the anxiety and disruption that accompany declining hormone levels. Everyone fears aging, but BHRT provides an answer; it is the "juice of youth."

The brain recognizes hormonal balance as valuable in perpetuating the species. This is nature's plan; we are hardwired to reproduce. But now, with the new life extension techniques, we can all enjoy and access true health and live longer than ever before. Today, we expect to spend an equal amount of time as nonreproductive people as when we were making balanced hormones; in other words, without replacing declining hormones, we will be *alive* but without a good *quality* of life.

As your hormones decline, you can become symptomatic for a wide range of problems. Your hair may get stringy, your sleep may become difficult, your libido may wane, your blood pressure may increase, and your immune system may no longer work optimally. This can accelerate the onset of one or more of the "big three": heart disease, cancer, and/or Alzheimer's disease.

Hormones are not to be taken haphazardly. What you need is different from what the next person needs. There is no "one pill fits all" as with the synthetic pharmaceuticals. By analyzing your lab work, your doctor will individualize your treatment, that is, prescribe the exact right amount of hormones for you and your deficiencies.

Every human on the planet has hormones. The hormones estrogen, progesterone, and testosterone make us men and women. They build bones, maintain muscle tone, and protect your joints. They regulate your heartbeat and breathing. They fight stress, calm anxiety, relieve depression, and allow you to "feel." They govern your sex drive and fertility. They stimulate your brain and immune system and relieve pain. They govern the menstrual cycle and enable pregnancy.

When your hormones are in balance, you feel perfect. When they are out of balance, your life quality diminishes substantially.

A hormone is a chemical substance produced in our body by our glands. Hormones are a complex combination of chemical "keys" that turn important metabolic locks in our cells, tissues, and organs. All of the 30 trillion to 40 trillion cells in our bodies are influenced to some degree by these amazing keys.

The turning on of the "locks" stimulates activity within the cells of our brain, intestines, muscles, genital organs, and skin. Hormones determine the rate at which our cells burn up nutrients and other food substances and release energy. They also determine whether our cells should produce milk, hair, secretions, enzymes, or some other metabolic (life) product. Hormones affect virtually every function in your body. They affect your mood, how you cope with stress, your sexuality, your sex drive.

All our hormones depend on one another. They have an interactive "language" and work as a team to maintain our health. At the end of our reproductive years, things start to go wrong for both men and women.

Many men are under the impression that hormones are the domain of women only. Nothing could be further from the truth. Men's hormones also influence who they are—or are not. No man wants to lose his "juice," so consulting a good antiaging doctor is crucial to maintain it (see appendix A for where to find testing) and to go forward. To accept the status quo is to live with the downward spiral of aging: becoming decrepit and frail and eventually succumbing to the diseases of aging.

Bioidentical hormones can be taken orally or by hormone cream. Your doctor can discuss these options with you and determine which form will work best for you. For those who find after a time that they aren't absorbing the cream or the pills, injections would be the route to take—again, based on your doctor's judgment.

CHAPTER 7

HOW HORMONES WORK

Hormones are one of the most incredible chemical symphonies on our planet: the human physiological response to danger. Your endocrine system dumps adrenaline and other hormones into your blood, which ratchets up your senses (enhance!), and tells your heart to start feeding your muscles extra juice. Your respiration increases to take in more oxygen. Coiled for imminent action, your body is primed to fight, or get the heck outa there. You are now super-human.

—Joe Brown, editor in chief, *Popular Science*

All our hormones, both men's and women's, depend on one another. They have an interactive "language" and work as a team to maintain our health. If one hormone is missing or insufficient, it will affect the other hormones. It's like a symphony; it is important that all the instruments be "in tune." Imbalanced hormones are a setup for disease and health problems. Notice that things start to go wrong at the end of your reproductive years. I'll say this again and again: biologically we are here to make babies (perpetuate the species) and then get out of the way when we are no longer able to do so. This worked well when we all died at the end of our reproductive years, but today that is no longer the case. We are all living much longer, like it or not.

We get sick when one or more members of the hormone team are not working at the same capacity as the other hormones. So when your doctor says, "Your thyroid is a little low," it's a big deal. It's a sign of imbalance. But why do our hormones decline or get out of balance in the first place?

Your hormones decline when your endocrine glands cannot maintain the same production of hormones they did in your younger years. The loss of hormones can begin as early as the midtwenties (though that is unusual), but generally around the age of thirty-five is when you first start to feel their loss. It never used to happen at such a young age, but stress and toxicity have accelerated hormone loss and thus accelerated aging. Without sufficient hormones, you will begin to age. Early-onset hormonal loss is equivalent to accelerated aging. Now I've got your attention, don't I?

> Mainstream medicine rarely connects common ill effects and toxicity with declining hormone levels.
>
> You want a qualified doctor who specializes in bioidentical hormone replacement. To go to a doctor who has not gone back to school to make BHRT his or her specialty is like going to a plumber for a heart bypass.

With hormonal decline come withdrawal symptoms. The symptoms vary from woman to woman and from man to man. But the symptoms are all part of the process and a very uncomfortable one at that. It's similar to puberty, when your hormone levels were rising, except that now the situation is reversing or has completely reversed, depending on your age.

At seventy-three my body makes very little sex hormones. According to biology, it is way past time for me to check out. But today's reality of new medical advances has enabled us all to have longer life. Imagine how differently I would feel (and look) were I not on these miracle medications. My age used to be the end of the line for most people, but because of my great health—or, as I call it, "juice"—and energy, I can entertain the idea of living for a very long time. The most exciting thing is that I will have this extended life with *quality*.

There are major and minor hormones. The majors include insulin, thyroid hormone, adrenaline, and cortisol. If any of these is too high or too low, you won't live very long.

The minor hormones (although why they are called minor I'll never understand, because when they are low, you feel awful) include estrogen, progesterone, testosterone, and pregnenolone. DHEA is often considered a major hormone because it is the most abundant steroid hormone produced in the body.

Now visualize a teeter-totter. On one end are the minors: estrogen, progesterone, testosterone, and pregnenolone. On the other are the majors: adrenaline, thyroid hormone, cortisol, and insulin.

Now visualize the teeter-totter going up and down. Optimal hormone health is when the teeter-totter is flat and balanced, with all the hormones lined up in a row and interacting with one another.

In hormone decline in both men and women due to stress, environment, or aging, the minors fall first. When this occurs, the majors often rise. A high cortisol level may be one reason you aren't sleeping well. A high adrenaline level combined with a low cortisol level can make you feel stressed yet at the same time fatigued.

ESTROGEN

In my book *I'm Too Young for This!: The Natural Hormone Solution to Enjoy Perimenopause* I explained the mystery of estrogen. Estrogen is one of the most powerful hormones in the human body: it is what makes a woman a woman.

Estrogen gives women their softness, their curves and breasts, and helps regulate a woman's passage through menstruation, fertility, and menopause. Both men and women make estrogen. To be a woman, you need high levels of estrogen and low levels of testosterone. To be a man, you need high levels of testosterone.

Estrogen is not a single hormone. It is a group of many separate yet similar hormones, which for simplicity's sake can be narrowed down to the "big three": estrone, estradiol, and estriol. These are produced in the ovaries, body fat, and other parts of the body and perform the functions we normally attribute to estrogen.

Approximately three hundred different tissues are equipped with estrogen receptors. This means that estrogen can affect a wide range of tissues and organs, including the brain, liver, bones, and skin. The uterus, urinary tract, breasts, and blood vessels also depend upon estrogen to stay toned and flexible. (Have you ever laughed so hard you peed your pants? Is this happening regularly now? It's because of the estrogen loss that comes with this hormonal transition from being reproductive to no longer being reproductive.) Estrogen works in concert with progesterone to nourish and support the growth and regeneration of the female reproductive tissues—the breasts, ovaries, and uterus—so the body will create eggs. In addition, estrogen imparts the characteristic female growth of body hair and distribution of body fat. It can also protect heart and brain function and promote bone strength.

The "new doctors" such as those featured in this book understand how to test for estrogen decline and determine replacement therapy according to your individual deficiencies. What is right for the next person is not necessarily right for you. We are individuals, unique and one of a kind. That is why it is called "the *art* of hormone replacement."

In chapter 2, you met Dr. Jonathan Wright, a pioneer in alternative medicine. He has a bachelor of arts degree from Harvard University and a medical degree from the University of Michigan. He was the first doctor in the United States to write a prescription for bioidentical hormones almost forty years ago; you can imagine the uproar. But as it caught on, both women and men started realizing that through these miracle hormones they could get back what they had lost in the aging process and begin to feel young and happy again. Who wouldn't want that? Again, bioidentical hormones are a "game changer."

Interview with

DR. JONATHAN WRIGHT

Dr. Wright is a wizard, and I say that with respect and admiration. He just knows things. An avid reader and researcher, he understands the need for nutritional balance, hormonal balance, and natural remedies for achieving optimal health. If you want to do yourself a favor, make an appointment for a full checkup at his clinic in Tahoma, Washington. It's worth the trip. Alan and I did this several years ago, and we are still amazed at the "detective work" that uncovered issues in each of us that would have plagued us going forward.

SOMERS: You wrote the first prescription for bioidentical hormone replacement therapy [BHRT] in the United States forty years ago. That took great courage, and you have paid a price for that. As a result, your office was raided and trashed by the FDA, who emerged "triumphantly" with vitamin B and carnitine, which still leaves me speechless. I always felt that was a terribly unfair thing to do to you simply because you had a new idea and a concept backed by research and knowledge.

It's similar to the famous quote about "the three stages of truth" by Schopenhauer: **"First it's ridiculed, second it is violently opposed, third it is accepted as self-evident."** You and I have talked about BHRT often, and I'd like your thoughts about going forward with the aging process relative to BHRT.

WRIGHT: There's so much incredible information on the benefits of replacement. Wait until you hear this: Over a decade ago research reported from researchers at Georgetown University Lung Biology Laboratory absolutely proved that:

A woman's lung health is dependent on estrogen!

Consider what happens after menopause. Your estrogen level drops dramatically. That is why, if you're not a tobacco smoker and you're a woman, unfortunately you have a six times greater chance of developing chronic obstructive pulmonary disease [COPD] than a man.

SOMERS: I did not know lungs require estrogen, but it makes sense. This is exciting and dramatic evidence of the necessity for estrogen replacement, especially when done correctly by working with a qualified doctor to create a complete replacement regimen of all the missing hormones individualized for each person, as all our needs are different.

WRIGHT: Yes, it's quite dramatic. When you look at women who don't smoke and men who don't smoke, the odds are that one man gets COPD to six women who get it because **lungs are estrogen dependent**.

If a woman is an athlete and in menopause, if she wants to maintain her lung function in order to continue her athletic abilities, estrogen will help her maintain her lung function.

There are so many benefits of estrogen replacement aside from removing the difficult symptoms of decline. For instance, here's another: I've heard from several choirmasters that women who took estrogen after menopause could now sing like when they were younger. You can always tell a young lady from an older lady on a call-in radio show. Hormones affect the voice; look at the way vocal frequencies change when young people go through puberty. That's all hormonal.

SOMERS: I remember years ago you told me my voice would remain in the same range for life because I was on a full complement of bioidentical hormones. My singing is still in the same key as always, and just the other day a friend came over and I called downstairs, saying I'd be right there. He said, "You sound like a girl!" Nice benefit most of us have never thought of. I guess Lauren Bacall didn't take hormones. Haha.

WRIGHT: She did have a very deep voice. To get hormone replacement right, the ratios are most important in achieving healthy hormonal balance. Urine testing is crucial to achieving correct balance and ratios—and of course, listening to the patient.

SOMERS: I agree. There's no one size fits all. My body "eats" estrogen. I require a lot to feel perfect, but you are always sure that the ratio of my estrogen to progesterone is in the right numbers. That's why a qualified doctor is so important. You can't guess at it.

WRIGHT: Yes, it's not just estrogen and progesterone; it's also the ratio of pro-carcinogenic estrogens and anticarcinogenic estrogens. We run a test for pro- and anticarcinogenic progesterone also because those do exist, but that test is not available anywhere at present. It will be available at Meridian Valley Laboratory in about six months. Getting back to these estrogens, I'm glad you mentioned testing.

Patients need to know saliva testing has too many drawbacks. There are many research papers that show if the hormones are being produced inside the body, the saliva is accurate, but if it's taken from the outside (meaning the patient is on BHRT replacement) saliva is not accurate.

Secondly, forget about blood testing because you can't get the free fraction of two of the three major estrogens, including the anticarcinogenic one—estriol—measured in a blood test.

The free fraction is the active fraction, and what we can measure of the estrogens with blood testing is the total, about ninety-nine percent, and that doesn't tell you about the active free fraction. Nobody ever measures free estriol in blood, and the only way you can measure all the free fractions of estrogens is with a urine test, which is why we only do the urine test because it's the most accurate and gives us the most information.

Women should also know the importance of iodine as a preventative for breast cancer. If breast cancer cells start to form, if iodine is present in that same breast tissue, the iodine combines with a particular fat that's in the breast cancer and kills the breast cancer. And that's just one way that iodine kills breast cancer cells. Other researchers reported that breast cancer cells—but not normal breast cells—can "take up" iodine, which kills them once it's absorbed. That's two ways that iodine kills breast cancer cells. Did he say iodine "kills breast cancer cells"? Yes, he did. Also, iodine, as well as iodide, causes the body to make much more of the anticancer hormone estrogen, called **estriol**. I actually had an article published about that.

SOMERS: I believe you saved me from a second bout of breast cancer by discovering through testing that my body wasn't making any estriol, the most powerful anticarcinogenic component of my estrogens. So thank you. I believe that was a lifesaver.

WRIGHT: It became so obvious; as the report published in the *Proceedings of the National Academy of Sciences* showed, if estriol is low, you must have her take iodine and iodide. With iodine and iodide replacement, the estriol will go up in nearly everyone, and that is so important because estriol is anticarcinogenic, so here's what I recommend: "A drop a day keeps breast cancer away." It's very important it be a drop of Lugol's solution, which requires a prescription for full strength. Full-strength Lugol's can't be sold online because of the DEA. She puts one drop on this breast over here today and one drop on that breast over there tomorrow. By doing this she cuts her risk of breast cancer dramatically because you already have the iodine ready and waiting inside your body for when (or if) breast cancer cells show up. If we use one drop only, we're never going to overdose. If we go to three drops, we might, so don't do that. Just use one drop a day, each breast. The full details about this, along with scientific references, were published in *Green Medicine Newsletter* in October 2018.

SOMERS: Why is there so much autoimmune disease?

WRIGHT: Yes, and women get much more autoimmune disease than men, much more. I'm sorry.

Oddly enough, autoimmune can go into remission during pregnancy. Ask any gynecologist. So, acting on that, Professor Nancy Sicotte of one of the southern California universities recruited six women with severe multiple sclerosis—so severe they were in wheelchairs—and when they did MRIs of their brains, they had all these MS lesions as well as extremely bad multiple sclerosis. They gave them all a very high dose of estriol. [Remember estriol, the anticarcinogenic estrogen that is made in giant amounts during pregnancy?] After a few months, they did another MRI on the women with MS, and they couldn't believe what had happened to their brains. Oh, my goodness, Suzanne, in seventy-five percent of those with MS [multiple sclerosis], their brain lesions had disappeared. No kidding, and that's with just estriol.

Then, for science, they took the patients off estriol, and guess what, the MS lesions came back. Yeah, so for women, estriol is anti-autoimmune.

SOMERS: Great to know.

WRIGHT: Remember I told you HCG takes away endometriosis? Well, researchers took white blood cells from women and men who had autoimmune disease. They found that HCG made the white blood cells "move away" autoimmunity in the women, but it did not do that in the men. Well, it sort of figures; us guys don't get pregnant, you know? And that's where HCG comes from; it's made in large quantities during pregnancy.

So the point is, ladies, if you happen to have an autoimmune disease—and women get it six times as much as the men—get your natural medicine doctor to try HCG.

SOMERS: Some publications are saying that HCG is dangerous. Is that true?

WRIGHT: No, that's false. There's a recent publication with people given thousands of units of HCG, and it didn't hurt them a bit. But you do have to work with your natural medicine doctor because it has to be injected.

You can learn to do your own injections, it's that safe, but you better learn the correct way. So HCG and estriol have enormous potential against autoimmunity for women, not for men, darn it. It's sexist and unfair, but that's the way it goes. It's worked for women with autoimmune disease.

CHAPTER 8

THYROTROPIN-RELEASING HORMONE (TRH)

You've most likely never heard of this one, but pay attention to this new breakthrough. It might just be what you need to get your hormonal "song" correct and into balance.

A year ago, I experienced a period of intense stress. The results on my body were devastating: trouble sleeping, hair falling out and breaking off, brittle nails, all indicators of a thyroid gone awry. It didn't make sense to me, because I was on thyroid hormone replacement according to my deficiencies determined by blood work. What was wrong? Then I heard about **thyrotropin-releasing hormone (TRH)**. For lack of a better explanation, it "wakes up" a lazy brain (in particular the hypothalamus) to shake things up and jump-start the hormonal communications system. Thyroid hormones are crucial to our health and quality of life.

Many people with hypothyroid conditions, including Hashimoto's thyroiditis, take either synthetic or natural thyroid hormone. In the alternative world, only natural thyroid hormone is given. I take Naturethroid. Most people have little or no understanding of why thyroid hormones are important.

The thyroid regulates the metabolism of the body, which is why low thyroid hormone levels frequently lead to symptoms such as fatigue, weight gain, and constipation. But thyroid hormones have many other important roles in the body and are extremely important in the growth, development, and metabolic function of just about all of the organ systems and tissues.

Thyroid hormones play an important role in the metabolism of protein, carbohydrates, and fats. With regard to protein, thyroid hormones stimulate the synthesis as well as the degradation of proteins. As a result, a deficiency in thyroid hormones can prevent protein synthesis, which is very important to body function.

Thyroid hormones also play a role in carbohydrate metabolism and affect the synthesis, mobilization, and degradation of fats. They also play an important role in regulating the expression of genes. They do this through thyroid hormone receptors, which are DNA-binding transcription factors whose functions can activate or repress gene expression. Thyroid hormones also play an important role in brain development and function. Triiodothyronine (T_3), as Dr. Wright explains in the following pages, is the active form of thyroid hormone and controls the expression of genes involved in myelination, cell differentiation, cell migration, and signaling. This is one of the reasons why a deficiency of thyroid hormones can cause cognitive problems.

T_3 plays a role in peripheral nerve regeneration. Having normal thyroid function is important for reproduction. Thyroid hormones are required for skeletal development and the establishment of peak bone mass. T_3 regulates bone turnover and bone mineral density.

Hypothyroidism (low thyroid) causes impaired bone formation and growth retardation, whereas **hyperthyroidism** (high thyroid) results in accelerated growth, advanced bone age, and decreased bone mass.

Stress blunts hormone production, and in my case clearly my thyroid was *hollering* at me to figure it out.

Dr. Wright suggested I look up the work of Dr. Walter Pierpaoli of Italy on TRH because thyroid replacement alone was not doing the job for me. This recommendation was my game changer. (We get our messages in mysterious ways.)

Dr. Wright recommends blood evaluation of **thyroid-stimulating hormone (TSH)** while on TRH. The expected result of TRH stimulation is an increase in TSH.

Dr. Walter Pierpaoli is currently the president of the Interbion Foundation for Basic Biomedical Research in Switzerland and the director of the Jean Choay Institute for Biomedical Research, also in Switzerland.

Dr. Pierpaoli is noted in the medical world for bringing TRH to light. Some call TRH a "miracle" because of all it does to promote body health and balance, including restoring normal thyroid function.

For me TRH was that miracle; after three months of taking it, my sleep pattern normalized, my hair grew back stronger, my nails became strong again, and my symptoms of low thyroid dissipated.

My brain, for lack of a better description, had gotten lazy, probably due to the stress I was experiencing at that time. My pituitary (located in the brain) was not sending the signals through TSH to the thyroid. TRH does not stimulate secretion of thyroid hormones such as T_3 and T_4 but may, as I experienced, "wake up" a lazy brain, revealing a deficiency of TSH in the pituitary gland.

I order my TRH, called Abaris, from International Aging Systems; see www.antiaging-systems.com.

Dr. Pierpaoli says TRH produces a regulation of lipid levels in the blood. **Blood lipids** are mainly fatty acids and cholesterol. **Hyperlipidemia** is the presence of elevated or abnormal levels of **lipids** and/or **lipoproteins** in the blood and is a major risk factor for cardiovascular disease.

Studies on TRH have shown improvements to cholesterol, triglycerides, phospholipids, albumin, aminotransferases, urea, testosterone, and glucose, to name but a few. And in animal studies it has helped restore healthy weights of the kidneys, thymus, adrenals, testes, heart, and liver. But weight loss is clearly the information that turned on the medical community.

> People become most excited when we mention weight loss with TRH!
> —Walter Pierpaoli

The mechanism behind the ability of TRH to induce weight loss is simple: it activates basal metabolism via regulation of anabolic hormones and proper release of insulin. With TRH, glucose is burned and fat is less likely to be stored. Only TRH can do that without any side effects. Dr. Pierpaoli says that it must be emphasized that TRH, even if injected intravenously in huge amounts, has not shown any side effects. However, he typically recommends taking a 5-milligram sublingual tablet of TRH first thing in the morning. He refers to TRH as a magic molecule of nature that knows what to do and how to do it.

The body weight of mice was taken before treatment with TRH, at thirteen days after treatment, and then again at thirty days. An average body weight loss of 13 percent within a month has been seen and substantiated in yet another animal trial.

Dr. Pierpaoli says his patients are happy that they feel so well when taking TRH and always ask for more. It's a natural molecule and cannot be patented. It is taken in cycles of one month on, one month off; thus it is taken for six months in a year.

TRH also induces the proliferation of insulin-producing cells, which could have great implications for advanced diabetics. This may be good for insulin-dependent diabetics, but most early-stage type 2 diabetics, along with overweight people who are not yet diabetic, produce too much insulin, which contributes to metabolic disorders.

More from

DR. JONATHAN WRIGHT

Dr. Wright has so much to say about everything that I've included him in two chapters. I asked him about the thyroid, its importance, and the complexities of the essential hormone it produces.

SOMERS: Dr. Wright, why do so many people have thyroid problems?

WRIGHT: Some Americans don't have enough iodine and iodide in their diets. The populations that have enough iodine or iodide in their diets are those who eat seafood regularly; the closer you get to the coast, the more iodine you're going to get in your diet. Unfortunately, you don't get much iodine from freshwater fish. A lack of iodine will affect your thyroid negatively, but if we get enough, our thyroid rates are going to stay healthy. The most active thyroid hormone by far at helping all the cells to make energy to keep us going happens to be called free T_3, which is the free fraction.

SOMERS: That's very interesting. So iodine is critical for the overall health of the thyroid, and when you don't have that element you have thyroid problems.

WRIGHT: Yes. Eastern Washington State is well known to be so selenium deficient that the selenium-deficient cattle actually get something called white muscle disease. Without enough selenium, we can't make enough free T_3. Without making enough free T_3, you're not going to be as energized.

SOMERS: Is that what happens on those days when I feel "dog tired," that I'm lacking selenium and iodine and my thyroid is taking the hit?

WRIGHT: Can't say that's the only possibility, but it's one possibility. Another thyroid disrupter, a big, bad one, is fluoride. Fluoridation does more harm than it ever did good. Fluoride is in the same family as iodide; so is bromide. Fortunately, we're not using bromide in conventional mainstream medicine anymore. We were doing a lot of that in the

1890s, but fluoride is now in just about everybody's water, and unfortunately fluoride will get into the thyroid and take the place of the iodide that should be there, so the thyroid gland simply can't work correctly or optimally; impossible with all that fluoride in there.

SOMERS: So were we sold a bill of goods when they told us that fluoride is a "public health achievement"?

WRIGHT: It actually has been a public health tragedy. There was a 2012 research article from Harvard, no less—I should emphasize it was the Harvard School of Public Health.

SOMERS: Your old alma mater.

WRIGHT: Yes. Dr. Grandjean and his colleagues pointed out that in fluoridated areas, the children could be expected to have seven less IQ points than the children from nonfluoridated areas on the average. Talk about a public health tragedy.

SOMERS: Have you ever experienced a patient with a thyroid so low [hypothyroid] that they just went crazy? I had a friend to whom this happened, and it was so serious, bordering on tragic.

> Low thyroid = **hypo**thyroid.
> High thyroid = **hyper**thyroid.

WRIGHT: Yes. And sadly, even doctors miss the body signs sometimes. And thyroid blood testing is very often not done comprehensively. They'll test for only T_4 sometimes, but even more often, they'll test for only TSH, a thyroid-stimulating hormone, which has its origin in the pituitary gland, not in the thyroid gland, and does not tell you what your thyroid should be doing.

Also, some don't measure the free fraction of the active thyroid hormones free T_3 and free T_4.

Now, with any hormone—thyroid, testosterone, estrogen, all the hormones—there is a "free fraction" and then there is a so-called bound fraction; researchers tell us that the free fraction is one percent or less of that hormone.

SOMERS: I'd really like you to explain for me and for my readers what "free T_3" means. It's so confusing.

WRIGHT: It's as if you put most of the hormones on this truck called a "hormone-binding globulin" running around the body doing nothing, and only one percent or so is not on the hormone-binding globulin truck but free in the bloodstream to do its job; that's the free component doing its thing.

You see, the thyroid hormone, as well as testosterone and estrogen, are all like very small "health keys." It's supposed to fit into what's called a receptor, and as we know, if we're going to put a house key into a lock, we need to have the key in our hand. But if that total of the bound fraction, which is called "total," on the blood test is normal, that doesn't mean that the "free" is normal. The "total" is this large protein that binds up 99 percent of each hormone. Comparatively speaking, it is like the size of a beach ball compared with a house key.

This hypothetical beach ball has got all these little keys attached to it, and then you try to unlock your door with that key attached to the beach ball. It's not going to work.

SOMERS: It's a great visual.

WRIGHT: So to make sure how much "free" hormone is available to fit into the lock, we have to measure our free T_3, and our free T_4. There's a terrific article by a Scottish doctor who points out that this whole dependence on TSH testing is not accurate because there never were correlations between the TSH test and the patient's clinical state. In conventional medicine they treat the test instead of treating the patient. That's why so much thyroid mistreatment is going on.

SOMERS: So that's what allowed my friend to find herself in a state of such deep depression, because the real thyroid numbers were missed until it was blatantly obvious. Shouldn't everyone, doctors included, worry about having a low thyroid?

WRIGHT: Yes, because what we want is optimal. We don't want to be told we're a little low. We want to have optimal function, and notice I didn't call it normal. "Normal" is being dead, too! What we want is optimal.

SOMERS: What is the far end of low thyroid and the far end of high?

WRIGHT: Well, one can have such a weak thyroid that one gets depressed. It's not common, but it can happen. It's about brain cells unable to produce energy inside the cells. Free T_3 is one very essential stimulus for cellular energy. We have to have that stimulation by the free T_3 molecule in every cell in the body for it to produce enough energy to keep itself going optimally.

SOMERS: A qualified doctor versed in bioidentical hormones will most likely know about the importance of free T_3. Would you say the thyroid takes orders from the pituitary, which is located in the brain?

WRIGHT: The pituitary gland is the conductor who gives the signal for the adrenal glands, the signal for the ovaries, the signal for the testicles, the signal for the thyroid, et cetera, et cetera, but then there's a "behind the scenes" conductor called the hypothalamus. It's the area of the brain right above the pituitary gland.

Here's an example of that: thyrotropin-releasing hormone, or TRH, comes from the hypothalamus, which then goes to the pituitary gland telling the pituitary to make TSH. I don't know why we need that multistep process, but that is the way that nature and creation decided, so I'm just going to respect that and copycat in my practice.

When your TSH is low, it can mean that it is not getting stimulated with the TRH from the hypothalamus. Dr. Pierpaoli pointed the way. For your issues we worked together to supplement a little bit of TRH, for there is no other way to turn the hypothalamus back on again. It usually happens when we're older. It's one of those things.

SOMERS: It's like the hypothalamus gets lazy as we get older and TRH wakes it up. That's the effect it had on me. Suddenly things started working again; my hair started growing again, it was thicker and shiny, and my nails improved. It made me realize that so many things we accept as normal aging are really caused by deficiencies. The TRH essentially turned my hypothalamus back on again, and now all is well and I feel optimal. It's very exciting when you think about it; in so many ways, we can literally turn back the clock.

WRIGHT: A lot of things happen when we're older. So now we can supplement with TRH, which stimulates the TSH, and that stimulates the thyroid gland, but doctors who rely strictly on TSH testing are going to tell people, "Well, look at that, your TSH is low, that must mean your free T_3 and free T_4 are enough for you." Excuse me; it often means your hypothalamus is malfunctioning.

It's crucial to look at all those hormones—free T_4, free T_3, TSH, all three—because if that TSH is low, and the T_4 is high or high normal, then as a doctor you'd expect the TSH to be low. But if both the free T_4 and the TSH are low, that usually means enough TRH isn't being made by the hypothalamus to stimulate the T_4 and free T_4.

SOMERS: So that's when the patient would need TRH replacement.

WRIGHT: Right. T_4 is not the energy-producing molecule; that's the signaling molecule, and it's called a feedback loop: TSH pushes the thyroid, T_4 goes back to the pituitary gland and says, "Hey, you're pushing me enough," and so the TSH goes down when the TSH is finally high enough.

SOMERS: That's a lot of initials. Haha. It's complicated and probably why low or high thyroid is so epidemic and not many patients are getting it fixed properly.

WRIGHT: Doctors usually rely solely on the TSH test, and it's just not enough.

SOMERS: The facts are: those of us who have been replacing hormones naturally are healthier. I've been on natural hormone replacement for twenty-five years, including replacing thyroid and TRH, and I feel fabulous, symptom free, and best of all, I almost *never* have to utilize pharmaceutical drugs. I firmly believe the less foreign molecules one puts into their body, the better off and healthier they are.

CHAPTER 9

THE HORMONE SYSTEM:
The Juice of Youth

Every human body on the planet contains hormones. Hormones build bones, maintain muscle tone, and protect your joints. They regulate your heartbeat and breathing. They fight stress, calm anxiety, relieve depression, and allow you to *feel*. They govern your sex drive and fertility. They stimulate your brain and immune system and relieve pain. They govern your menstrual cycle, and they enable pregnancy. When your hormones are in balance, you feel perfect; when they are out of balance, your quality of life and health diminish substantially. All our hormones depend on one another. They have an interactive "language" and work as a team to maintain our health. If one is missing or insufficient, this will affect the other hormones. Imbalanced hormones are a setup for disease and health problems. As I explained earlier, there are major and minor hormones.

The majors are insulin, thyroid hormone, adrenaline, and cortisol. The minors are the best known: estrogen, progesterone, testosterone, DHEA, and pregnenolone. When the minor hormones fall or decline, you get the symptoms associated with menopause: low estrogen, mood swings, inability to sleep, inability to think clearly, memory lapses, weight gain in all the wrong places, wrinkled skin, age spots, a general lack of "juice."

Below is a brief overview of the majors and the minors. I have also listed the hormones that are equally important to the "hormonal song"; remember, all of them interact with one another. When one is "off," they are all off. The hormonal system is a symphony, and it's important that all the "players" show up; otherwise the music will come off discordant.

THE MINOR HORMONES

Estrogen

Estrogen is one of the most powerful hormones in the human body. It is what makes a woman a woman. Estrogen is not a single hormone; it is a group of many separate yet similar hormones. For simplicity's sake these can be narrowed down to "the big three": estrone, estradiol, and estriol. These are produced in the ovaries, body fat, and other parts of the body. There are approximately three hundred different types of tissues that are equipped with estrogen receptors. This means that estrogen affects a wide range of tissues and organs, including the brain, liver, bones, and skin. The uterus, urinary tract, breasts, and blood vessels also depend on estrogen to stay toned and flexible. Estrogen works in concert with progesterone to nourish and support the growth and regeneration of the female reproductive tissues—the breasts, ovaries, and uterus—so the body will produce eggs. It can also protect heart and brain function and promote bone strength.

Progesterone

Progesterone is one of the two main hormones produced in the ovaries. The other is estrogen. It is produced primarily in the second half of a woman's menstrual cycle. It is also produced in small amounts in the adrenal glands in both sexes (men also produce some progesterone in the testes), where it acts as a precursor for other steroid hormones. All hormones are considered steroid hormones: testosterone, progesterone, estrogen, DHEA, pregnenolone, aldosterone, and more. The term *steroid* refers to both hormones produced by the body and artificially produced medications that duplicate the action of the naturally occurring steroids. Progesterone has many functions, and without it we are left with unopposed estrogen, which will leave you pretty defenseless against disease, including cancer. When progesterone declines severely, we are at risk of having our bodies in an unhealthy hormonal state of imbalance.

Estrogen is carcinogenic, and progesterone is *anti*carcinogenic. Nature has it figured out beautifully: women in the fertile years make estrogen every day of the month in varying amounts and progesterone fifteen days of the month. Just when we are reaching our estrogen "peak," progesterone, which is anticarcinogenic, comes in to balance everything out. That is why it is so important to go to a qualified doctor who understands the importance of balance.

"Estrogen dominance" is simply not having enough progesterone. Just when estrogen gets too high and could be dangerous, progesterone flies in to the rescue (nature is perfect). At the end of those fifteen days, either you have a period or you are pregnant. We menopausal women don't have to worry about getting pregnant; our eggs are gone.

I am convinced I got breast cancer in my forties because, looking back, I had all the hallmarks of estrogen dominance: fuller breasts, starting to gain weight, mood swings, inability to sleep, and no understanding of the hormonal system. My body was like so many women's bodies in midlife: we drain out of progesterone first, leaving us with too much estrogen and no protection from cancer. No wonder I got breast cancer. My body was a perfect setup. Also, progesterone is a "feel good" hormone. Without it come the mood swings, loss of bone density, weight gain, and other symptoms of premature aging.

Natural progesterone is also associated with reduced incidences of certain cancers; it's your protection. It is the anticarcinogenic component of your "hormonal song." Without enough progesterone, you are left without the built-in protection from cancer that nature provided.

Ever notice that we woman get our first cancers around the end of our reproductive years? This is nature's way of clearing the deck for the young, reproductive ones. It's all about perpetuation of the species. Nothing personal.

Some women don't want to reinstate their period when they go on bioidentical hormone replacement, but beware; I understand the inconvenience, but the only time in nature you made estrogen and progesterone simultaneously (every day of the month for both of them) was when you were pregnant. But nature never expected that you would be pregnant for the rest of your life. That's what happens when you tell your doctor you don't want to reinstate a period; it is called "continuous combined therapy," and I personally am adamantly against it. You will gain weight this way (your body will think it's pregnant), you will not get the full benefits of balance, and you will be putting yourself into danger because you will be going against nature, and whenever we do that, it rarely goes well.

Testosterone

Testosterone is our sex "driver" and an anabolic steroid that builds bone and muscle. Testosterone is necessary in both the woman's and the man's hormonal song. Men make high amounts of testosterone and smaller amounts of estrogen. Women make more estrogen and lower amounts of testosterone, which is essential for strong bones and a strong heart. In fact, the heart has plenty of androgen receptors for testosterone. It is your "pumping power," and of course you need it for "that ol' feeling" of romance. But to limit this important hormone to its effect on the sex drive alone would be underrating its value. It has many other functions: it maintains bone density, affects muscle size and strength, and is responsible for skin oil secretion. Testosterone is essential to a woman's hormonal song, although in lower amounts than in men. It can help with the symptoms of hormonal loss such as hot flashes and vaginal dryness. It lessens the risk of osteoporosis by improving bone density, reduces body fat, improves mood and lessens depression, improves muscle mass, decreases the risk of autoimmune disorders, fights fatigue, improves symptoms of diabetes, reduces the risk of heart disease, and helps in the treatment of lupus. Testosterone supports the brain by increasing blood supply and increasing the connections between neurons. It increases the potency of your memory, normalizes your mood, and reduces anxiety. The traditional way of taking bioidentical hormones is by rubbing each hormone cream on your skin daily; this generally produces the best results. It's what works for me. My husband needs testosterone injections because he doesn't absorb cream well.

Danish researcher and pediatrician Dr. Niels Skakkebæk published a paper in 1992 showing male fertility declined between 1940 and 1990, and also commented on the findings, saying:

These two new papers add significantly to existing literature on adverse trends in male reproductive health problems . . . Here in Denmark, there is an epidemic of infertility. More than 20 percent of Danish men do not father children. Most worryingly [in Denmark] is that semen quality is in general so poor that an average young Danish man has much fewer sperm than men had a couple of generations ago, and more than 90 percent of their sperm are abnormal.[1]

Think of the awesome negative connotations of this information. I fear that the rest of the world will follow suit. Our men will no longer be able to procreate if things continue status quo. Endocrine-disrupting chemicals have undoubtedly contributed to the dramatic decline in reproductive ability among men. Excessive microwave radiation from wireless technologies, obesity, and inactivity also play a significant role.

According to a study reported on *Scientific American*'s Environmental Health News site, a decrease in male fertility was linked to environmental estrogen exposure, and the magnitude of these findings was summarized as follows:

They observed adverse effects starting in the first generation of mouse lineages where each generation was exposed for a brief period shortly after birth. The impacts worsened in the second generation compared to the first, and by the third generation the scientists were finding animals that could not produce sperm at all.

This latter condition was not seen in the first two generations exposed. Details of the experimental results actually suggested that multiple generations of exposure may have increased male sensitivity to the chemical.

Sex hormones are what drive the differentiation between the sexes. When synthetic chemicals that mimic these all-important hormones enter into the mix, it confuses the process and interferes with the biological process of turning the fetus into a male. Think about this: suddenly the most natural processes in our bodies relative to conception and reproduction are getting confused. Can't be good. The survival of the species is at stake. It's imperative that we understand the devastating effects of toxicity and take the steps to unload our individual toxic burdens.

Clearly testosterone is a very important hormone for both women and men.

Dihydroepiandrosterone (DHEA)

Dihydroepiandrosterone (DHEA) is abundantly produced in healthy young adults, but the level declines dramatically as we age. DHEA is made by the adrenal glands and converted into testosterone and estrogen. DHEA is involved in critical body functions: mood, sexual desire, bone density, weight. It has positive effects on the brain, immune system, reproductive organs, muscles, and other organs and tissues. It's important in the prevention of heart disease and cancer and in weight loss. It also helps maintain collagen levels in the skin and therefore smooth, younger-looking skin. It is known as the antiaging hormone. DHEA helps alleviate depression, helps prevent atherosclerosis, helps increase bone mass, slows osteoporosis, improves insulin resistance, and assists in wound healing. DHEA levels stimulate **insulin-like growth factor 1 (IGF-1)**, which maintains new bone formation; also, healthy DHEA levels suppress the production of **interleukin-6**, an inflammatory cytokine that causes excessive bone breakdown.

One of the things older people are often warned about is not to fall, because aging brings about brittle, frail bones, so keeping DHEA at healthy levels is vitally important.

Other minor hormones that play important roles in keeping our "juice" and moving forward are **oxytocin** and pregnenolone.

In the interview with Dr. Thierry Hertoghe in the following pages, he explains the magic of oxytocin, HGH, and other lesser-known hormones. Suffice it to say that oxytocin causes people to feel natural happiness and love and reduces anxiety; it also causes women to feel more orgasmic. (Now I've got your attention.) It also helps with insomnia and your general feeling of vitality. And did I say it makes you want to have a lot of sex?

Pregnenolone

Pregnenolone, another hormone made by the adrenal glands, is a little-known sexual stimulant. A pregnenolone supplement taken on a daily basis increases sexual arousal and promotes better orgasm.

You now see how all the hormones are constantly communicating with one another. Pregnenolone is a "mother hormone" because it helps make so many other hormones in the body. It can gently boost low progesterone and can help correct the progesterone/estrogen ratio, a huge factor in protecting oneself from cancer. It is also a memory hormone. In higher doses it reduces fatigue, fights depression, protects the joints, relieves arthritis, and speeds healing.

Without enough pregnenolone, you are sure to have memory problems and poor concentration. You will be at risk for stress, depression, and chronic fatigue plus a reduced capacity for physical exertion, and if you don't have sufficient levels, you will experience a host of symptoms.

The good news is that pregnenolone is available over the counter. Nature has it all worked out. As we go forward, it is our job to replicate the perfection of nature as best we can by putting back that which is missing to make our bodies operate at peak.

In my book *I'm Too Young for This*, I went into great depth about all the hormones and how to take them, and the doctors who "get it" are in this book or can be found at www.foreverhealth.com.

THE MAJOR HORMONES

Insulin

Insulin has many functions in the body. It is a major hormone secreted by the islet cells of the pancreas that helps to move glucose from the blood into the cells for use as energy. The level of insulin in your body determines whether nutrients taken in will be burned off as energy or stored as fat. This is why insulin is called the fat-storing hormone. High insulin tends to impede the release of other hormones involved in the body's ability to burn stored body fat. You don't want high insulin. A pattern of high levels of glucose and insulin in the bloodstream will cause glucose to be stored as fat. Insulin is designed to fall while you are sleeping, but if you have high cortisol, you may gain weight even if you aren't eating much. Nature is on alert and trying to keep your cells constantly supplied with glucose. To learn more, read the interview with Dr. Thierry Hertoghe in the following pages to find out his thoughts on insulin and why it is such an important hormone in the "hormonal song."

Thyrotropin-Releasing Hormone (TRH)

The interview with Dr. Jonathan Wright in chapter 8 explained in depth about **thyrotropin-releasing hormone (TRH)**, but here's a thumbnail: The thyroid affects virtually every system in your body. To understand unexplained weight gain, fibrocystic breasts, joint pain, hair loss, loss of sex drive, and so many other complaints, you need to understand the thyroid. If your thyroid isn't "right," you won't feel "right." It's that simple.

Adrenaline

Adrenaline is our engine. It pushes us forward. It's what gives us a surge of boundless energy. If we are living a balanced life, our bodies release adrenaline when we need that surge and afterward return to a

calmer baseline. It's when we get addicted to adrenaline and put ourselves into situations that continually require our bodies to want more
and more of it that problems arise. Eventually you flatline. Then a host
of symptoms occurs and for lack of a better description you are "running on empty." Busy people are likely running on adrenaline, nature's
best energy bar. But like a caffeine bump or an illicit drug's high, it's addictive and dangerous to your health. When your adrenals are burned
out, you have no energy and you feel a racing inside that makes sleep
impossible, which further hurts the function of your adrenals. Lack
of sleep makes everything worse, and now you are in a vicious cycle.
People with adrenal insufficiency are not calm. They live with the feeling every moment that the sky is going to fall. Symptoms include ex-
haustion, heart palpitations, recurrent infections, achiness, low blood
sugar, and inability to sleep. It can also cause anemia, hormone imbalance, and inflammation.

Cortisol

Cortisol is the stress hormone. It is released by your adrenal glands.
When you encounter a stressful situation, you quickly release cortisol to
raise your blood sugar level and give you energy. Cortisol is the only hormone the lack of which will cause you to die from the first body stressor,
such as an infection. Cortisol is needed for mood enhancement, dyna-
mism, work capacity, stress resistance, stimulation of immune defenses,
and the reduction of joint and other pain. If you do not have enough
cortisol, your immune system will eventually degrade. **Cancer patients
with low cortisol have little ability to fight the cancer, which increases
the chances that the cancer will metastasize throughout the body.**

It's crucially important to do lab testing to determine your cortisol
levels. The remedy is simple: cortisol replacement (mine is in the form
of capsules), as determined by your individual deficiency.

OTHER HORMONES

Human Growth Hormone (HGH)

Human growth hormone (HGH) is controversial and for no good reason. Our own bodies make it until around age thirty-five, and then it starts to decline. It's part of the "hormonal song," so it stands to reason that as you replace other missing or low hormones, you should also replace HGH, as determined by your deficiencies according to your lab work. As with all hormones, too little is not enough and too much is too much. What you are striving to achieve is a "just right," perfect balance. When all is well and balanced in the body, the feeling of well-being is indescribable.

HGH is responsible for so many bodily functions and deficiencies, and a lack of it can result in premature aging. (Now I've got your attention! Haha.)

According to Dr. Hertoghe in his book *Reversing Physical Aging*, HGH deficiency signs/symptoms in *adults* include:

- Baldness (in men)

- Decreased muscle mass and strength

- Dry, thin skin

- Fatigue and/or tiredness

- Lower tolerance to exercise

- Reduced bone density

- Weight gain, especially around the waist

In Dr. Hertoghe's book *Atlas of Endocrinology for Hormone Therapy*, he explains the physical ramifications of a lack of HGH. He describes GH deficiencies relative to your appearance that HGH is responsible for:

- **Back:** A bowed back, shorter stature, reduced height with aging on the face, tensed shoulder muscles, droopy muscles

- **Face:** A small, deeply wrinkled forehead, droopy upper eyelids, thinner nose, thin lips, small cheekbones, deep nasolabial folds, receding gums, sagging cheeks, jawbone atrophy, small chin

- **Chest:**
  - **Men:** Gynecomastia
  - **Men and women:** Sagging breasts

- **Abdomen:** Overweight/obese body, abdominal obesity, droopy belly, pregnancy stretch marks in women

- **Buttocks:** Fatty buttocks, sagging muscles, atrophy, stretch marks of rapid weight loss

- **Thighs:** Cellulite, sagging inner thighs, fatty cushions above the knees

- **Knees:** Deformed knees (osteoarthritis)

- **Legs:** Thin, dry skin

- **Feet:** Muscle atrophy in the soles; reduced arch, flat feet

- **Behavior:** Nervousness, anxiety, tendency to dramatize stressful situations, excessive emotional reactions, sharp verbal retorts

- **Neck:** Loose skin folds under the chin

- **Shoulders:** Atrophying muscles

- **Arms:** Droopy triceps, thin muscles, decreased muscle strength, high systolic and diastolic blood pressure

- **Hands:** Backs of the hands: thin rigid, prolonged pinched skin fold, palms muscle atrophy (soft when pressed)

- **Fingers:** Deformed finger joints, thin fingers

- **Nails:** Longitudinal lines

These are the physical manifestations.

In the following interview with Dr. Hertoghe, he explains the internal ramifications of *all* declining hormones. You are going to be amazed when you read how easily we fall apart and how simple it is to put us back together again.

Melatonin

Melatonin is a hormone and also part of the body balance "song." Dr. Pierpaoli's work covers all hormones, but I thought you would like to know the following: he says that all women, in particular those who show low nighttime levels of melatonin in their saliva, show a remarkable improvement of latent and unsuspected conditions of low thyroid function (hypothyroidism) by taking my melatonin formula that includes zinc and can be ordered at aging-matters.com. In fact, it was observed in studies that a significant increase of the active thyroid hormone triiodothyronine (T_3) occurred in all women independently of their nighttime levels of melatonin by taking my particular formula of melatonin plus zinc.

This is probably why my sleeping patterns were restored to normal when I started taking a combination of TRH and melatonin. Dr. Pierpaoli's version of melatonin, called Melatonin MZS, is unique because it includes zinc and selenium. It is time released into the bloodstream between 1:00 and 3:00 a.m. This is important because hormones work best when they are given not only as the right molecule in the right dose and format (for bioavailability) but also at the right time. Since melatonin has a peak during the early hours of 1:00 to 3:00 a.m., this is an important factor in the efficacy of taking this particular form of melatonin. As you will read in this book, zinc has many hundreds of functions in the human body, and almost all of us who do not supplement have less-than-optimal zinc levels. He claims that sleep is deeper and more profound with this combination.

In the course of a six-month study, taking 3 milligrams of melatonin nightly produced a clear-cut decrease of the pituitary hormone luteinizing hormone, or LH (which increases progressively in the course of aging), in the bloodstream. This was most noticeable in younger women forty-three to forty-nine years of age. The recovery of pituitary function is more pronounced and rapid in younger women. This equaled an arrest and even reversal of brain aging and restoration of reproductive functions in the women taking evening melatonin.

As a result, 96 percent of women who had taken melatonin in that study reported a total disappearance of morning depression, which is typical in perimenopausal and menopausal women.

His results show that nighttime use of melatonin produces an improvement of thyroid function (synthesis of T_3 and T_4) and pituitary sensitivity to ovarian hormone output, as demonstrated by decreases in LH and follicular-stimulating hormone (FSH).

The concluding sentence of the study was "These findings seem to show a recovery of pituitary and thyroid functions in melatonin-treated women, toward a more juvenile pattern of regulation."

I obtain my MZS from IAS via www.antiaging-systems.com (you can save 15 percent by using the code ANWA-15 at the store).

I cannot place enough emphasis on the joys of achieving perfect hormone balance. It takes some patience, but the payoff is more than worth it.

What I've given you here is an insight into bioidentical hormone replacement. A qualified doctor will work with you as an individual and through lab testing as well as self-reporting of your symptoms to your doctor, who can then fine-tune your prescription to your individual requirements. I am so "in tune" after all these blissful years of hormonal balance that I know when the stresses of life or a bad diet affects my levels. Hormone replacement is truly the magic pill, and it will give you your edge.

Sometimes I wonder if when I was growing up I was ever in perfect balance. I experienced so much stress as a child: an alcoholic father who ranted and raved, a teenage pregnancy, and raising a child alone when I was a child myself, all of which was very stressful. Stress blunts hormone production. Was my early hormone imbalance the seed of my breast cancer? It's something to think about.

In many ways, menopause saved me. I felt so bad (as in awful) when my hormones began to decline and drain out that I had to do something to fix myself. It wasn't easy twenty years ago. The solutions for women at that time were what I call the "menopause cocktail" of antianxiety pills, sleeping pills, synthetic so-called hormones (which have nothing to do with a woman's physiology), and more. I found those "solutions" unacceptable, and that was what put me on the quest to find true relief. My search for an answer was my ticket to peace and balance. I've never looked back. I feel great every day; I rarely feel anxious or moody. In fact, it's difficult to remember the "old days" of unexplained mood swings, all because of hormone replacement.

It's great to feel upbeat all the time!

Interview with

DR. THIERRY HERTOGHE

My goal as a doctor is to see the person rejuvenate. The person has to have a firmer face, firmer body, and look and feel younger. It's not sufficient just to look ten years younger than other people of the same age. You should look fifteen, twenty years or more younger. Then you know your treatment is on the right track.

—Thierry Hertoghe

Dr. Thierry Hertoghe is the president of two important medical societies: the World Society of Anti-Aging Medicine (WOSAAM), one of the leading international antiaging/life span scientific societies for physicians, with more than 7,000 members, and the International Hormone Society (IHS), the third largest international hormone society counting over 2,800 physicians around the world.

But that's just for starters. Dr. Hertoghe has been at the front of the pack of the healthy aging movement. He understood long before most others that there was a new way to age. In writing this book it was paramount for me to introduce him (again) and bring to my readers his incredible expertise and understanding of the hormonal system and how to rejuvenate. He is also a caring, compassionate man and doctor. His goal is not only to treat illness but also to optimize the health of each patient, while trying to delay and even reverse aging.

Dr. Hertoghe is focused on hormone treatments, nutritional therapies, lifestyle and dietary improvements, and antiaging medicine with the fundamental aim to optimize your health and lifestyle. He is focused on patients who want to take care of themselves, live better, longer, and healthier, and be part of the healthy aging movement no matter what their age.

I am proud to call him my friend, and it is with great pleasure I bring him to you, my dear readers.

SOMERS: The quote at the beginning of this section is extremely provocative. Dr. Hertoghe's goal is to make you years younger through his breakthrough therapies. Is this the fountain of youth we have all been looking for? It's a very exciting option to entertain.

I want to thank you for your time, Dr. Hertoghe, and I am excited to present you to my reading audience. This is the second time you have honored me with an interview for my books. You are a pioneer and always have so much to say about cutting-edge advances in health. You have written several books, and your latest book, all two thousand pages, called *Reversing Physical Aging*, is remarkable. You write mainly for doctors, but I found myself devouring the information because of your unique writing style and clever technique: each human health issue is accompanied by a photograph. My husband had chronic red, irritated eyes he developed later in life. I compared his picture with a photo in your book illustrating the same and was able to discern that he had low adrenals and very low cortisol. Brilliant.

We laypeople like to have visuals. As a result, I increased his cortisol intake to 25 milligrams daily taken early in the morning, and it has made a significant difference, along with Dr. Jonathan Wright, who suggested a vitamin A and vitamin C deficiency. The combination of both protocols has given him back his youthful clear eyes.

I always thought aging is aging, and as the years go by things change significantly. The possibility of reversal seemed pretty much impossible unless it was done surgically, and most often with surgery there is usually some negative price to pay. So here you are explaining and illustrating with this fantastic book the simple theory that you replace that which is declining. It's something I have fully understood relative to hormone replacement, but you have gone much further and deeper.

You were one of the first to tout the benefits and joys of replacing HGH [human growth hormone]. You say so many of your patients were averse to injections—fear of pain, et cetera—so you found a solution by putting three important antiaging and health substances together in one vial. What are those substances?

HERTOGHE: Patients can combine several major hormone therapies that need to be injected together so they only need to inject once under the skin. Thus, growth hormone, which gives more elasticity, and IGF-1, which thickens the skin, hair, and muscle, can be injected together.

SOMERS: You also had me add thymosin alpha-1 to my "three-shot" to keep my immune system strong.

HERTOGHE: Yes, and in some patients, I also add insulin into this same shot.

SOMERS: Why insulin?

HERTOGHE: Insulin allows amino acids to absorb better, and in most people these three supplements are necessary. Insulin deficiency produces typical signs of aging like droopy triceps and buttocks that are no longer firm, and by mixing these three injections together, they work better than injecting them separately. I saw amazing results. Really, I never thought it could be possible in such a short period of time to get the body so much firmer. It was actually evident in the first week in my first patient.

SOMERS: In one week?

HERTOGHE: Yes. We got results in one week's time. By adding these hormones together, they become much more potent. A dose given on its own would be normal, but a combined injection works much more quickly, because by combining them together, each treatment becomes more efficient. The first results I saw were with my wife; in one week, we saw her whole body get much firmer. In most patients, it takes more time.

SOMERS: You are making my readers want to run to Belgium to get some!

HERTOGHE: Yes, it was remarkable. Her face took longer to react because she kept eating grains, which counters the beneficial effects of a hormone treatment. I was so surprised by her results that I did this treatment myself, and I loved the results.

SOMERS: Well, being with you this summer, I have to say your face and your age do not correlate, so whatever you are doing, again, I wanted some and that's why I am taking this three-shot. I also love that it is nondrug.

HERTOGHE: Thanks. I started applying this same technique to much older women, like seventy-year-olds.

SOMERS: Hey, who says seventy-year-olds are "much older"? Haha.

HERTOGHE: Sorry, but it's a fact, at seventy your triceps begin to get droopy and also your buttocks get droopy. In several seventy-year-olds, I saw the same results in three to six months. When they came back, they were all very happy because these were results we didn't get with the other hormones individually, but just by adding these three hormones together, the difference was remarkable.

SOMERS: Can a patient go to your clinic in Belgium to be assessed and then you make up the vials for your patients? Can a qualified doctor in the United States order these ingredients if the patient's lab results indicate deficiencies?

HERTOGHE: We don't make the vials. Your antiaging-qualified doctor in the States can prescribe the combination. We explain to patients' doctors in different countries where to order and how to make the mixtures because we have patients coming from all over the world, making it very difficult to make enough mixtures until the next consultation, and if there's an interruption in the program, that's not so good. It's not dangerous, but if the treatment is interrupted, you lose the effects.

SOMERS: Clearly, hormones are more than what we think of as estrogen, progesterone, DHEA, testosterone, HGH. *How* we take them makes a difference, right?

HERTOGHE: Yes. Hormone creams are for fat-soluble hormones such as the sex hormones. Subcutaneous [under the skin] injections are for water-soluble hormones such as HGH, insulin, and IGF-1.

Injecting HGH, insulin, and IGF-1 is the best mode of transport because you're assured it's in the body. Otherwise these hormones may not be sufficiently absorbed because water-soluble hormones are very big. (Growth hormone is very large—it's 191 amino acids; insulin and IGF-1 are between 51 and 80 amino acids.) So absorption through the skin is much more difficult because of the length of the hormone molecule and because it's water soluble.

For this reason, it is better to inject these water-soluble hormones subcutaneously, and subcutaneous injections are very comfortable.

SOMERS: I am fascinated by this information, and I can feel my readers feeling the same. For sagging skin your concoction is IGF-1, insulin, and in some cases HGH, and also, I read that you prescribe the hormone relaxin, correct?

HERTOGHE: Yes, the problem with relaxin is its availability. I may be one of the only physicians in the world to have relaxin in injectable form for personal use, so I'm working hard to make it more available. It's extremely expensive.

RELAXIN

Relaxin belongs to the same family of hormones as insulin. Over the last decade, several relaxin-like peptides have been discovered, although the function of these peptides remains unclear. Recent studies have revealed effects of relaxin on other systems in the body. Relaxin decreases tissue fibrosis in the kidney, heart, lungs, and liver and promotes wound healing. Tissue fibrosis is the formation of hard tissue as a result of inflammation, which can lead to scarring and loss of organ function. This has made relaxin of interest to scientists studying how the heart heals after it has been damaged, which may help to treat heart failure in the future. In addition, relaxin can influence blood pressure by relaxing blood vessels; promote the growth of new blood vessels; and it is also anti-inflammatory. All of these properties could make it a potential therapeutic target for the treatment of certain diseases.

So that's a problem. The other three products are much easier to get, and it works unless your diet is not good. If you're a vegan, for example, you are not taking in animal amino acids, and these are the building blocks that exist in mammals and humans to make many hormones work.

SOMERS: A lot of people feel going vegan is the optimal way to live your life, but I remember when I was interviewing Dr. Nick Gonzalez, the late, great Nick Gonzalez, he said, according to science, vegans don't live as long. Have you ever heard that?

HERTOGHE: Yes. Yes. What I also say when asked, there's almost no centenarian, certainly no supercentenarian, that is a vegan. Meat has vitamins you almost don't have in vegetables, like vitamin B_{12}, that are extremely important for the cardiovascular system. There's a marker for increased risk of atherosclerosis in our blood called homocysteine, and that is higher in vegans because of the lack of vitamin Bs.

So if you're a vegan, you should certainly add all the vitamins you are lacking because of your diet. This includes all the fat-soluble vitamins, vitamin A, vitamin D, and vitamin K. (Vegans also cannot make vitamin D very easily, because they don't have the precursors coming from animal fat.)

SOMERS: What's a precursor?

HERTOGHE: The human body makes hormones from precursors, smaller or bigger molecules to which it adds or takes out atoms. Cholesterol, for example, is a precursor to sex hormones. Vegans are low in vitamin Bs and specifically B_{12}, so it's vital to add these supplements to lessen the burden and the cost to the body to be a vegan. A vegan (any person, actually) also can only absorb about ten percent of the amino acids you find in vegetables or grains, but from meat, it's about seventy percent of the amino acids.

SOMERS: Why do we care about amino acids?

HERTOGHE: **Amino acids are what makes your body tight, what makes your skin firm. When you look at a person, mostly what you see, his or her appearance, is the effect of amino acids—the skin, the muscles. Not the brain, which is mostly made of fat. You really need to have enough amino acids to look and feel great.**

SOMERS: That can only come from animals?

HERTOGHE: The best form of amino acids is from animals. Amino acid profiles, i.e., the ratio of arginine to lysine, found in vegetables are often not optimal/ideal. When you don't have all of what you need, it's difficult to make a muscle or muscular structures. For example, if you're missing amino acids, you can't make muscle fibers.

SOMERS: Let's talk vegetables: I grow my own, which is such a luxury. You can almost feel the power of vegetables when they are freshly cut and consumed immediately. It's amazing. You talk about sprouted grains, give me some examples.

HERTOGHE: Well, for instance, you have to sprout soy. You can put all sorts of grains in water so they have the ideal medium to sprout. We explain to our patients the timing needed to sprout. Even rice can sprout. I firmly believe this is the better way of preparing grains. Eating rice that is not sprouted is unhealthy. You will have a bloated belly, and it's mostly the lower belly that will bloat in that case.

SOMERS: I thought it was interesting that you said generally, if someone has a puffy face, they've got a bloated stomach.

HERTOGHE: Yes. [Laughs.] And you will see that this is really the case. It's not me, actually, saying that. There's a famous late German physician named Dr. Mayr, and he created the Mayr Cure and had a center in Austria.

SOMERS: What is the Mayr Cure?

HERTOGHE: With the Mayr Cure you don't eat much. Dr. Mayr showed the relationship of puffy face to bloated belly. He took pictures of his patients' belly and face before and then after a cure of partially fasting. By eating less and differently, the face became firmer and the belly flatter. Every time I see in a patient a bloated face and what is called the nasolabial folds—that's the folds that go from the nostrils down to the corner of the lips, that person is bloating in general, particularly on the belly.

SOMERS: Gluten, though, is also an aggravator, isn't it? Gluten makes the face puff up if you're gluten allergic?

HERTOGHE: Yes, gluten. But even if some grains are gluten free, if they are made from grains that are not sprouted, you will still have the presence of enzyme inhibitors from grains blocking your digestive enzymes.

SOMERS: Why is that?

HERTOGHE: These enzyme inhibitors function to block life in a grain, a seed, until the right conditions arrive for it to sprout. Soaking grains in water breaks down these enzyme inhibitors. The reason we should avoid ingesting the enzyme inhibitors present in unsprouted grains is that by blocking our digestive enzymes, these inhibitors reduce the digestion of our food, allowing for it to remain too long in our intestines, providing a bloated belly. A good digestion is very important to ensure hormone efficacy. This is the reason why I put so many pictures showing the impact of food on our appearance in the textbook *Reversing Physical Aging*.

Once you understand the effects of food on yourself, you are pushed to improve your diet and make the hormone treatment we discussed work much better. If the food is good, you get double or three times better results: a firmer body, for example.

SOMERS: I'm in one hundred percent agreement with that. I believe it's about the food, and today's food is damaged. It's very good you mentioned soy, sprouted soy, but it's hard to find soy anymore that's not genetically modified.

HERTOGHE: Yes. So we're survivors of that. [Laughs.] My newest book is a textbook about the face and the senses. If as a woman you have a bloated face, it could also be that your estrogen is too high and progesterone too low.

Progesterone has great importance as a protector of the breasts and the prostate, which I will discuss in the second volume, still to be published.

SOMERS: We have to keep you alive a long time to get all the information out of your head. [Laughs.]

HERTOGHE: I will have to eat some of your vegetables, then. I'll live longer. [Laughs.]

SOMERS: Exactly. The other question I have about insulin is that we are all reminded of the *dangers* of high insulin, and yet you're injecting insulin. Can you explain to me what I'm not understanding?

HERTOGHE: When insulin is excessive or deficient, it has adverse effects. You need to be in the middle range. If the reference range for insulin in the fasting state is, for example, between 3 and 27 IU per milliliter of blood, you should be around 7, but if it's lower, it's not good. Higher is also not good. If it's a reference range between 20 and 120 [that's the new range in a different unit], then you should be in the lower end of the reference range—not lower and not higher.

Insulin is very important because it is the main hormone that actually helps absorption not only of sugars but also of amino acids. So if people are extremely deficient in insulin, even without developing diabetes, then they are usually extremely thin; their skin becomes very, very thin, their muscles don't develop, nor do their bones develop naturally. It's because they never had enough amino acids.

People with low fasting insulin will usually not respond to treatments like growth hormone or testosterone to improve their muscle mass. They need insulin to get more volume in their skin and muscles. I'm talking of using very small doses of insulin, not the high doses used for diabetes treatment.

SOMERS: What is the average diabetes dose, or is there one?

HERTOGHE: Diabetics use doses around 70 units a day, but for insulin-deficient people who are not diabetic, the efficient dose is about 1 or 2 units a day before a meal, or sometimes even as little as 1 unit a day. For example, I had a patient who was extremely thin and extremely weak. She could only get out of her bed six hours per day, and she could walk maybe sixty or a hundred yards and then was exhausted. She was completely handicapped by terrible fatigue, so I said, "You need to take growth hormone." She said, "I don't have the money for growth hormone." Then a miracle happened. I said, "Well, I know that growth hormone increases the level of IGF-1 [insulin-like growth factor 1], which produces most of the physical effects of growth hormone." Most of the patient's thinness could be attributed to IGF-1 deficiency. I knew that insulin also increases IGF-1. So I said, "We'll give you a cheaper treatment, and we'll do it very cautiously." So she took insulin before each meal, 1 to 2 units. And then the wonder happened: she completely recovered her energy, so she was no longer confined to her bed during the day, she could walk for about four and a half miles, or six kilometers, a day.

Her energy returned, she put on twelve pounds—six pounds of fat, six pounds of muscles—and it changed her body, it became much more beautiful. She was able to take on a full-time job again as a tax consultant. It was tremendous. I've also seen men who never could have muscles—they were skinny, no muscles, atrophy—who with insulin, very small doses before each meal, greatly improved.

Actually, when you see very old people who lose their muscles, a great part of the loss is usually due to an insulin level that is too low. I'm not talking about people who are obese with a lot of insulin. That's also not good. So too much or too little is not good.

SOMERS: I guess, as with everything in the hormone world, it needs to be "just right."

HERTOGHE: Yes. The right dose for every person.

SOMERS: That sweet spot. It was interesting [laughs], my ego, when I saw you recently, I was thinking to myself, I bet he thinks I look pretty great for seventy-three years old. [Laughs.] And then you started picking up the skin on my hands and said, "Wow, that takes five seconds for it to go back into place!" There went my ego! Haha. So you suggested taking my cortisol all in the morning, because I had been doing it in four doses of 5 milligrams throughout the day.

Well, you're a wizard, because that dog-tired fatigue that I had been experiencing in late afternoon has completely gone away since I've loaded up with cortisol in the morning. And is it my imagination, but my hands are starting to look better? How much is too much cortisol? Because I know you can overdose on cortisol, and then you'll never go to sleep again.

HERTOGHE: On the average a woman's body makes about 20 milligrams of cortisol a day and a male's body 30 milligrams. So if you're of average size, that's the amount that you generally need. You only absorb about half of the cortisol, so when you take it, half will be broken down by your gut bacteria, and the other half will be absorbed. You need fifty percent of the endogenous production, but to get that, you need to give the whole dose, 20 to 30 milligrams, depending. Now, 20 to 30 milligrams per day is the amount produced by people who have a sedentary life. If you have an extremely active life with a lot of stress, you need more. The body doesn't make cortisol alone when it comes into action confronting stress. We also make other hormones like DHEA and **androstenedione**, but mostly DHEA, to protect you against the side effects of cortisol. If you have to take more cortisol, you need to take more DHEA to protect yourself. Otherwise, your skin can atrophy.

SOMERS: Why would you have skin atrophy with excess cortisol?

HERTOGHE: Because cortisol is a hormone that takes down inflammation. Cortisol decreases inflammation to block tissue overconsumption of cortisol, so then another hormone that builds up tissues is required, and that hormone is DHEA.

SOMERS: That DHEA level would be determined by lab work or just by looking at your wrinkled and droopy skin?

HERTOGHE: Lab work is always best to be accurate to determine the dose of DHEA. On average, a dose that is more or less equivalent in milligrams to the dose of cortisol that a person needs; a young adult human body makes 20 to 30 milligrams of both cortisol and DHEA daily.

SOMERS: So if I am understanding, that would be the measure: if you're taking 25 milligrams of cortisol, then take 25 milligrams of DHEA?

HERTOGHE: Yes. If you're taller, you need actually more of both hormones. If you're smaller, thinner, you need less. That is revealed in lab tests.

SOMERS: How interesting. So what you do is intuitive. You look at a patient, and before you do any lab work, you're assessing their deficiencies just by their appearance?

HERTOGHE: I almost know exactly what is the dose I need to give just by looking at a patient, but I still need the lab test, because they can make some corrections on my reasoning. It helps me fine-tune the treatment by doing the lab test.

SOMERS: This must be very exciting work for you, truly healing and refining.

HERTOGHE: Yes, the final results and final effects of the treatments are seen on the body. For certain hormone deficiencies, even the voice, its tone, can give me information on how intense the deficiency is or not.

SOMERS: Yes, years ago Dr. Wright told me I would keep my singing voice and the sweetness in my voice by taking bioidentical hormones. You told me you pay attention to the "reasoning" or good sense of the person. In America we might call that woman "scatterbrained."

HERTOGHE: If the person is confused or not making sense, it's usually a person with low cortisol, and that's not normal. If she or he has low energy at all times, it can be due to low sex hormones.

I teach other doctors to look for actual physical signs of hormone deficiency. Physical signs of hormonal decline on the body often give me a good idea of the intensity of a hormone deficiency, because whenever they are more pronounced, more intense, the deficiency is greater. That means that the patient needs a higher amount of the hormone and vice versa if it's too low. If it's a very light sign, then the patient may need a very small dose.

SOMERS: I'm a huge admirer of you and the work that you've done and what you've had to go through to achieve this respectability and recognition. You're dabbling in an area that's not pharmaceutical, and that's always difficult. I know this to be true from my own personal experience. One of the many great things you do is you travel around to different parts of the world and you teach doctors. In fact, in this two-thousand-page book, you specifically state at the beginning that it's meant for doctors. The problem I find as a writer about health and hormones and the effects of chemicals on the human body is the inconsistency with treatment. For instance, a friend wrote me yesterday, "I'm on an estradiol patch, and I've gained so much weight. I weigh two hundred pounds now and I diet and I don't eat grain and I don't drink alcohol and I don't have sugar. And I just keep gaining weight and gaining weight. Then I took some testosterone, but I didn't like the way I felt, and it made me perspire, so I gave it to my son."

Frankly, I thought, what kind of doctor are you going to that gives you a one-size-fits-all patch and then a little testosterone? It's frustrating for me, because I know the joy, the benefits, the beauty and quality of life enhancement from replacing deficiencies. Is there anything that can be done to create a consistency in the way doctors are treating?

HERTOGHE: I know what you are talking about, especially with American doctors. They don't look sufficiently at the physical signs, despite the fact that the examination of these physical signs helps to fine-tune the treatment. I was just speaking with an artificial intelligence [AI] firm about producing for physicians a software I've programmed that analyzes physical complaints, medical history, lab tests, and physical signs determined by the physical exam and that helps physicians in correctly individualizing hormone treatments.

SOMERS: That's fantastic. It's a way of standardizing so doctors can stop guessing.

HERTOGHE: Yes, I'm very excited to have this program to help me in my own practice, and it makes sense.

SOMERS: What are you looking for in your patients?

HERTOGHE: My goal is to see the person rejuvenate. The person has to have a firmer face, firmer body, and look and feel younger. It's not sufficient just to look ten years younger than other people of the same age. You should look fifteen, twenty years or more younger. Then you know your treatment is on the right track.

SOMERS: Well, my readers can't see you, but let me vouch for Dr. Hertoghe. He looks twenty, twenty-five years younger than he is. I mean, it's quite remarkable. But what is interesting about the way you are aging is that it looks "right," not cosmetic or false or plastic like so many who are chasing youth today. It doesn't look contrived, just a young, healthy man, which is what we're all looking for—I mean, I don't want to be a young, healthy man. [Laughs.]

HERTOGHE: No. But a young, healthy woman, yes. No? [Laughs.]

SOMERS: Exactly. [Laughs.] Let's talk about the brain: the hypothalamus, the pituitary, the pineal, all the essential parts of the brain which I believe are under attack. Do you think the attack on the brain actually originates in the GI tract from toxic contaminants we are all exposed to?

HERTOGHE: The gut is one of the factors; the other factor, like you say, is the pollutants that overwhelm us. For example, I recently read a study in men where they checked for plastics called phthalates. There are many different phthalates, but in this study they just checked for eight. On the average, at least six of those plastics were in every one of those men.

SOMERS: What do you mean by plastics?

HERTOGHE: Yes. Plastic. Chemicals.

SOMERS: Yes! [Sighs.] It's just terrible what we've done.

HERTOGHE: The more plastics they found, or phthalates, the lower the testosterone levels, in fact, up to twenty, thirty percent decrease in levels. However, we don't only have plastics that accumulate in our body, we have heavy metals and other materials. Many of us are also polluted by mycotoxins, which are toxins produced by yeast that proliferate in our gastrointestinal tracts and wreak havoc with our health. This is one of the reasons why I always start my patients' programs by explaining the importance of making the right choices and avoiding pollutants in the food. Studies show that eating a paleo diet that includes only or mostly organic foods decreases the toxic load. Just by doing that your hormones are already getting better. After age forty, you need hormones, but if you eat the right foods and avoid chemicals, you'll respond better to hormone treatments and you will preserve your youthful hormone levels longer.

SOMERS: My understanding—and I agree with you—is the more toxins you take in through the skin, the food you eat, and the air you breathe, the more likely it is to not only invade the GI tract but eat through the GI barrier wall, causing leaky gut, allowing them to get into the bloodstream and make their way to the fattiest organs and glands.

The brain is the fattiest organ, and it is exposed to many toxins that may predispose to neurodegenerative disorders. I worry about brain shrinkage and the impact of aging and toxins on the pituitary and other glands in the brain. I guess what I'm asking is how do you detox the brain and wake up the pituitary and pineal gland to start operating again at normal or max, if possible?

HERTOGHE: One of the only ways is to create hormone balance. For example, when my father was still living, we were treating a lot of people who were toxic, but we didn't know about that problem at that time and with thyroid hormones they did fine, in fact, much better. But once we began to understand what Dr. Bill Rea in Dallas and many of those Americans who were pioneers in the field of environmental medicine were describing, we realized toxins were playing a big part in making people sick.

Once we started checking the chemical levels in our patients, we found a tremendous amount of toxic burden in each person. We realized many of our patients we were treating for hypothyroidism [low thyroid] were hypothyroid partially or completely because of pollutants.

The thyroid treatment we gave permitted them to depollute more easily and to feel much better. When you depollute people—we saw that in Bill Rea's center, where they keep those toxic people in a sort of hospital on the outside of the city—we saw that after treatment these people were much lower in pollutants but didn't improve anymore because their bodies had been broken by pollutants. They weren't dealing then with hormone replacement, which has to be a part of the solution.

SOMERS: What I admire about the way you've set up your clinic—and I say this over and over when I've spoken at doctors' conferences—is that there needs to be an "alpha" doc. In your clinic you are the alpha doctor, and then you've got your "sub" doctors all the way around—and I don't mean sub in any kind of negative way, just in that they all report to you, and you are the one who has all the information in front of you in order to have a complete overview. Am I understanding correctly that that's what you do?

HERTOGHE: Let's say I supervise the other treatments, but each doctor has a certain autonomy. The doctors here are enthusiastic people. They like this medicine. We all work well together, and they're very open to new ideas. We try to have people who really take the time with the patient, because if you don't take enough time, you can't personalize the treatment, and that's fundamental for the efficacy of the treatment and the safety.

SOMERS: You mention MSH a lot. What is MSH?

HERTOGHE: MSH [melanocyte-stimulating hormone] is the hormone that stimulates the darkening of the skin. So if you're black, light brown, or whitish, it depends on your level of MSH or the number of receptors you have that make you respond to MSH. This hormone protects you against the sun, UV radiation. But it also has additional effects in that it stimulates your sexuality much more than any other hormone.

SOMERS: **This is the Peptide sex shot; PT 141.**

HERTOGHE: It actually stimulates the brain to become sexually rambunctious. I obtained it from my compounding pharmacy by prescription. I tried it several times, and I don't know if I have gotten any tanner, but my libido goes off the charts with this peptide. Finally, a nondrug sex stimulant for women *and* men! To me it seems more logical and safer than Viagra, which is a stimulant for men only.

We know that when we go on a sunny vacation, sex will be much more stimulating and will even feel better. Even our skin gets sexually more sensitive. That's the effect of MSH. When men have difficulties in erections, and it takes three minutes even with a good product that can stimulate erections like Viagra or Cialis, with MSH derivatives they may have fuller erections that hold on maybe twenty to twenty-five minutes.

SOMERS: Wow. I can't wait for my readers to learn this!

HERTOGHE: The problem is it's not so available. You're luckier in the United States, because you have compounding pharmacies that can offer it with a doctor's prescription. There are also websites, but a doctor like me cannot ever recommend a website, because it doesn't have the control you have with a compounding pharmacy, which is safer.

SOMERS: Well, I think the line you just gave me, that for a man to want a twenty-minute erection, MSH is their friend. [Laughs.] There's going to be a run on MSH in this country.

Does one take MSH daily for overall well-being, or does a man take it only when he wants a strong erection?

HERTOGHE: An MSH derivative can be taken one week before and during a vacation to have a greater tan and get protection against sunburn. To boost sexuality, a very little dose of approximately 0.1 milligram per day is taken one to three times a month. A higher dose of around 0.5 milligrams, subcutaneously injected, can be taken for the sexual-enhancing effects; it remains active for seventy-two hours with a climax starting six hours later, so do not inject the higher dose just before bedtime but six hours before. For women, an MSH derivative can turn on sexuality as no other, creating a strong physical desire and sensitivity all over the body that at overdose might feel pleasantly uncontrollable.

SOMERS: How long does it take to work? Any other benefits of MSH?

HERTOGHE: Some patients say it tightens the inner sides of the thighs. It also can increase sexual scent; however, there are possible side effects. If you slightly overdose, your skin can excessively darken. If you suddenly overdose, you can get terrible nausea. In men at very high doses it can cause an excessive and painful erection. In patients with no or insufficiently corrected cortisol deficiency, MSH derivatives can darken existing pigment spots and create new ones that take nine to twelve months to disappear after stopping.

SOMERS: What else is going on in the antiaging world that people don't know about yet? What are you excited about?

HERTOGHE: What excites me are the **peptides**. In healthy aging medicine, the new big improvements in rejuvenation are peptides, which are smaller proteins that the organs of our body produce for their local use to keep working well. For instance, muscles make peptides for the muscles, the liver makes peptides for the liver, and the brain makes peptides for the brain.

SOMERS: You mean you can target a specific organ or organs?

HERTOGHE: Yes, exactly. They have now been able to isolate those peptides that our body makes naturally and attach them to a longer molecule, so they remain active in the blood for a longer period of time. Normally, many of those peptides would stay one or two minutes active in blood, but by injecting peptides you can rebuild muscles or rejuvenate the liver or have better brain functioning.

SOMERS: What's the catch?

HERTOGHE: Each peptide only works for that organ, and each peptide is specific to that organ. Most hormones work on many different organs simultaneously, such as bones, muscles, brain, et cetera, all over. With most peptides, you can target one type of organ that has stopped functioning perfectly due to aging.

SOMERS: Do you have a way to test all the different organs to see peptide deficiencies?

HERTOGHE: There is to my knowledge no test yet on the market, but a physical examination can reveal the existence of a peptide deficiency. Looking at your muscles, for instance, allows me to see if they are in good shape or not. If not, taking specific muscle-enhancing peptides will improve them.

SOMERS: What is the method of delivery for peptides?

HERTOGHE: It's usually subcutaneous, an injection under the skin.

SOMERS: What if several different organs were deficient in different peptides? Could you put that all into one injection?

HERTOGHE: Yes, you could certainly put them into one injection. For me personally, I have, on average, seven peptides or hormones I inject simultaneously all at the same time with the same injection once a day in the evening, before bedtime. It's easier that way and has a synergetic, more potent effect when you put them together. They increase energy levels and stimulate the mind. With hormones, you get positive effects on your mood and things like that. Peptides improve your physical body or just individual organs. I have experienced peptides that improve muscle tone, and they're quite efficient for that. But not in everybody, because again, if you don't have enough insulin, you don't have enough amino acid getting into your body and your muscle tone may not improve. Everybody needs a different dose of the peptides, and you can only know the best dose by trial and error.

SOMERS: This is exciting alchemy. I caution that too much is too much. The first time I tried it, I felt like a howling animal, and it was not fun. We have now found the right dose, once a week a teeny bit—should be according to your doctor's recommendations. It is made by compounding pharmacies.

HERTOGHE: It is exciting, because the effects can be very powerful.

SOMERS: I'm anxious to experience all of this. It's just fantastic.

What about chronic high cortisol? It seems to me if the minor hormones are too low for too long, then the cortisol goes too high. Is that why we women die of heart attacks?

HERTOGHE: Physicians can decrease the severity of a myocardial infarction [heart attack] by giving an overdose of cortisol, because of its anti-inflammatory actions.

But what is not good to have in the long term is a persistently high cortisol level with not enough anabolic hormones, because studies in animals have shown that the more DHEA they get, the more they're protected against tissue wasting caused by increasingly higher cortisol levels. Cortisol is safe if the levels in the body are adequately balanced by protective hormones such as DHEA, sex hormones, and growth hormone. It depends on the right balance. It's true that with aging, most individuals have lower cortisol production, but only twenty percent lower, while the anabolic hormones [the hormones that build up your body] make muscles, good skin, good hair, and those hormones decrease from fifty to eighty percent.

Imbalance of hormones makes you age quicker. It's unsafe to have high cortisol when you have low anabolic hormones. If your cortisol is excessively high, the way to lower it is to take supplements of hormones that decrease cortisol, such as growth hormone, oxytocin [the "love and sex" hormone], anabolic hormones, and thyroid hormones.

SOMERS: We didn't talk much about oxytocin; my husband and I take three sniffs at night and our dreams are always pleasant. I'm in a happy mood most all the time. I believe oxytocin is a big part of my inner "hormonal song" operating optimally. Balancing the treatment protocol is the "art" of hormone replacement. You need to work with someone who understands how to replace all hormones so everything is in the "hormonal symphony" and is in balance and all communicating with one another. I know at times when I have my body running at peak, where I can feel everything's in balance, wow, what a difference. It's like being alive while you're alive.

The planet is lucky to have you with us. We will all benefit. Thank you.

HERTOGHE: Thank you, Suzanne.

CHAPTER 10

TESTOSTERONE

Testosterone is a hormone attributed to the male of the species, but women also make testosterone and it is crucial for the balance of the "hormonal song." Men make more testosterone than estrogen, and women make more estrogen than testosterone.

That's what makes us male and female.

Most people don't realize that testosterone levels affect the entire body system. For instance, coronary heart disease is associated with low testosterone levels; they don't cause just erectile dysfunction and libido. To stay healthy, a man has to have adequate testosterone levels. If estrogen dominance is an issue (yes, this happens to men), he may then get cancer of the prostate, because that is likely to be caused by the estrogen rather than the testosterone.

New approaches to prostate cancer through bioidentical testosterone replacement not only keep the patient protected but are an antidote for prostate cancer.

Interview with

DR. ABRAHAM MORGENTALER

Dr. Abraham Morgentaler is a maverick doctor who has written several bestselling books. My particular favorite is the bestseller *Testosterone for Life: Recharge Your Vitality, Sex Drive, Muscle Mass, and Overall Health*.

Dr. Morgentaler is an associate clinical professor at Harvard Medical School. He was born in Montreal, Canada, and graduated from Harvard College in 1978 and Harvard Medical School in 1982. He completed his residency in 1988 in the Harvard Program in Urology and then joined the faculty of Beth Israel Deaconess Medical Center and Harvard Medical School.

In his book and this interview, he debunks the myths about the safety of testosterone, including the controversial link between testosterone therapy and prostate cancer. I love having the chance to speak with him. He is always on the cutting edge and has improved the quality of countless men's lives. Dr. Morgentaler is one of the "good guys," who happens to be crazy smart.

SOMERS: Thank you, Dr. Morgentaler. You have been ahead of the pack in the treatment of prostate cancer for many years. What seems obvious to you—and through you to me—has not caught on in so many doctors' offices around the country. The whole notion of testosterone as the antidote to prostate cancer is still not front and center in mainstream medicine. Can you dispel the notion that testosterone is the culprit in prostate cancer?

MORGENTALER: Can I dispel it? Yes, absolutely.

SOMERS: For instance, if my husband takes testosterone replacement, is he going to get prostate cancer?

MORGENTALER: Certainly not because he takes testosterone. The whole idea of testosterone as the culprit for prostate cancer was based on a misunderstanding and came about decades before we had any real way of looking at any of this. Modern data show that testosterone either has no association with increased risk or has even decreased risk. In one recent study involving more than fifty thousand men, the group of men taking testosterone had a significantly lower risk of developing prostate cancer than men who did not take testosterone. Interestingly, the longer the men took testosterone, the lower their risk of cancer!

Prostate cancer happens to men when they're older and their testosterone levels have declined; it almost never occurs in younger men in their twenties with peak lifetime testosterone.

The idea that testosterone causes prostate cancer and makes it grow rapidly took hold a long, long time ago and went unquestioned for sixty years. I hate to say it, but doctors are often like ducklings: they follow in line once they are taught something, even if what they were taught was wrong. Physicians pride themselves on being skeptical; however, they are only skeptical about new issues that are not part of their core beliefs or training. The unfortunate upshot is that once a concept takes hold, it takes a very long time to undo it.

SOMERS: Like the now-debunked low-fat myth. It's now been discovered that the concept was wrong and the truth was the reverse; every cell in our body requires protein, *fat*, and carbohydrate. Without fat our cells lose one of their essential building blocks. I am happily eating butter again!

You conducted an important study on testosterone and prostate cancer at Harvard, and a few years ago you called me and said, "I have something I think you'll find interesting. I've conducted a study on men with prostate cancer who come to my office. It doesn't seem to matter how elevated their PSA, when I put them on testosterone, their PSA numbers regress and, most importantly, the cancer regresses."

I'm paraphrasing and simplifying it. You were much more eloquent, but that was the gist and I thought the information fantastic, a true breakthrough.

MORGENTALER: Thank you. The study you're referring to was groundbreaking, and I'm very proud to have played a role in moving our understanding forward.

We now offer testosterone in my practice at Men's Health Boston to individuals who are symptomatic from low testosterone, and this includes certain men with a history of prostate cancer.

When I first spoke with you about this, probably around 2011, it was considered radical to offer testosterone therapy to men with any history of prostate cancer, even those who appeared to have been cured many years after surgery. The fear of testosterone's actions on prostate cancer was so strong that it was believed testosterone treatment would cause the cancer to come roaring back, *even if there were no remaining prostate cancer cells in the body*.

Imagine, then, how scary it was when my colleagues and I took a giant step further by offering testosterone therapy to men with untreated prostate cancer sitting inside them. These men were on a program called active surveillance, in which they underwent no immediate cancer treatment because their cancers did not appear aggressive and were carefully monitored with follow-up prostate biopsies, with the understanding that they would undergo treatment if their cancers grew in size or revealed a more aggressive grade.

In 2011, my colleagues at Baylor Medical College and I published in the *Journal of Urology* the results of follow-up biopsies in thirteen men on active surveillance who had been treated with testosterone. All the men had improved energy, sex drive, or erections. And *none* of the cancers had progressed! In several, cancer couldn't even be found in the follow-up biopsies.

That study, although small in number, was the first time that anyone had bothered to investigate what happens to prostates with cancer when testosterone is raised. And although thirteen men is too few to conclude that testosterone could never cause any prostate cancer to grow, it was more than enough to conclude that the prevailing belief for so many years—that higher testosterone must necessarily cause prostate cancer growth—could not be true.

Recently my team presented our results from the last five years at the annual meeting of the American Urological Association, in which we studied 190 men with prostate cancer who had been treated with testosterone. This included men treated with surgery, men treated with radiation, and almost 49 men on active surveillance. Some men did, of course, have recurrence of their cancers or progression; however, the key point is that our rates of cancer recurrence or progression were lower than results from large published studies in men who did not receive testosterone.

At this point, I believe the vast majority of men with prostate cancer are candidates for testosterone therapy, regardless of the grade or stage of their cancer. The only exceptions are some special cases with far-advanced disease. Testosterone therapy is not only *not harmful* to men with prostate cancer but may be beneficial.

SOMERS: It just seems as the man's testosterone levels decline, the prostate seems to enlarge. I imagine the reason is because the prostate is looking for its essential building block. Does testosterone make "food" for the sperm?

MORGENTALER: Yes, testosterone is essential for sperm growth and development.

SOMERS: If you are losing testosterone, your prostate's going to enlarge, looking for essential ingredients—like making a cake but not having any eggs.

MORGENTALER: I'd like to tell you a story. A ninety-four-year-old man, let's call him GS, calls me from another state with his daughter on the line. He's an accomplished scientist. His daughter is a nurse practitioner. They've both read my research, and he says, "I'd like to come see you and have you treat me with testosterone." He had had metastatic prostate cancer for quite a few years already. I wasn't able to promise him anything on the phone but agreed to meet with him. I had never treated anyone with testosterone who had metastatic disease.

The standard treatment for men with metastatic prostate cancer is to lower testosterone with medications like Lupron. He had undergone a short course of that but became so weak he couldn't walk or get out of the house. What he was asking me to do by *raising* his testosterone was radical. I had treated hundreds of men with testosterone and prostate cancer by then but not someone whose cancer had spread to the bones.

The fear, drilled into all physicians who deal with prostate cancer, was that testosterone could make prostate cancer in the spine grow and collapse a vertebra, causing compression of the spinal cord and paralysis.

When he came to see me, he had tubes coming out his back on each side to drain urine from the kidneys because his ureters were obstructed by cancer-swollen lymph nodes. These nephrostomy tubes, as they're called, drain into small plastic pouches that fill with urine and are then emptied when full. When he came in, he was wearing a tweed jacket with one of the bags of urine in one pocket of his jacket, the other bag in the other. He walked with a cane but got on and off the exam table by himself. After examining him, we went to the consultation room with his daughter, the nurse practitioner, and I asked, "How can I help you?"

"I want you to treat me with testosterone," he said.

The standard blood test marker for prostate cancer is called PSA, and PSA levels above 4 [nanograms per milliliter] are considered abnormally high. GS's PSA was over 500, which at the time was the highest PSA I'd ever seen. Here he was, ninety-four years old, cancer in his bones, tubes carrying urine out of his body, and a PSA greater than 500, and he was asking me to treat him with testosterone.

I said, "What are you hoping to get from testosterone treatment?"

He replied, "Well, I used to exercise every day, and it made me feel good. I'm too tired and weak to do that now. And I don't feel like my mind is sharp. I used to correspond by email with colleagues from around the world, and I just don't do that much anymore. I'm too tired to do much of anything."

I told him, "I've never treated anybody like you. The standard belief among physicians is that your cancer could worsen rapidly with testosterone, you could end up being paralyzed, and you could die tomorrow or in a week."

He said, "Doctor, I've read all your work, and I know you're the only one who would even consider treating me. I've never lived my life in fear and I don't intend to now. I'm ninety-four years old, I know I've got cancer all through my body, and I know I'm going to die sometime, but while I'm here on this earth, I want to live as well as I can."

So I treated him. I gave him his first testosterone injection in the office, and his daughter injected him every two weeks at home. Within a month he was exercising regularly and corresponding again with his friends and colleagues around the world. He was happily working on another of his many patents. At seven months, now ninety-five years old, his daughter sent me a picture of him looking fantastic, sitting and smiling in the waiting room of his dentist. He and his daughter knew they were making medical history and gave me permission—in fact, encouraged me—to tell his story.

GS died at ten months when one of his nephrostomy tubes fell out and he developed a serious infection. His daughter refused hospitalization, and he died several weeks later. Before his death his PSA had risen above 2,000, yet he never experienced bone pain or any of the terrible things I'd been taught would happen if a man in his situation received testosterone.

SOMERS: I admire your courage for taking a chance with him, and in the biggest picture I admire him for the gift he's given to mankind.

MORGENTALER: Thank you. My patients are always impressing me with their bravery and often with their clear thinking about life—something sorely lacking among many of my medical colleagues. He understood that we're all going to go sometime and there is enormous value in living well while we're here.

SOMERS: What a wonderful story. He allowed you to learn with his case. What he wanted was quality of life. I call it being alive while you're alive.

MORGENTALER: I confess I was really worried that something terrible would happen to him in the first days after I gave him that initial testosterone injection. His story gave me the courage to start treating some other people who are younger and in similar situations. I now have about a dozen men in my practice with metastatic prostate cancer who are receiving testosterone therapy, some for as long as three years. We have entered a brave new world with this.

At this point I've come to believe that men with prostate cancer, regardless of grade or stage, can reasonably be offered testosterone therapy. The main exceptions are some men with advanced metastatic disease who already benefited from androgen deprivation, meaning their bone pain improved or they had masses that shrunk. Those men are likely to see those symptoms return with normalization of testosterone.

In 2006, I published a paper called "The Saturation Model." The idea was, at that time, that prostate cancer would grow faster and more aggressive as testosterone levels increased. So even if somebody was mid-range of normal testosterone and we raised it higher, the belief was their cancers would get worse, *and that turns out to not be true.*

SOMERS: Why have doctors been so mistaken about the dangers of testosterone?

MORGENTALER: In the 1940s, it was first discovered that an older blood test for prostate cancer called acid phosphatase was often elevated in men with metastatic prostate cancer, and it would decline after various treatments that dropped testosterone, including estrogen treatment or castration— removal of the testicles. Physicians concluded testosterone makes prostate cancer grow and depriving the cancer of testosterone makes it shrink.

This was the prevailing belief for sixty years, but it was never challenged during that time, and it turned out to be too simplistic. It turns out that prostate cancer cells do require a certain amount of androgen [a testosterone-like substance] for optimal growth, but they can only use a little bit of it. Once they've had their little bit, more doesn't do anything; the cancer cells can't use it. We can say that the prostate cancer cells become "saturated" with testosterone, just like a sponge gets saturated with water and then can't absorb anymore. This is the Saturation Model, which I first described in 2006. Most men walking around, even if they have low levels of testosterone, have saturated or nearly saturated the ability of the prostate cancer cells to use testosterone. This explains why depriving the cancer completely of testosterone can cause the cancers to shrink, yet raising it in someone whose testosterone is near or above the saturation point won't do anything to the cancer. As a result, the vast majority of my men with prostate cancer never experience progression of their cancer with testosterone.

I use the analogy of a plant and water. Think of a houseplant as prostate cancer and water as testosterone. If you deprive the plant of water, it will shrink, it will lose its volume. If the water-deprived plant is given water, it will grow. But once the plant has all the water it needs for optimal growth, running a garden hose into it twenty-four hours a day will never cause that houseplant to grow to the size of a sequoia tree! It has *saturated* its ability to use water. That's how it works with testosterone and prostate cancer.

SOMERS: I get it. The plant has reached its capacity, its saturation point. Great description. Switching gears: A lot of women are now on full bioidentical hormone replacement, including progesterone, testosterone, and estrogen. Those of us replacing with BHRT are very happy women. If a woman rubs her hormone cream on where it can "rub off" on her husband, can this elevate the man's DHT?

MORGENTALER: I don't worry too much about DHT in the bloodstream for men. DHT stands for dihydrotestosterone. It's one of the two key active metabolites of testosterone, the other being estradiol. The concern about DHT is that it is the primary androgen in the prostate. When there appears to be too much androgen, in this case DHT, it can cause prostate cancer or stimulate growth of a small cancer into an aggressive one.

The reason I don't worry much about DHT measured in the blood is that, one, I'm not worried about androgens of any type causing prostate cancer and, two, circulating DHT measured in the blood has little to do with DHT concentrations within the prostate, which creates large amounts of DHT itself. Concentrations of DHT within the prostate tremendously exceed what is measured in the blood, and blood levels can't tell us what's happening within the prostate.

However, one action of DHT that guys don't like is that in the scalp it contributes to male-pattern baldness. Medicines that block DHT, like Propecia, help to prevent hair loss in men and in women and may even promote new hair growth.

SOMERS: Is it good to block DHT with a drug like Propecia? Seems to me if the body makes it, there is a reason for it being there.

MORGENTALER: That's a philosophical question, Suzanne! There are many unpleasant or even dangerous things that happen to our bodies "naturally" as we age, but in my opinion that doesn't mean they don't merit treatment. Aging sucks! Age-related conditions, namely conditions that become increasingly common as we age, include bad eyesight, bad hearing, bad teeth, bad blood vessels, heart disease, diabetes, arthritis, and cancer. One could argue all of these are natural, yet we interfere with nature with surgery or medications to improve the quality of our lives or to prolong life. The question as I see it really becomes how to weigh the benefits versus the potential harms for any treatment, recognizing that not treating something may have its own risks.

SOMERS: Doctors often get freaked out over elevated DHT. For some the antidote is progesterone suppositories for men.

I try to put my estrogen cream in a place on my body Alan never seems to touch (which took some creativity on my part). Turns out he doesn't spend too much time behind my ear. Haha.

Okay, switching gears again. The heart: my understanding is the heart is arguably the most important muscle in the human body and it has plenty of androgen receptors. How important is testosterone replacement for heart health?

MORGENTALER: I'm so glad you brought it up. The heart is a muscle, and testosterone has important beneficial actions on muscles. For twenty years, the data showed testosterone was good for the heart, study after study. Then, in 2013, a paper was published in *The Journal of the American Medical Association* [*JAMA*]; it was a look back at over eight thousand men in the VA system, all of whom who had undergone cardiac catheterization and had low levels of testosterone. Some eventually went on to get a prescription of testosterone, and others did not. Those were the two groups: one that got T and one that didn't. What the authors reported was that men who received prescriptions for T had more adverse events than men who didn't, specifically heart attacks, strokes, and death.

But this study turned out to be deeply flawed. The authors misreported their data, which actually showed there were fewer adverse events in the testosterone group by half! Not only that, but months later the authors discovered—and admitted—that nearly ten percent of at least one study subgroup of their "all-male" study population was comprised of women!

SOMERS: Women? In a testosterone study?

MORGENTALER: Crazy, isn't it? It's hard to find a less credible study. Twenty-nine medical societies petitioned *JAMA* to retract the study, but they declined.

Here's a quick update on testosterone and cardiovascular risk. My colleagues and I recently published a review of all the articles that reported major cardiovascular events since 2015, when the FDA added a weakly worded warning to all testosterone products. These "events" include heart attack, stroke, and death. Although one can obviously die from things that are unrelated to the heart, most deaths are cardiovascular in nature, and so deaths are usually included in analyses like this. Out of twenty-two studies, not one showed an increase in major cardiovascular events with testosterone.

SOMERS: This confusing misinformation could be enough to discourage a man who might otherwise reap such enormous benefits as quality of life with T replacement.

MORGENTALER: It's been terribly confusing. And physicians are as confused as anyone. Soon after the *JAMA* paper was published, the *New York Times* ran an editorial that was called "Overselling Testosterone, Dangerously." Basically, it said, "These men taking testosterone are dumb suckers who can't deal with getting old and are willing to take snake oil in the form of testosterone in the vain hope they can regain their lost youth. And now, ladies and gentlemen, researchers have found that the treatment is not only ineffective, but it is dangerous, too."

SOMERS: So were they mocking men who wanted to take testosterone?

MORGENTALER: Yes! Mocking men who take testosterone, shaming physicians who prescribe it, and promoting false information about cardiovascular risk. The cumulative effect of media's coverage of two outlier studies has been devastating to the field. As you know, testosterone therapy is beneficial to men in so many ways—sexually, physically, cognitively—and it has even been shown to improve mood. We have high levels of evidence for so many of its benefits. Yet people are now afraid of testosterone because it has been alleged to cause heart attacks. It's interesting to me that just as the fear of prostate cancer was subsiding, this new fear of heart attacks has risen to take its place.

SOMERS: Tell me about testosterone relative to the brain. One of the most alarming things happening today with aging people is brain conditions, brain diseases: ADD, ADHD, OCD, dementia, Alzheimer's. It's almost as though people are expecting that their last years are going to be fraught with being decrepit, frail, and end up in a nursing home not knowing who they were or who they are. Does testosterone play a role in helping to, for lack of a better way of asking, save the brain, keep the brain firing?

MORGENTALER: I'm convinced it does. We still lack the requisite types of studies to say this definitively, but based on my experience treating thousands of men over thirty years, I have no doubt that testosterone can help stave off dementia and keep the brain working well. It's part of what keeps us young and alive.

I had a patient not long ago with low levels of testosterone, a successful business executive. I treated him with testosterone, and at his follow-up visit he was so happy. I just love how he described the feeling. He said, "Before I started testosterone treatment, I felt like I was seeing the world in black and white. Now I feel like I see the world in color."

SOMERS: That's beautiful, it's like your ninety-four-year-old patient, the scientist, who said (and I'm paraphrasing), "If I don't have anything, I want to have my brain." He wanted to be able to keep thinking and writing.

MORGENTALER: Right. How we experience the world defines us. This is all about the brain: what we experience, what we see, how we think, and *how well* we think.

Moreover, testosterone routinely improves the mood of men who take it. Clinicians have observed this for a very long time. However, mainstream medicine doesn't believe things until they have a large, randomized controlled study. Well, finally we have one. A good one.

In 2016, the first results of the largest prospective study with testosterone to date, called the Testosterone Trials, were published. I followed 790 men sixty-five years and older who got either a year of testosterone gel or a year of a placebo gel. At the end of the study, all the things we expected to get better with testosterone did, as in sexual interest, sexual activity, physical activity. But one thing that was great to see was improved mood. Positive aspects of mood were increased, and negative aspects of mood, like depression and irritability, were decreased.

SOMERS: Try to think of another medication other than an antidepressant that actually improves mood and also allows you to go through the same activities of your day.

MORGENTALER: Excellent point. You can get dressed in the morning, eat your breakfast, drive to work, do your work, come home at the end of the day, and if you are in a positive frame of mind, you might say, "This was a good day." If your brain is in a different state, you can do exactly the same things, and it all feels like a misery.

SOMERS: Before testosterone replacement was even on the radar, they were doing a very popular movie with Walter Matthau and Jack Lemmon called *Grumpy Old Men*. When I was a kid, there was a television series called *Hazel*, and Hazel the maid was this scatterbrained, "couldn't remember anything" older lady. We took scatterbrained for granted back then. It just was what happened to a lot of older women. I realized *Grumpy Old Men* was about lack of testosterone, and Hazel the maid was in menopause; she couldn't remember anything because she wasn't on replacement.

MORGENTALER: There are so many benefits with testosterone therapy. There are new data showing that men with higher testosterone levels are less likely to get dementia than men with low levels. Having a robust testosterone level is a normal condition for men and frankly also for women, although the levels between men and women are different.

There are also data from several studies showing that the metabolic syndrome, which is a collection of risk factors like diabetes and high blood pressure, can actually be reversed in some of these men with testosterone. And insulin resistance, a key feature of type 2 diabetes and a cardiovascular risk factor, improves with T therapy.

SOMERS: Testosterone stimulates muscle strength and growth, right?

MORGENTALER: Yes; when men have low testosterone, they lose muscle and gain fat. There is a stem cell that can go in two pathways: toward the muscle cell lineage or toward adipose or fat lineage. Low levels predispose these cells to develop toward fat cells and normal or high levels toward muscle.

SOMERS: Look at the many advantages of testosterone replacement. Do you think all men in hormonal decline would benefit from T replacement?

MORGENTALER: We have an epidemic of low testosterone in men that has been underrecognized, underappreciated, and undertreated. There's no doubt in my mind that the way for people to live well into their late years is to have the robust levels of hormones they used to have, especially testosterone.

SOMERS: So testosterone is good for sex, vitality, even mood, but most importantly for general health.

MORGENTALER: A big resounding yes to that! Research shows testosterone improves the risk of diabetes, metabolic syndrome, and obesity. It helps to maintain normal nerve cell size and function. When T is lowered, those neurons [nerves] shrink in size and become testosterone receptors, so it is no surprise that nerve- or brain-mediated functions are all improved by healthy levels of testosterone. In the end, what exactly is quality of life? I would say that quality of life is impacted enormously by our facility to perform physically, to experience a sense of wellness, and to be able to experience ourselves and our interactions with others in a way that allows the full range of human emotion.

SOMERS: Without quality of life, you aren't really living. It's a pleasure to speak with you. I love your passion, and you seem to enjoy your work so much.

MORGENTALER: I've been blessed to have worked my entire career with interesting research projects and with generous and often brave patients willing to take a risk with me as I developed new ideas that might benefit them. We have a divine opportunity to help men and women find their inner *chi* and to take important steps toward a healthier, more engaged you.

We are walking miracles, all of us.

Information on how to find Dr. Morgentaler can be found in appendix C, "Doctor Contact Information."

PART III

TOXINS AND THE GUT

CHAPTER 11

THE DEVASTATING EFFECTS OF TOXICITY ON AGING

If you choose to perish, do so with full knowledge of how cheaply how small an enemy has claimed your life.

—Ayn Rand

I have written extensively about the devastating effects of toxins on our hormonal and endocrine systems. We drink water to do something good for our health, yet the chemicals from the plastic bottles the water comes in negate its good effects.

My book *TOX-SICK* went in depth to explain how toxins enter the body. We have three points of entry: our skin, the food we eat, the air we breathe. Each of us has the capacity to control these pathways if the message is taken seriously and we make some changes in our lifestyle and diet.

Whatever we put onto our skin—the body's largest organ—eventually ends up in the bloodstream. Think about this: skin, under a microscope, looks as though it has large holes in it. Those holes are our pores, and the creams and chemical potions you apply to your skin eventually enter the bloodstream. Imagine rubbing toxic creams on your skin day after day; it stands to reason that eventually the buildup will wreak havoc on your health.

Unexplained weight gain can often be attributed to your toxic burden also. The brain in its wisdom understands that our organs and glands need protection from the environmental assault, so to protect us it stores the toxins in our fat cells. **The more toxins you take in and are exposed to, the more fat cells are required for storage**—until the brain realizes there is no more "room at the inn," then the brain can no longer help. At that point the toxins go on a rampage, looking for fatty organs and glands. Now you've got a lot of extra fat filled with toxins; that's your cellulite—and so much more.

The second pathway is through our gut; thus the food we eat is vitally important. If you eat processed, fake (heavily processed) foods, poor-quality oils, and nonorganic food, your gut (GI tract) will take the hit.

> It is clear that the more you abuse your body by insulting it with toxic substances, the more likely one of your repair systems will undergo an early breakdown.
> —David A. Kekich

The longer you live, the higher your individual toxic burden will be unless you go out of your way to unload the toxins.

A recent study demonstrated that after people die their bodies are not decomposing as quickly as they used to because we are consuming on average eight pounds of preservatives a year in the food we eat. Shocking!

You can reduce your chances of getting serious illnesses by balancing your hormones, metabolizing them properly, keeping your vitamin D levels high enough, and supplementing with nutrients in which you are deficient.

Omega-3 fatty acids (found, for example, in fish oil) enhance your brain function. Good-quality oils and good fats have more to do with your health than you ever imagined.

Something I say often in TV interviews and lectures is that we are under the greatest environmental assault in the history of humanity.

Let that sink in.

If that is so, it is crucial to understand that the object of living a long life of high quality is to take toxicity seriously. It's at the base of most human conditions, be it disease or a body that is in a state of dis-ease.

As I say over and over in this book, a human being is made up of about 37 trillion cells. When cells need to repair themselves, some of the components necessary to allow this to happen are stored in the fat of the cell membrane. Without an adequate amount of good fat, the cell membranes can't function and thus the cell can't function.

Cells replace themselves frequently. If you don't give the cell new building materials, including adequate amounts of good fat, the body will have to make the cells with materials from the worn-out cells it is replacing. Building new things using worn-out parts creates a new thing that doesn't work much better than the old one did.

For cells to function well, their membranes must be made with good fats or phospholipids. Cell membranes made of bad fats—I sometimes refer to them as "plastic fats"—impair cellular function.

Hydrogenation of unsaturated vegetable oils produces trans fatty acids (e.g., traditional margarine), which have documented adverse health effects.

Americans today ingest far too many omega-6 fats (such as soybean and corn oils), which deprive cell membranes of healthy amounts of omega-3 fatty acids.

Since all of the brain and nervous system, the liver, and every cell membrane are made of fat, you need to eat lots of good fat to keep making good cells.

Though the amounts of trans fats have been reduced in typical diets, Americans are consuming far too many omega-6 fats.

Refined omega-6 vegetable fats, such as corn oil and soybean oil, are used in cookies, crackers, sweets, salad dressings, and most fried foods. An astounding percentage of calories is estimated to come from omega-6 vegetable fats.

Poultry, which many people eat in lieu of red meat, is also a rich source of omega-6 fats due in large part to the high amounts of corn fed to the animals. A chicken leg contains about 1,800 milligrams of omega-6 fatty acids.[1] Turkey contains almost as many omega-6s, while duck contains less.

When chicken is fried in vegetable oil and eaten as part of a fast-food chicken sandwich, the amount of omega-6 fats surges to over 12,000 milligrams. If you add a salad with 2 tablespoons of a soybean oil or omega-6-rich safflower oil dressing, you will be ingesting about 7,200 milligrams of additional omega-6 fats.[2] So a meal from a fast-food restaurant consisting of a fried chicken sandwich and salad can result in the consumption of more than 17,000 milligrams of omega-6 fats.

The ideal ratio of omega-6 to omega-3 consumption is about one to one. This means you should ingest about the same amount of omega-3 fatty acids as omega-6s. This one-to-one ratio is difficult for most people to attain. Fortunately, there is evidence that if you are able to maintain a dietary ratio of four omega-6 fatty acids to every one omega-3 fatty acid, you should be in good shape.

Ingesting sufficient omega-3 fats while not overdoing omega-6s is a major challenge. That's why the low-fat movement was so detrimental to our health. The introduction of "fake fats" such as Crisco and the overconsumption of omega-6 fats—what I call "plastic fats"—are having serious deleterious effects on the health of our nation.

Think of a cell with a plastic membrane. It's like wrapping the cell in cellophane. The cell sends out the signal that it is hungry, and in response the body sends glucose and insulin to the cell. The trouble is, insulin can't efficiently bind to unhealthy cell membranes to prompt cells to pick up glucose from the blood. The result is a buildup of excess glucose in the blood that your cells are less able to utilize for energy. Soon the cell is surrounded by insulin and glucose that is not fully available for important functional cells but is readily stored in fat cells. This is known as insulin resistance, which so often evolves into type 2 diabetes.

This happens as cell membranes are damaged by excess omega-6 and trans fats and deprived of the omega-3s needed for healthy functionality. This impairs optimal glucose utilization and contributes to unwanted weight gain as glucose (blood sugar) begins to off-load into fat cells. If this isn't enough to make you want to reduce your intake of omega-6 fats and hydrogenated oils, some research suggests that excess amounts of omega-6 and trans fats in red blood cell membranes are a risk for developing heart disease![3]

Insulin resistance is the decreased ability of cell membranes to respond to the insulin signaling needed to utilize glucose properly. Your cell membranes endure structural damage if you consume more bad fats, especially in the presence of an omega-3 deficiency.

In lay terms, the structural damage caused by bad fats on cell membranes is like turning them into "plastic." The more "plastic" you eat in the form of bad fats (with insufficient omega-3s), the fatter you will get.

Guess what happens to a brain full of plastic. It doesn't work well, and it becomes prone to depression, chronic fatigue, attention deficit, "brain fog," and more. Guess what happens to a liver that's full of plastic. It can't clean the toxins out of our systems, and the toxins build up. Without a well-functioning liver, you will develop a myriad of chronic health problems.

Healthy fats such as olive oil, flaxseed oil, and quality fish oils are all vitally important to the formation of the human body, which contains approximately 30 trillion to 40 trillion cells. Nature knew we would need these healthy, glorious fats, so she made them taste scrumptious.

All the great cuisines of the world depend on the local fat of their regions. The French refer to it as *terroir*: perfect soil and clean water, making excellent grass for the cows that eventually give us their delicious meat, butter, and cream.

The olive trees in Tuscany are a source of pride for the precious oil they produce, which is then used liberally in Tuscan cooking. Just thinking about the flavor makes your eyes roll up in ecstasy.

Why did we villainize these perfect and delicious foods?

We were told that eating fats would make us fat, but the real truth is that by eating what I call plastic fat, you will get fat. If you continue making cell membranes from eating these plastic fats, you will keep on eating more and more because your cells are starving. Even though the cells are coated with glucose, it can't get into the cells because the "plastic" is in the way. Eating plastic fats makes a liver that won't work, leading to the inability to manage your metabolism and causing weight gain. And eating plastic fats makes a brain that can't control your endocrine system, causing your thyroid, adrenals, pancreas, and sex organs to malfunction.

In reality, eating more good fats and stopping eating all "plastic fats" will help you achieve a normal weight.

Every choice you make to eliminate toxins of any kind, be they in food, skin care products, home cleaning products, laundry detergent, even perfume, will move you forward toward living a long life of high quality and optimal health while thriving and surviving this massive chemical assault.

Despite the assurances of safety from both industry leaders and government entities, a staggering number of products contain hazardous chemicals that are toxic to humans. Whether from BPA-ridden canned goods, toxic personal care products, or harmful cleaning chemicals, there is no shortage of toxins in the average home.

Worst of all, most of these toxins go unnoticed; we casually invite them into our homes, never taking heed of the harm they cause. Toxins can be hiding even in your furniture, your children's toys, and the pans you cook your food in. Whether in the form of building materials or consumer products, we are basically surrounded by them.

Fortunately, you can take steps to eliminate the presence of toxins in your home and reduce your exposure to them.

Let's start with food. Organic food is not negotiable. Most of us got sick from the processed, pesticide-sprayed food we were led to believe was safe. It wasn't. Today organic food is plentiful, affordable, and delicious and is the right fuel for the human body. Be aware that the phrase "conventionally grown" is false advertising. The only thing conventional is the pesticides the food is sprayed with. Studies show that GMO foods typically contain higher levels of pesticides and herbicides.

The body "engine" requires vital nutrients that many people can't absorb because of gut imbalances. Here are some of the main offenders.

Topping the list, of course, is pesticides. These can be found in an array of fruits, veggies, and even grains. The Environmental Working Group (EWG) found traces of glyphosate—the active ingredient in Monsanto's Roundup (a glyphosate herbicide)—in a host of breakfast cereals and other goods.[4] According to Natural News:

> *Popular oat cereals, oatmeal, granola, and snack bars come with a hefty dose of the weed-killing poison in Roundup, according to independent laboratory tests commissioned by EWG.*
>
> *Glyphosate, an herbicide linked to cancer by California state scientists and the World Health Organization, was found in all but two of forty-five samples of products made with convention-*

ally grown oats. Almost three-fourths of those samples had glyphosate levels higher than what EWG scientists consider protective of children's health with an adequate margin of safety. About one-third of sixteen samples made with organically grown oats also had glyphosate, all at levels well below EWG's health benchmark.[5]

Glyphosate is the most commonly used herbicide in the United States.

PHTHALATES

Phthalates, chemicals produced by plastic bottles and many other things, outgas and have been found to cause poor testosterone synthesis by disrupting an enzyme required to create the male hormone.

Women with high levels of phthalates in their system during pregnancy were found to have sons that had feminine characteristics.

Phthalates are also found in vinyl flooring, detergents, automotive plastics, soaps and shampoos, deodorants, perfumes, hair sprays, plastic bags, and food packaging, among a long list of common products. They include:

- **Bisphenol-A (BPA).** This is common in plastic products such as reusable water bottles, food cans, and dental sealants. BPA can alter fetal development and heighten breast cancer risk in women.

- **Perfluorooctanoic acid (PFOA).** This is a potential carcinogen commonly used in water- and grease-resistant food coatings.

- **Methoxychlor** (an insecticide) and **Vinclozin** (a fungicide). These have been shown in studies to induce changes in four subsequent generations of male mice after initial exposure.

- **Nonylphenol ethoxylates (NPEs).** These are potent endocrine disruptors that can interfere with your gene expression and glandular system. They are also referred to as estrogen-mimicking chemicals. They have been implicated in unnatural sex changes in male marine species.

- **Bovine growth hormones.** These estrogen-mimicking and growth-promoting chemicals are added to commercial dairy products.

- **Monosodium glutamate (MSG).** This food additive can impact reproductive health and fertility.

- **Fluoride.** This potent neurotoxin, found in certain US water supplies, has been linked to endocrine disruption, decreased fertility rates, and lower sperm counts.

- **Pharmaceuticals that provide synthetic hormones.** Pharmaceuticals such as contraceptives can provide you with synthetic hormones that your body isn't designed to respond to and cannot detoxify properly. Chronic illnesses may result from long-term use of these drugs.

- **Metalloestrogens.** This is a class of cancer-causing estrogen-mimicking compounds that can be found in thousands of consumer products. Included in the list of potent metalloestrogens are aluminum, antimony, copper, lead, mercury, cadmium, and tin.

The United States Food and Drug Administration permits more than 84,000 chemicals to be used in household products, cosmetics,

food, and food packaging, and a majority of these have never been tested for safety. According to the US Government Accountability Office, **85 percent of new chemical applications include no testing whatsoever.**

We are under the greatest environmental assault in the history of humanity. And it is being played out right before us. Cancer used to be rare. Now either you've had it yourself or you know many people who have or had it. We are accepting this as normal as opposed to asking the question "Why?"

The answer is a no-brainer. **Whoever thought it was a good idea to spray poison on our food? And then tell us it was safe? Why would we accept that?**

Interview with
DR. JONATHAN WRIGHT

SOMERS: Let's talk about sleep. All the boomers are paddling around their houses at three a.m. Is waking up at three a.m. due to a deficiency?

WRIGHT: Only sometimes. I, too, hear from my patients about waking at three a.m.; I also hear about four and five a.m., and that is likely to be the low point of cortisol and of course the low point of blood sugar, and there is a relationship.

Insulin drives blood sugar down, and it does so by putting the sugar in the cells. It has to have some opposition, because otherwise you'll have low-blood-sugar attacks. Cortisol, from the adrenal glands, can in some situations help balance blood sugar again.

If you have a deficiency of cortisol, then the blood sugar might go too low. I read a paper written by a neurologist years ago that pointed out that when sugar goes too low in the middle of the night, we wake up.

It's the darndest thing. It's the opposite of what happens in the day-time, so sometimes it's not enough cortisol, and that is not uncommon in people whose blood pressure is low normal or low; that's one of the ways of telling you might not have enough cortisol. Without enough cortisol, you can't keep the blood sugar up, so the blood sugar goes down, and we wake up.

SOMERS: So the antidote seems to be to have your doctor order lab tests for cortisol levels and replace according to your particular deficiencies with bioidentical hydrocortisone, which is cortisol. If cortisol is high, it's impossible to sleep, and chronic high cortisol can lead to heart attack or stroke.

WRIGHT: One of the ways of dealing with waking up at three a.m. is eating protein at bedtime, because when there's not enough sugar around, our body will take some of the amino acids from protein and turn them into sugar. I am not going to tell you it works for everybody, but it works for some folks by just eating protein at nighttime; that keeps the sugar levels up.

People who need the extra protein are a very select group, only one-third of the population of the United States. These are people who have the genetic tendency to type 2 diabetes. If it's anywhere in your family—and you can easily find out if you're genetically predisposed even if you're seventeen years old—there's a test called the **Kraft Prediabetes Profile**. It checks the insulin levels along with the sugar levels. You can read about this test for free at the Meridian Valley Laboratory website, www.meridianvalleylab.com, because they're one of the few in the country to do the test. It was pioneered by Dr. Joseph Kraft, who ran it on fifteen thousand people over his career, and through this test he was able to tell you precisely who has the tendency to type 2 diabetes and who doesn't, and which are the people who need the higher protein.

SOMERS: Why would it be the ones with the genetic tendency?

WRIGHT: One-third of the population of the United States have the genetic tendency to type 2 diabetes. Is it because of all that sugar? No, because the other two-thirds *can* eat sugar. It's going to be bad for them in other ways, but it's not going to give them type 2 diabetes.

While lifestyle, diet, environment, and physical activity are known risk factors, some people's type 2 diabetes is caused by a genetic mutation, and that's what Dr. Yudkin identified.

This select group has the ability to make three times as much insulin in response to sugar and carbs as other people, but it's not known why so many people have that mutation. I presume it goes back to the cavemen: in the summer they ate berries and fruits, and those have a limited season, most of the time the summer and fall. So for survival, if you can get fat quicker, let's say this tribe gains nine pounds and this tribe gains three pounds and here comes the cold winter and there isn't enough food around, guess whose tribe survives better to have little babies next year? The one that got fatter, that's all.

SOMERS: Luck of the draw. Some people have paleo ancestors that ate too much. I have an uncle like that. Haha.

So to recapitulate, if you can't sleep:

• Have the Kraft Prediabetes Profile done to find out if your blood sugar level is low.

• If so, then check your cortisol level to see if that is too low also. By adjusting and balancing these two levels, your sleep should return to normal.

When a person comes to your clinic for the first time, what tests do you ask for ahead of time?

WRIGHT: Well, I don't. I read the person's application form: their concerns, what their mom and dad had in the way of health problems, if they did, here's the surgeries I've had, et cetera, et cetera, and then it's individually specific according to those forms and their issues. So there is no one test that fits all, no way.

SOMERS: I get it, I understand. It's individualized, as it should be; no human has the same needs as the next human. In your comprehensive exam and consult, do you offer a toxicity test?

WRIGHT: Yes, there are several labs, but the one I happen to like is done by a lab called Great Plains Laboratory.

It's called GPL-TOX; you can google it online. This test checks for most of the toxins we are most commonly exposed to, and it details your levels. Most toxins are stored in fat cells, so heavy sweating is one detoxification strategy which helps rid us of those particular toxins. Whatever it is that causes the heavy sweating—exercise or sauna—initially you need to do it often. There was research from one of the southern California universities in which they actually biopsied the fat and then sent the results off to the toxicology lab. One particular participant test revealed that he was loaded with toxins. It was suggested he do thirty episodes of heavy sweating for between thirty and forty minutes daily. Afterward they biopsied him again and found that after thirty episodes of heavy sweating, the toxins were down by two-thirds. Now, it didn't say one hundred percent, but they were down by two-thirds.

SOMERS: That's impressive. Detoxification is not a fast remedy; it takes time. But worth it; sweat the poisons out. Makes sense.

Are you a fan of far-infrared sauna?

WRIGHT: Yes, I am, because it induces heavy sweating. Initially, I have a hard time getting men to try it until I explain the following: men like chasing the ladies, and they can do that better if they have higher levels of nitric oxide. The drug Viagra raises your nitric oxide levels by stopping the breakdown of nitric oxide, which helps dilate blood vessels everywhere, including that key place for guys. Japanese research found that infrared penetrates right to the blood vessels and induces the formation of more nitric oxide, so when I tell guys about that, they're on their way to the infrared sauna store.

SOMERS: **So far-infrared sauna makes for better erections?** That should be a banner headline! I suppose that would be good for high blood pressure, too?

WRIGHT: Of course, anything that will dilate your blood vessels is good for lowering blood pressure; magnesium dilates blood vessels, as does eating beets, and sweating from taking infrared sauna detoxifies the additional nitric oxide. Infrared "frequencies" from infrared saunas are "bonus points" in terms of lowering blood pressure, and don't forget that sunshine contains infrared frequencies, too.

SOMERS: When my blood pressure went so high last year, you told me about the supplement Carditone being effective. Was it ever! I was going through some terrible stress, and my BP went to a frightening 171 over 110. I was told I "had" to take blood pressure medicine.

I don't take drugs, but I'm not stupid. I have too much to live for. But when I started taking Carditone, a natural supplement, my BP lowered to a lovely 116 over 80. Thanks.

WRIGHT: Yes, Carditone does something called "depletes," which means lessens, as in it lessens the adrenaline, specifically, and specifically noradrenaline; those are two versions of adrenaline. Adrenaline is manufactured in the adrenal glands, and noradrenaline is almost the same thing, but it's manufactured in the nerve cells. These two substances constrict blood vessels. Adrenaline and noradrenaline are the hormones present when we get all excited, but they constrict blood vessels, and the constriction of blood vessels drives up the blood pressure.

Carditone is based on an Ayurvedic remedy; it's a botanical, and people have known about this herb for literally a couple thousand years. Carditone depletes the adrenaline so that the blood vessels can't be as constricted. Now, there is good news and bad news: most women tolerate it perfectly. I have run into some men, when they take Carditone, and, oops, things no longer work as well in the bedroom. For a guy to get aroused, he has to have a little bit of adrenaline happening there, but if his adrenaline is depleted, he can't get as excited. So guys need to know about that, but that's not every guy, and most guys with high blood pressure can use it and not get into trouble.

> Carditone is a combination of a patented extract of rauwolfia, which has traditionally been used to support blood pressure levels already within the normal range and also has calming properties, several other herbs, and magnesium.

You must know, one of the things about Carditone is it is possible to overdose and drive one's blood pressure down too low. I am not kidding you. One person came in, his blood pressure was down to 80 over 45, depleting himself of too much adrenaline and noradrenaline. We don't want to drive it that low.

SOMERS: I love the idea that I have my BP under control without taking any drugs.

WRIGHT: Also, it's good to order nitric oxide test strips from the drugstore. Those are little strips of plastic with a little patch of sensitive material on the end. On the tube there is a color code which will give you an indicator of your nitric oxide levels. All important. Take that little strip, put it on your tongue first thing in the morning, and it turns anywhere from no color at all to a little bitty, bit pink, or it can go all the way up to a bright pink, and when it's a bright pink, that person's body is making an optimal amount of nitric oxide. Why do we want to do that? Because nitric oxide dilates blood vessels, and when we dilate blood vessels, guess what? Our blood pressure comes down. This allows you to check yourself: Is my body making an optimal amount of nitric oxide? If you aren't making enough nitric oxide, then take food into consideration; beets are number one, and spinach is number two. That explains why Popeye was always carrying that can of spinach when he was chasing Olive Oyl! Yep, he knew something.

THE TEN BEST FOODS TO INCREASE NITRIC OXIDE PRODUCTION

1. **Arugula (rocket)** is the richest plant source of nitrates. It contains 480 milligrams of nitrates in 100 grams of the vegetable. Eating it regularly will help your body increase production of nitric oxide. Arugula also contains vitamins A, C, and K, folic acid, thiamine, vitamin B_6, and pantothenic acid, besides minerals such as copper, iron, calcium, zinc, and magnesium.

2. **Rhubarb** is a rich source of nitrates, calcium, and vitamin C. Eating 100 grams of rhubarb will provide you with 247 milligrams of nitrates.

3. **Garlic** is a known sexual health aid and one of the most beneficial herbs. It works by supporting the synthesis of nitric oxide synthase (NOS). Garlic also contains allicin, one of the most beneficial high blood pressure remedies, which creates greater blood flow throughout the body. Another amazing benefit of garlic is that it contains the chemical diallyl disulfide, which stimulates the body to release a hormone that spurs the production of testosterone.

4. **Dark chocolate** is known to support heart health. It also helps increase the production of nitric oxide. It is worth noting that dark chocolate refers to unprocessed cocoa and not to popular chocolate bars. Processed chocolate contains sugar and other ingredients and is low in nitrates.

5. **Watermelon** contains citrulline, an amino acid that changes to arginine, which is a nitric oxide precursor. Not many foods contain a large amount of citrulline, which is why it has become very popular in supplementation form.

6. **Swiss chard** contains 151 milligrams of nitrates per 100 grams. It is also a rich source of vitamins A and C, providing 44 percent and 18 percent RDA per serving, respectively.

7. **Beetroots** are a rich source of nitrates. The root can be consumed in salads and in the form of juice. Beet greens also contain nitrates and can be eaten in salads for maximum nitrate content. Drinking 100 grams of pure beet juice provides you with 279 milligrams of nitrates. Beets also contain vitamins A and C, several B vitamins, and minerals such as manganese, magnesium, iron, potassium, and zinc. Beetroots are one of the most reliable nitric oxide–boosting foods and are now very popular in supplement form.

8. **Pomegranate** boosts nitric oxide and is a tremendous anti-inflammatory. It also reduces oxidative stress, a leading factor in the production of coronary artery disease. The polyphenols in the pomegranate help to convert dietary nitrite to nitric oxide. They also keep nitric oxide from converting back to nitrite.

9. **Celery** contains nitric oxide precursors. However, the amount can differ depending on where it is grown and the fertilizers used. Try some celery and orange juice to kickstart your libido.

10. **Shrimp** is a rich source of L-arginine, an amino acid that is a precursor of nitric oxide. L-arginine is synthesized into nitric oxide. Eating shrimp regularly helps increase nitric oxide production.

NITRIC OXIDE–BOOSTING FOODS

Nitric oxide helps maintain good blood circulation, which is essential for overall good health and sexual health in particular. Inadequate production of nitric oxide leads to various cardiovascular problems and is one cause of erectile dysfunction. The good news is that some foods boost the production of nitric oxide. It is worth noting that besides increasing the production of nitric oxide, eating a wide variety of these foods supplies your body with vitamins and minerals, in addition to their antioxidant and anti-inflammatory properties.

So you can either chow down on a lot of those until, when you put the test strip in, it comes out bright pink, or some people need to take a supplement, and there's a supplement out there called **L-citrulline**; anywhere from 1 gram to 3 grams a day, sure enough, that test strip is going to turn bright pink.

I always recommend that people start with the food, and then you test yourself once. Then let's say you start eating a lot of beets, and give it four or five days before you test again, because it takes your body some time to adjust its nitric oxide production. It doesn't happen overnight. Test yourself every four or five days until you've optimized your nitric oxide.

SOMERS: I believe it's all about the food regarding today's health. What you eat is what you become. Eat real food. Organic food. Grass-fed protein, organic chicken. It's the Hippocratic theory: "Let food be thy medicine, let medicine be thy food." Hippocrates was right, and today it's more important than ever.

Most of my friends who have been on the road for years, eating processed and fast foods, are either dead or have Alzheimer's or cancer.

How important is fish oil in today's health?

WRIGHT: These days, it's much more important than ever. Fish oil contains omega-3 fatty acids, which are anti-inflammatory. Fish oil helps control inflammation all through the body; it also happens to help to improve the population of brain cells in the memory area of the brain, and we can all use having our memory cells improved. Fish oil is a huge help and a very good idea.

SOMERS: Talk about keeping memory. I believe deep down, all of us fear losing our minds. With the toxic assault, it seems that most people are now expecting to end up with Alzheimer's at some point, housed away in a nursing home. What an awful thought. What can we do?

WRIGHT: First we've got to separate ourselves into families with type 2 diabetes, and families without type 2 diabetes. The ones who have type 2 diabetes in the family have that niacinamide issue again, Suzanne, and here's why: in families where there's type 2 diabetes, research shows that those people cannot make very much niacinamide internally. Back in the 1930s, when niacinamide was first discovered, it wasn't known that some people can make it in their own bodies. It was called a vitamin, and the official definition is supposed to mean that nobody can make it in their own body, but that is not true about niacinamide. Two-thirds of the population that has no tendency to type 2 diabetes can convert tryptophan [an amino acid found in proteins] into niacinamide. Professor Oxenkrug, a psychiatry professor, has written extensively about tryptophan to niacinamide conversion and how if you have type 2 diabetes, you don't have that conversion. In families with type 2 diabetes, their bodies don't make enough niacinamide, and over time, that leads to arthritis, and a large percentage of those with type 2 diabetes have one or more "brain issues," because the brain needs niacinamide, too.

If you don't naturally make enough niacinamide, you're not going to have enough energy. If your body is making niacinamide, inside every cell it stimulates that mitochondrial complex that turns out ATP [energy], and now that cell is energized.

SOMERS: So if your body isn't making niacinamide, then supplementation is crucial?

WRIGHT: We have put niacinamide in our brain formula called ReMIND (www.tahomadispensary.com), and there's another product out there called Sage Memories, and that one's got niacinamide in it, plus sage and rosemary, which have been found to help with memory, plus a little bit of over-the-counter lithium.

SOMERS: Over-the-counter lithium is amazing for memory. I've been taking yours for years from your Tahoma Clinic, 20 milligrams daily, and people joke about my memory: "Don't tell Suzanne, she remembers everything." I have to think that the lithium has something to do with it. I also take your ReMIND, six capsules daily.

WRIGHT: Going to lithium for a moment, one of the things that has been flat-out proven for lithium to do is to stimulate the formation of new brain cells. No kidding, new brain cells, and that's also in ReMIND, along with carnosine, found in meat. (That's where it gets its name, from *carne*, Spanish for "meat.") Carnosine protects the body's proteins from toxic glycation reactions. These occur when glucose binds to a protein in the body and forms a nonfunctioning structure. The accumulation of damaged proteins generates chronic inflammatory problems. Carnosine can help prevent this. So does the quercetin that's in ReMIND.

The fourth ingredient happens to be **taurine**, and, oh, boy, do I love taurine. Taurine has been found to do several things. These are for sure, Suzanne. Taurine is an amino acid which does not participate in the formation of protein at all; it's an electricity regulator in the brain and heart. For example, it helps to control seizures in small children.

But it also helps with heart rhythm disturbances. But let's get to what it really helps with: new brain cells!

SOMERS: Wow, so both the lithium and the taurine make new brain cells!

WRIGHT: And here's some more fun research. I love reading these research papers. Taurine not only makes new brain cells, but there's a study done in thirty-six countries, and what they found uniformly in every country is the more taurine in the urine, the less cardiovascular disease!

SOMERS: That's huge! The more taurine in the urine the less cardiovascular disease.

WRIGHT: But here's the capper that's going to get everybody's attention: taurine helps you to lose weight!

SOMERS: Now you're talking.

WRIGHT: Several grams of taurine a day were the only factor that led to a slow, steady weight loss in the group of people they were studying, who happened to be ladies. Taurine helps a person to lose weight. Oh, my goodness. How can you beat that? Losing weight, cardiovascular disease, new brain cells, taurine, yeah?

Taurine supplementation:

- Helps make new brain cells

- Reduces the risk of developing cardiovascular disease

- Helps you lose weight

WRIGHT: Mm-hm, there's carnosine and quercetin; those two substances go around in the body looking for those "senile cells" and getting rid of them, and by the way, that's also the way that nature gets rid of them.

CHAPTER 12

THE GUT

Aging is caused by worn-out body parts. Our hearts stop working perfectly; our cells get filled with debris; our mitochondria (the energy center of our cells) get tired and lazy; the brain shrinks, often due to toxic exposure; the pituitary gets lazy. These and many other declines are what we will be exploring. The great news is that everything can be regenerated, depending on how far you want to go.

My friends complain about aging issues; it seems that with each passing year, we face problems with various body parts that never bothered us before.

My first aging issue was hormonal decline. I was able to solve that dilemma through bioidentical hormone replacement therapy (BHRT). I've never looked back. What a joy to wake up each day feeling energetic and upbeat.

My second aging issue was acid reflux. I had never had that before, and when I mentioned it to friends, I realized it was epidemic. The pain and discomfort I experienced as a result of my acid reflux was exacerbated by radiation treatments for breast cancer. The radiation (unbeknownst to me) caused inflammation (esophagitis) in the tube that connects the mouth to the stomach (the esophagus) in my body. Reflux of stomach acid into my esophagus was caused by an impaired ability of my lower esophageal sphincter valve to seal. Then the radiation treatments impaired my body's ability to produce stomach acid. Why is that important?

Because without hydrochloric acid (HCl), I could not start the process of digestion of food in my stomach, in particular proteins. The "mouth" that connects the stomach to the intestines felt clogged, and everything I ate seemed to get "stuck" between the stomach and the opening of the small intestine. It was extremely uncomfortable. Then my food and my stomach contents refluxed back up into my esophagus because of the loss of my stomach muscle tone. I am committed to taking hydrochloric acid (HCl) supplements with every meal for the rest of my life as my remedy for balancing my gut issues that were caused by radiation damage.

Many of us lose HCl with aging, which impairs the body's ability to begin the process of digestion of proteins.

This brings me to the next section, an understanding of the gut and why it is going so wrong for so many. It's important to note that if your gut isn't healthy, you aren't healthy.

> *All disease starts in the gut.*
> —Hippocrates, the Father of Medicine

GASTROESOPHAGEAL REFLUX DISEASE (GERD)

As we age, we can develop many health problems, from bacterial overgrowth to inflammation, from small intestinal bacterial overgrowth (SIBO) (that's what causes your bloated intestines) to acid reflux. More and more people are suffering from esophageal cancer, probably as a result of acid reflux. Acid reflux, otherwise known as **gastroesophageal reflux disease (GERD)**, is rampant. You see it in the swollen and irritated bellies of so many people, causing, pain, bloating, discomfort, and belching. The powerful antidote for most reflux recommended by allopathic doctors is **proton pump inhibitors**, a drug class that powerfully suppresses gastric acid production. However, long-term use of these types of powerful acid-suppressing drugs has been potentially linked to significant problems, including kidney disease, bone fractures, low magnesium levels, diarrhea, vitamin B_{12} deficiency, and even dementia![1]

Many of you have the condition because you don't make enough stomach acid, and now your doctor gives you a drug to take away even more acid. It soothes momentarily, but notice the people who are sucking on antacids; they are sucking on antacid lozenges all day long. Or they are regularly taking proton pump–inhibiting drugs. There's got to be a better way.

Aging often brings poor digestion, especially of high-protein foods. In fact, aging is linked to a gradual decline in the amount of stomach acid your body produces. This is a problem because stomach acid is necessary to help activate enzymes in the stomach that help digest proteins. So by replacing lost acid in the stomach, you may start to fix the problem by restoring the body to balance. When all was well, you made plenty of hydrochloric acid and digestive enzymes. You don't usually hear children complaining of acid reflux, do you? Heartburn is a result of the sphincter muscle between the esophagus and stomach not closing all the way. This allows acid and other stomach contents to reflux back into your esophagus. Add to this not enough digestive enzymes and hydrochloric acid, and you set the stage for chronic digestive issues.

Acids, digestive enzymes, and bile are essential for digestion. When you suffer from reflux, you frequently swallow air as a reflexive action to the discomfort and pain related to the reflux, which makes you feel bloated and uncomfortable. When you don't have enough stomach acid, the stomach produces gas bubbles. According to Dr. Jerry Tennant in his book *Healing Is Voltage: The Handbook*, "These bubbles are coated with stomach acid much like soap coats a bubble. The gas bubble causes you to belch or simply rises up into your esophagus where you taste the acid. It burns your esophagus so you feel discomfort or overt pain. This is called GERD or gastroesophageal reflux disease."

So you need stomach acid to help begin the process of digestion of proteins, especially in the stomach. In addition, you need to avoid doing things that will weaken or reduce the tone in the lower esophageal sphincter so that stomach acid does not reflux back into your esophagus, causing pain and inflammation. Logically, then, as we get older, it makes sense to replace the loss of acids and digestive enzymes, as well as to avoid activities that make GERD worse.

Factors that worsen and intensify heartburn or GERD include:

- Heavy meals

- Excess alcohol consumption

- Excess caffeine consumption

- Obesity

- Eating two to three hours before bedtime

- Hiatal hernia

Without sufficient stomach acid, healthy digestion and absorption of vital nutrients can be severely impaired.

Stomach acid activates digestive enzymes in the stomach primarily for the purpose of protein degradation. Specifically, stomach acid activates pepsin, which is the chief enzyme in your stomach that breaks down protein foods.

Acid and enzymes break down our food and enable the extraction of its minerals and nutrients. When you eat a protein, your stomach acid and enzymes must break it down into amino acids. As the digested food reaches the small intestine, the amino acids are (1) absorbed so the body can make and repair proteins, (2) used to generate biomolecules, and (3) utilized as an energy source. If you don't have enough stomach acid, partially digested proteins reach the small intestine and are absorbed there. Some emerging research suggests that the body may mistakenly recognize these as foreign particles and potentially mount an immune response to neutralize the perceived threat, even though it is really not a threat. Some scientists believe this is one way that food allergies may occur. So to jump-start the digestive process in the stomach, you may need to replace the lost stomach acid as well as the digestive enzymes that drop off with aging.

You can obtain hydrochloric acid in a form called Betaine HCl, which includes pepsin, as well as digestive enzymes called Enhanced Super Digestive Enzymes, from Life Extension and other websites.

Why do we lose stomach acid? Most often the problem is age related; it's the beginning of the breakdown of the body. If you aren't digesting your food and extracting the nutrients it will be the beginning of a cascade of poor health. If your gut isn't healthy, you aren't heathy.

Putting back the substances that you have lost in the aging process will restore your gut and GI tract to normalcy and help restore gut health.

If you've had radiation therapy to your chest, as I did for breast cancer, it inhibits your body's ability to make sufficient hydrochloric acid for life!

Without stomach acid, you can't absorb the zinc in your food. No stomach acid equals zinc deficiency. Why do you care? There are more than 350 biochemical reactions that rely on zinc, including the production of neurochemicals in the brain, so taking drugs that shut down your stomach acid may make you become depressed by altering your serotonin signaling. This depression can lead to chronic fatigue (feeling dog tired) and allergies. You go to your regular doctor, and what does he give you? Antidepressants. These drugs are a temporary Band-Aid but have been shown to increase the frequency of depression when taken long term. Now your sexual performance diminishes, and essentially you are on an emotional roller coaster, plus the allergies bring a runny nose, migraine headaches, explosive diarrhea, and an emotional and physical downward spiral.

Think holistically; this may all have started because of a lack of vitamin B_1, iodine, zinc, and other nutrients known to enhance emotional well-being, all because you weren't digesting your food due to a lack of HCl. If you stop the drugs, the issues and symptoms reappear because you never really fixed them, you just covered them up with what I call "Band-Aid medicine."

The human body is a system, a sophisticated, highly intelligent communication system. It requires balance to operate at optimum. When you were a kid, if you were healthy, your system worked perfectly, even with dietary abuse. But as we age, an imbalance here and an imbalance there start to add up, until one day you go to the doctor saying you feel like crap and testing shows all your imbalances.

Body imbalances need to be rectified. This is not normally the domain of mainstream doctors. It's not how they think. The answer in their world is the latest pill. The "new doctors," such as the ones I present in this book, are in the trenches working with biochemicals all day long; they all report how exciting it is to bring a body back from imbalance. They often say that this work is rewarding because they see such major improvements in health and rarely have to rely on pharmaceutical drugs. Plus the fact that their patients hug them and bring them thank-you gifts says it all.

I presume that if you are reading this book you want to outwit the environment and the mess we call our medical system.

The allopathic-only protocol we have all been force-fed has tried to convince us that pharmaceutical pills are "the only way," but we have hit a wall. Taking pills and more pills is not working, and the result is a steady downward spiral of our individual health. I asked Dr. Herbert Slavin of Florida, "How did it get this way?" He explained, "The issue had to do with the influence of the drug companies and their taking control of health care in this country. It dates all the way back to 1910, when the Flexner Report was published. Abraham Flexner was representing, directly or indirectly, the Rockefellers and the Carnegies. His job was to go around to all the schools that taught health care, which back then included chiropractic, osteopathic, naturopathic, homeopathic, whatever schools they had. What they didn't have was allopathy, which is what is practiced today, essentially the use of drugs and surgery to treat disease.

"Flexner was hired because both the Rockefellers and the Carnegies owned—you guessed it—pharmaceutical companies, and they had to figure out how to market their products," he says. "They came up with this idea that the best way to market pharmaceuticals was to teach the doctors to use them. Flexner went around to the various medical schools, such as the Mayo Clinic, Johns Hopkins, and others, and offered financial incentives to these institutions to change their curriculum to educate their doctors on the use of pharmaceuticals. The schools in turn received a huge influx of money and changed their curriculum so that now today when patients come into their doctor's office with a chief complaint, which is a symptom, they are given a prescription for a drug or drugs."

As patients we got used to this fast reaction, and that has become the problem: we want immediate results.

And that's how this happened: medical students were no longer taught the "art of medicine"; rather, they were taught to write prescriptions, and here we are: that original offer of funding (which was accepted) was the end of the natural "pathics" and the beginning of "allopathic" (pharmaceutical drug) therapy. This became the accepted way, and all the other "pathics" were dismissed as quackery.

If there isn't a pill for a condition, doctors are stumped. The tragedy of this protocol is that the primary role of physicians as healers depended upon the delicate balance of patient care and research, but today the science (drug) approach to medicine eclipses the active hands-on witnessing of patients.

But things are changing after more than a hundred years of allopathic care and the resulting poor health of so many people (because, after all, pharmaceutical drugs *do not heal*; they are essentially symptom relievers). There is now a huge move to alternative and integrative therapies, using, as Dr. Wright says, "nature's tools." Millions of people in this country and around the world are looking for a new way, which ironically was the old way. Remember when the doctor told you to go to bed and rest and drink plenty of liquids for a few days? Now you are told to take your pills and make sure you take them all for seven days, otherwise they won't work. Sleeping, drinking plenty of liquids, and resting for seven days would do a better job in most cases, but make sure you talk to your physician before stopping prescribed medications.

The other tragedy is the fact that so many children are being put on drugs. I mean, did you take drugs when you were a kid? Now it's accepted: drugs for allergies, runny noses, colds, and flu; strong cough medicines; amphetamines (imagine) to counteract their chemical exposure in today's environment. No one has any idea of their long-term consequences. And then there's the overuse of antibiotics, which shred their little stomach linings, with never a warning to take probiotics simultaneously.

Remember: "anti"-biotic takes away, "pro"-biotic puts back. Simple.

The fewer foreign molecules you put into your body, the less you are going to confuse it.

The doctors in this book think differently, outside of the box; they use natural therapies and turn to Western medicine only as a last resort.

It's amazing how many people say to me, "I just want to feel good again." Lack of energy and frustration as to what to do going forward can cause people to feel hopeless and give up.

Take your heart cells, for example. According to Dr. Russell Blaylock, a renowned neuroscientist and dear friend, "Your heart never takes a day off. To beat strongly over an entire lifetime, your heart demands adequate nutrients, such as vitamin D, vitamin E, vitamin C, folate, calcium, plus the mineral magnesium, which is critical to ensure a normal heartbeat and blood pressure." These simple supplemental additions offer preventive changes by "putting back" adequate nutrients and can positively affect the paradigm of your aging and how well you are going to do it.

Dr. Blaylock goes on, "Take your brain cells; your brain has very high requirements for energy. That's why it needs a constant supply of micronutrients to meet its demand.

"In order to maintain brain health, researchers have documented the importance of vitamin E, the B vitamins, vitamin C, zinc, magnesium and other nutrients for healthy memory, cognition and mood."[2]

To minimize the effects of an aging brain, supplementation is essential.

Dr. Jonathan Wright has already explained the proper way to determine your mineral and nutritional deficiencies through lab work that you can have your doctor order on your behalf.

It's time to be your *own contractor*, meaning telling your present doctor what tests you want him or her to order for you so you can bring yourself back to optimal health and energy.

The better educated you are, the better contractor you will be.

Interview with

KENT MACLEOD

Kent MacLeod is the founder and CEO of NutriChem Compounding Pharmacy & Clinic in Canada. An international thought leader, he is also an award-winning pharmacist with more than thirty years of clinical experience in delivering patient-centered health care. He describes ways of improving the gut microbiome.

Under the guidance of Kent MacLeod, NutriChem protocols help people understand how to rebalance their gut microbiome. The human population in general is out of balance due to toxicity, processed foods, and pharmaceutical drugs.

His book *The Biology of the Brain: How Your Gut Microbiome Affects Your Brain* is a must-read to understand the damage that has been inflicted on our GI tracts by the environmental assault. He makes the argument that imbalanced microbiome in the gut will negatively affect your brain. He argues that all gut issues affect the brain.

> *It's not pretend anymore. We now know that destroying the microbiome has extreme effects on your brain, your immune system, and increases your risk for deadly infections.*
>
> —Kent MacLeod

MACLEOD: We keep treating acid as a problem in the stomach, but most of the time, gastrointestinal disease is a problem of a thin mucosal lining of the GI tract. A functional mucosal lining requires a healthy microbiome and can easily handle stomach acid. If you just turn off the acid with antacids, the bacteria in your gut shifts toward unhealthy bacteria, which can be a disaster for your microbiome.

One of the easiest things to do for someone's general health is to get them off of their long-term protein pump inhibitor [PPI] drugs if it is being used inappropriately. NutriChem pharmacists actually sit on the

Canadian Deprescribing Network, and one of our major areas of focus is helping patients to come off of inappropriate PPIs.

Your microbiome is a community of living organisms, which is interconnected with the rest of your body and brain. Just as stress damages and leads to other symptoms or diseases, it also plays an integral part in aggravating your microbiome.

A few PPIs that you might be familiar with or have been prescribed at some point include:

- Omeprazole (Prilosec, Prilosec OTC, Zegerid)

- Lansoprazole (Prevacid)

- Pantoprazole (Pantoloc, Protonix)

- Rabeprazole (AcipHex)

- Esomeprazole (Nexium)

- Dexlansoprazole (Dexilant)

Taking PPIs gives relief but at the cost of your well-being and microbiome, which suffer in the long term. Taking any of these medications is an indicator that your microbiome needs recalibration.

The hardest thing I've learned over the years with the thousands of patients I've helped is their struggle with understanding and knowing the full picture of the gut. Chances are you are not a gastroenterologist, nor do you have any educational or professional training in the area.

This is actually a good thing and a bad thing. It's bad in the sense that you're unaware of the true importance of each of your bodily functions and how to take care of them. It's good because you're starting from square one and can learn afresh, without any preconceived biases.

It's better you have no prior knowledge; sometimes it's just easier to move forward with PPIs and other medications that are so detrimental to your gut's well-being, but at what cost to your health?

There is a misconception of what the stomach does. Common knowledge might lead one to believe the stomach is where digestion of food and liquid takes place. And though this is partially true, meaning digestion *begins* in the stomach, it would be missing the mark.

The acids in the stomach aid in the digestive process. Full digestion really takes place in the small intestine, where food and liquid are broken down and absorbed. If you take PPIs, you're altering the pH levels of the stomach acids, which in turn lead to increased pH [lower acidity] of the small and large intestines, increasing risks for infections.

PPIs dramatically alter the pH of the GI tract, changing the populations of bacteria in the small intestine. This can shift the gut toward unhealthy bacteria, such as *C. difficile*.

Maybe you've heard of *E. coli* and salmonella. But you might not have heard of a more dangerous infection caused by a bacterium called *C. difficile*. The reason this infection is so dangerous is that it's almost untreatable. Virtually no antibiotic will kill it. And when you increase your PPI intake, you increase your risk of *C. difficile* infection. It's important to note that your gut normally contains a healthy amount of *C. difficile*. Just as "good" bacteria are necessary for a balanced and healthy gut, so too are "bad" bacteria necessary. The importance is balance. By maintaining a healthy microbiome, you reduce or completely eliminate your risk of infections and other diseases.

PART IV

THE HEART:
How to Keep It from Breaking

CHAPTER 13

DISPELLING MYTHS ABOUT HEART HEALTH

Deep down inside, everyone worries about his or her heart. It's the wild card. We know diet affects heart health, but what about random fatal heart attacks? Where do they come from? The ones where everyone says, "Geez, he plays tennis every day. How could this happen?" Why did someone as young and in the prime of life as John Ritter drop dead from an aortic dissection? What if he had known about EECP? EECP is explained in this chapter.

The body has a language, and we need to pay careful attention to the signs of poor heart function: shortness of breath, momentary chest pains, stiff legs, stiff hands and arms, dizziness. All these things are the body talking. It is up to us to listen.

The triad of heart disease, heart attack, and stroke has become one of the biggest killers of humans. Men and women are at equal risk. Stress is at an all-time high; lack of understanding of diet, medications, and hormonal imbalances is a huge contributor to weakening the heart.

The low-fat movement was a disaster leading to an increase in heart disease. In reality, healthy fat is essential for your body. **Without fat in the diet, cognition diminishes.** Low fat consumption is one of the major reasons we have an epidemic of Alzheimer's disease. According to Dr. Stephen Sinatra, "When I did the research, I found that cholesterol is found at the scene of the crime, but it's not the perpetrator. In other words, cholesterol plays a very small part in the genesis of inflammation, and it is inflammation that is the root cause of heart disease." So we've been barking up the wrong tree ever since the flawed study in 1941 by Ancel Keys declaring that fat consumption was the reason for the development of heart disease. We gave up fats, and people got fatter and sicker. But the low-fat diet that was promoted by our government, the media, and most food manufacturers was not only **DEAD WRONG** but downright **DEADLY!**

Let me take a moment to show you what went wrong in our food supply. This might make you a little angry, but if you have hypertension, it explains why you have it and also how to fix it.

The problem started in 1955, when the influential Dr. Ancel Keys presented his thesis connecting dietary animal fat to heart disease to a World Health Organization conference in Geneva, Switzerland.

Keys had studied the diets of people in twenty-two countries, but for his presentation—and to make his thesis stronger—he showed data from just seven countries.

Keys showed that people in Japan and Italy had low animal fat consumption and low rates of heart disease, while Australia, Canada, Great Britain, and the United States had high animal fat consumption and higher rates of heart disease.

It was all too easy. And nobody should have drawn conclusions from it. But the results of Keys's Seven Countries Study, which he put into a simplistic chart, raced around the world.

Keys made the cover of *Time* magazine and perhaps got the fame he wanted. But his theory that animal fat—and the cholesterol in it—causes heart disease was wrong. The really unfortunate part is that rather than reducing heart disease, his ideas increased it!

That's because in 1977, a committee headed by Senator George McGovern, after holding hearings on our national diet, issued a set of dietary guidelines designed to reduce the consumption of animal fat and, hopefully, heart disease. That caused a world of trouble. If only we had known . . .

The dietary guidelines led food manufacturers to replace animal fats with processed vegetable fats. The labels on foods containing them say "low fat" and "heart healthy." But they're not healthy at all, just the opposite: they're disease makers!

The heart requires healthy fats such as omega-3 essential fatty acids to function well. All those years well-intentioned professionals bought into the myth that fat was the culprit, when in fact the opposite was true. As a result, we gave up our beloved butter and switched to omega-6 vegetable oils (often carcinogenic), eschewing the bounty of beautiful fats nature provides, such as extra-virgin olive oil. We opted instead for flavorless foods and worse, for example using chemical-laden margarine instead of butter. But such foods trigger a chemical reaction in your body that causes inflammation and oxidation—the drivers of disease.

Interestingly, according to the American Heart Association, NAD+ supplementation, which you will read about in the interview with Bill Faloon in chapter 16, may improve heart function.

Stabilizing the intracellular NAD+ level is a promising therapeutic strategy to improve myocardial bioenergetics and cardiac function. The AMA also suggests that supplementation with an NAD+ precursor, nicotinamide riboside (NR), reduces cardiac dysfunction in preclinical models of heart failure.

The unfortunate result was that this change in our food supply dramatically increased the rates of heart disease, hypertension, arthritis, diabetes, and even cancer. Remember McDonald's French fries from three or four decades ago? They were really tasty, and that's because they were fried in beef tallow. But because of the dietary guidelines that called for reducing the consumption of animal fat, McDonald's gradually phased out the beef tallow and replaced it with processed vegetable oil, which it has used since 1990.

Okay, now, stick with me—because this next part is pretty shocking.

After Keys wrongly named animal fat and cholesterol as the cause of heart disease, pharmaceutical companies developed cholesterol-lowering drugs . . .

. . . and then, to sell them, they promoted the heck out of Keys's bogus theory—and even manipulated the results of statin drug studies to make them look effective, when in fact they helped less than 1 percent of users.

Unfortunately, the flawed cholesterol theory got into our medical schools, where drug companies hold great sway, and a whole generation of doctors learned it. And then those doctors became the teachers of the next generation.

You could call it a comedy of errors, except that it was no laughing matter. **Statin drugs can damage muscles and even weaken your heart because they block an essential heart nutrient called coenzyme Q10 (CoQ10).**

Today we know better. Refined vegetable (omega-6) fats and sugars are primary culprits.

Clearly, nature wanted us to have a high-fat diet. In our first year of life we were provided an extremely high-fat diet of breast milk until the baby formula lobby got ahold of the literature. Think about this:

Butter has almost the same percentages of polyunsaturated, monounsaturated, and saturated fats as . . . BREAST MILK!

I gave birth one month after my nineteenth birthday. I was a child and knew nothing. Immediately after delivery, I was asked if I was going to nurse. I didn't know what they were talking about, so I said no. I was immediately given a "dry-up" shot, and I was handed my baby, wrapped in a soft receiving blanket, with a bottle of formula. Two weeks after his birth, I had an overwhelming urge to nurse, but of course I couldn't. The damage had been done. I remember the sadness I felt.

Nature is profound, and the nature in me inherently knew we had both lost out on something. As a result, both my baby and myself were denied all the protection afforded by breast milk: protection for me from breast cancer and the same protection from cancer and disease for my son. We were denied prolactin and oxytocin, the "love and sex" hormone, and we were denied the bond created by that mother/child experience. When did we decide to outthink nature?

Interestingly, my son has had a lifetime of asthma and breathing issues, and I had breast cancer.

We do the best we can with the information we have at the time, so with maturity and therapy I have been able to forgive myself, but it truly was a shame and one of my few life regrets.

In this part, I introduce you to a cutting-edge cardiologist and surprisingly a jaw specialist. They are integrative, meaning that they take the best from both kinds of medicine. Neither of them hands out medications like candy; each has his own unique approach. These are the doctors I trust with *my* heart.

There are new approaches to heart disease both before the fact (preventively) and after heart disease and damage have occurred, and luckily for us there are now shifts in the way doctors are looking at heart disease.

If what you want is bypass surgery, stents, blood pressure medicine, and statins, then this is probably not the section for you. If, on the other hand, you are looking for true healing and cures, a life without statins and blood pressure meds, then I believe you will find the next interview riveting.

As stated, I am a patient of these professionals. My family dies of heart attack and stroke. As an Irish woman I genetically have a tendency to high homocysteine levels, most likely the cause and effect of the heart conditions in our family, although with today's stress levels, environmental insults, and hormonal decline, its effects have been magnified. The professionals I have interviewed are Dr. Stephen Sinatra, a leading integrative cardiologist/author in the United States and most likely the world, and Dr. Leonard Feld, a jaw specialist who makes the connection between misalignment of the jaw and heart disease. In between these two interviews, we'll also discuss EECP, a nondrug therapy with outstanding results for saving one's heart.

Interview with
DR. STEPHEN SINATRA

When my blood pressure skyrocketed due to unusual stress a few years ago, it was Dr. Stephen Sinatra, a top-of-his-field integrative cardiologist, in conjunction with EECP, that helped me normalize without drugs. In today's world, doctors reach for the prescription pad too quickly, and then you are part of the pharmaceutical merry-go-round.

You are reading this book to avoid that, so listen to what Dr. Sinatra, a cutting-edge heart doctor, is doing. He is integrative, meaning that he employs the best of both kinds of medicine. I believe this is what we all want to do: go natural, but if a catastrophic event occurs, you want a doctor who knows when to go allopathic.

As a result of his guidance, I needed no drugs to return my blood pressure to normal.

SOMERS: Thanks once again, Stephen, it's always a joy to speak with you. I'm honored to pick your brain and thrilled to access your great knowledge as well as experience your humor and warmth.

You are a heart doctor, a cardiologist, unusual because your approach is integrative; a doctor who doesn't reach for the prescription pad first. This is our connection and why I have returned to you over and over. We both know the answer does not always lie in pharmaceuticals, and I believe more and more people are responding to taking charge of their health, utilizing new information to try "a different way."

The facts are that as we age, everyone worries about their heart. I'm worried about *my* heart. My family dies of heart attack and stroke. It's the wild card. It's as though you can do everything right, but the heart holds the cards. I've always found it interesting that as a cardiologist with an integrative approach, you are also a psychotherapist. You must love school! Haha. But psychotherapist? Why?

SINATRA: Thanks, Suzanne. I realized early on that there are emotional risk factors that lead to heart disease. I needed to understand my profession from that point of view. I deal with the "heart." I became certified as a bioenergetic therapist after two years of Gestalt therapy training facilitated by founder Fritz Perls' disciples. To become certified myself, it was required that I do my own personal therapy. As a result, I went through years of psychotherapy with some of the world's best therapists. I came to believe in personal therapy wholeheartedly. During psychotherapy, we explore our lives instead of looking through a rearview mirror, so to speak.

SOMERS: What do you mean?

SINATRA: We have so much resistance built up that we're not experiencing our true selves. You see, many of us unknowingly live in a "false self" as a way of protecting our belief patterns. It's about taking responsibility for all your problems. That's the whole key. We must understand that we all create some cause in the way we interact with the world. For example, one of the reasons I wrote the book *Heartbreak and Heart Disease* is that as a cardiologist/psychotherapist, I realized that **many cases of heart disease often originate from deep hurts and disappointments that we all experience in childhood**.

SOMERS: How important is forgiveness?

SINATRA: It's all about forgiveness. You aren't free or healed unless you can find true forgiveness. Holding on to old hurts and anger is never good for the heart.

SOMERS: What's new in the "heart world," medically speaking?

SINATRA: Many things. For instance, there's interesting new research on women and heart disease. Twenty years ago, I authored a book called *Heart Sense for Women*. It had always been believed that women didn't get heart disease. Now we realize that heart disease is the number one killer of women! While one in eight women will contract breast cancer[1]—the most feared diagnosis for women—sadly, almost twenty-five percent of women will perish from heart disease.[2] Those are tough statistics. So we have started seriously looking at heart disease evaluation, treatment, and prevention specific to women.

SOMERS: How much do hormones factor into heart disease?

SINATRA: There's no question that when women hit menopause, their incidence of coronary disease goes up as much as four times.[3] That's a significant statistic. Women are protected by estrogen in their premenopausal days and at lower risk than men during those years. But about ten years into menopause, women catch up with their male counterparts.

Now, what's also changed in our society is that many more women are out in the workplace and competing well with men in workplace environments. I've lectured on this trend. And as a heart specialist, I honestly believe this scenario predisposes a woman to heart disease. If a woman becomes more like a man, such as a corporate executive in the workplace—performing, being the breadwinner—and at the same time, she continues her female roles—nurturing her children, taking care of parents, cooking, maybe driving the kids to school, appointments, and all of that—she's literally working like a dog.

I remember one of my cardiologist mentors, the late Dr. Bob Elliott. He used to say that maintaining her femininity and softness while acting like a man at work and working like a dog on all fronts represents what I call the "unholy trinity" for a woman that can lead to heart disease. And yet that's what many women expect to be able to do, especially the generations after ours. Of course, if a hardworking woman has a husband or partner who assists her in childcare and on the home front, that can balance things for her. I love seeing this new generation of more hands-on dads!

SOMERS: It sounds like a country song.

SINATRA: Be a woman, act like a man, and work like a dog? Suzanne, write that song. I'm telling you, write that song.

SOMERS: I have another theory relative to heart disease and hormones. Correct me if you think I'm wrong. As we women age, our minor hormones drop—estrogen, progesterone, testosterone—and our major hormones rise: adrenal, insulin, and cortisol. Chronic high cortisol leads to heart attack and stroke. So it could very well be that another reason we women are dying of heart disease is a drop in the minor hormones, leading to a rise in the major hormones, and cortisol is a major hormone. And now we are living longer, so it's a lethal combo?

SINATRA: That could definitely be a factor. We see high cortisol levels in people under prolonged, chronic stress. In fact, cortisol is so strongly associated with emotional distress that it has even been measured in one's tears. And many of us strongly feel that stress—psychological distress—is a risk factor for developing heart disease. I have seen plenty of folks have their heart attack during a peak emotional event, when their cortisol was most likely skyrocketing abruptly. So high cortisol can be a provocative tipping point.

The other biochemical thing that has tweaked my interest is something new relative to heart disease: the chink in the armor of the protective benefits of HDL cholesterol. HDL stands for "high-density lipoprotein." Newer research shows that an HDL blood level of 40 to 60 milligrams per deciliter is ideal. Too much HDL, say, nineties or higher, could represent a dysfunctional HDL, which does not have a protective impact and may even be harmful.

After being dubbed the "good cholesterol" for so many years, we now realize that too much HDL can be dysfunctional: it fires the inflammation I believe to be the real cause of heart disease. So again, that new research concluded that it now looks like there is that "sweet spot" for HDL: 40 to 60. When HDL is too low, it's not good, and when it's too high, it may not be good. That target "sweet spot" from 40 to 60—and around 50—is one of the current major treatment goals of traditional cardiologists. And I concur.

Total cholesterol numbers around 180 to 220 are good. As for low-density lipoprotein, LDLs of 100 to 140 are also in a good range. Remember, many cardiologists may agree or disagree with these numbers. I still believe the most ominous cholesterol is the small, highly inflammatory Lp(a) particle. Lipoprotein a—nicknamed "Lp little a"—is also an independent risk factor for heart disease when out of range. And elevated Lp(a) can run in families. So if you have a family member with high Lp(a), you should check your own. In fact, if you have a strong family history of heart disease, you should check your Lp(a). We did not check for Lp(a) years ago, so you would not know if it's a culprit cause of heart disease in your family. Trouble is, Lp(a) does not respond well to the traditional pharmaceutical drugs.

We've talked about inflammation in your other books, Suzanne. And what I am most concerned with is this secondary component of LDL—the subfraction called Lp(a), which is the small-but-stealthy-and-sneaky particle. It's the SS factor! Like our initials: SS. Lp(a) is the *real* cholesterol story. Though very small, this highly inflammatory particle is like that little red head of a match that starts the firestorm of inflammation inside what we call the endothelial layer. Small things can wreak havoc, for sure!

SOMERS: But most doctors miss this. High Lp(a) is like little razor blades on the inside of the arteries, right?

SINATRA: Exactly. And high Lp(a) causes blood clotting as well. That's why I have always been in favor of offsetting high Lp(a) levels with natural blood thinners, such as lumbrokinase [brand-name Boluoke in Canada] and nattokinase. The problem with typical cholesterol-lowering drugs—the standard-of-care statins—is that they can increase that very dangerous component of LDL called Lp(a), which is counterproductive. Statins lower coenzyme Q10 levels, as well. Also counterproductive.

As you well know from working with me—and this is where I wear my traditional hat, and it's true—I'm not a big believer in the cholesterol theory of heart disease. So I would not routinely prescribe statins, were I still in practice. But there are some subsets of the population that are more vulnerable than others when it comes to the aggressive secondary prevention of heart disease. For me, that population is males under the age of seventy-five with documented coronary calcification.

Today we can see what's going on with new innovative noninvasive testing. I prefer not to use these measures if not absolutely necessary. EBCT [electron beam computerized tomography] is technology which, like CT scans, means exposure to a lot of radiation, which is not a good thing. But should you have a malignant family history of heart disease and sudden death at a young age, the radiation risk is justified. If you've had blood-related family members die young and suddenly from heart disease, then it's a good idea to get that EBCT scan.

Should EBCT results show calcification in a young male, I would pull out the prescription pad and employ a statin for its profound anti-inflammatory and blood-thinning properties, not to target cholesterol. I'd also recommend 100 to 200 milligrams CoQ10 daily to offset the depleting effects of statins.

But here's the catch-22: statins have some potential to increase coronary calcification as well.

SOMERS: Frankly, it doesn't seem to me that statins do the job except in rare or genetic cases. The side effects are frankly frightening. Coronary calcification? Increasing Lp(a), the most dangerous component? There's also muscle wasting [rhabdomyolysis] and brain fog. My friends on statins have brains that aren't "firing." I understand what you are saying when a life is at risk but only in those rare cases. I would much prefer to go with a natural blood thinner. Would treating inflammation naturally be your first choice?

SINATRA: Yes, absolutely. Take your son, for example. He had a targeted risk factor that I recognized, being an integrative cardiologist.

SOMERS: Yes, he is fifty years old, and his blood work showed very high Lp(a). We both appreciated the direction you gave him, which was to take the natural blood thinner lumbrokinase. It took several months to normalize his numbers, and he is grateful he was able to accomplish this with your help, without drugs. So thank you.

I've read that statins create forgetfulness and muscle degradation. What does that indicate?

SINATRA: It's true, statin side effects are troublesome for many. Statins do lower cholesterol, but you *need* cholesterol for your thinking, for your memory. You need cholesterol in the brain: it's vital for the brain. And cholesterol also makes sex hormones. Some men become impotent on statin drugs. I saw it in my own practice as a young cardiologist, when I used to prescribe statins, even in young forty- and fifty-year-olds. So often they'd come back to me and say, "Doc, I'm having problems with sex, thought, and memory," yet another danger of too-low cholesterol. And that's what statins do.

Brain function is vitally important: this is your mental health. There was a study at Duke University where they looked at 120 healthy women and found that low cholesterol levels, under 160 [millimoles per liter], were associated with higher levels of anxiety and depression. Even immune system dysfunction becomes more apparent when cholesterol falls to very low levels.

SOMERS: Clearly statins have had a brilliant marketing plan. Everyone including the doctors bought into it.

SINATRA: Yes, what marketing! Doctors are prescribing statins like candy—with little attention to their downsides, I might add. Cholesterol has been vilified—which is so wrong—that we ignore everything it does *right*. Cholesterol actually protects our health, and I truly feel the most vital aspect of cholesterol is the support of proper brain function. Also, when LDL cholesterol goes too low, below 70, you may sacrifice some protection against cancer.

SOMERS: Brain health is quality of life; losing your brain or diminished brain function alters who you are.

SINATRA: Yes, having a healthy brain and using alternative ways of combating inflammation for continued quality of life are essential for us as human beings. There are a lot of things you can do to support the brain—supplements like phosphatidylserine (PS), astaxanthin, and wild blueberry, for example.

I got involved with a PS study years ago. I gave it to older men and was amazed, Suzanne. I remember older men telling me they were now doing crossword puzzles again. One was tying flies again. They said their brain function came back.

Losing one's memory or faulty brain function is the unwanted dinner guest, and it's from an accumulation of things. The older we get, the more toxic the environment, and that is now penetrating our brains: radiation, insecticides, pesticides, BPA, the amount of mercury in the environment. All contribute to Alzheimer's and dementia. The list goes on and on and on, but having a healthy brain to me is more important as a heart specialist than having our hearts working perfectly. I mean, brain function is vital.

Now, the good news is that there's a heart-brain internal body hotline—conversations that go back and forth between the two organs. And there are a lot of nutrients that help the heart that also help the brain.

SOMERS: Tell me what they are.

SINATRA: Omega-3 essential fatty acids do a lot for the brain and a lot for the heart. Certainly, coenzyme Q10 is vital for the heart and brain and is the magical spark plug. You mentioned this in the Facebook Live event we did together for drsinatra.com [https://www.facebook.com/SinatraMD/videos/1978557142195473/].

You offered a brilliant metaphor, comparing CoQ10 to a rip cord on a power motor. You are so right on! My own simple analogy is that CoQ10 acts as the spark plug that sets off the whole machinery driving ATP—adenosine triphosphate, the energy of life, or our *chi* energy—in a preferential direction.

So if CoQ10 is the spark plug of the ATP process, it makes sense that the more CoQ10 you have in your body, the easier it is to generate that spark to get your *chi* energy going or your life going. I've heard from so many people who say these exact words: "Doc, I got my life back!" When you keep hearing that from people, you realize that there's something special about CoQ10.

Not only is it like the spark plug that gets everything going, it's also a membrane stabilizer—a very important perk for each and every cell in the body to enhance the transportation of energy into and out of the cell.

If you are over the age of fifty, take 100 to 200 milligrams daily. CoQ10 is best taken after meals over the course of the day in divided doses. If you're compromised with heart disease and/or high blood pressure, then more, perhaps up to 200 to 300 milligrams daily. If you have severe heart failure and/or are waiting for a heart transplant, then 300 to 600 milligrams. It depends on how sick the person is; the sicker the person, the more CoQ10. But for most healthy people, 100 to 200 milligrams is usually quite adequate.

But the problem is, because of the toxic environment, our memories are failing, inflammation is skyrocketing, and blood sugar is off the charts sky high. It's an unholy trinity. People really need to focus on not only their heart health but their brain health at the same time.

The sine qua non of aging—or accelerated aging—is leaky membranes. You're familiar with leaky gut. So if you have leaky brain membranes, where vital nutrients can't get in and toxins can't get out, there's a problem. CoQ10 stabilizes those membranes. That stabilization translates into more efficient shuttling of nutrients into and waste products out of the cells.

I am also a firm believer in pure, uncontaminated squid oils for the brain, like **docosahexaenoic acid (DHA)** and **eicosapentaenoic acid (EPA)**. I must admit I do prefer DHA over EPA because the brain, the retina of the eye, and the heart rely so heavily on DHA. But joints are another thing. If you have arthritis in your fingers, then you need more EPA. So it makes sense to use more EPA in that situation.

SOMERS: I would say, not to do so is at your own peril. Imagine how stupid you will feel when you realize you've lost your brain health because of bad lifestyle and dietary habits. Same for heart health. Would you say we are actually in control of our health by the choices we make over a lifetime?

SINATRA: Absolutely. It's up to us to do right by ourselves. Choices matter, and over a lifetime there is a cumulative effect. There's so much you can do to preserve your precious organs and glands.

For example, take astaxanthin supplementation for eye health. We have been focused on heart and brain, but vision is so essential. There are over 1,400 published articles on astaxanthin research showing it not only helps the brain and the heart but also helps the eyes. This supplement is essential for the retinal health of women and men, and for women especially. It also improves the skin.

So to summarize, I would encourage such patients—and everyone—to get on the right track, look at their risk factor profile to target interventions, and live a healthy, "higher-vibration" lifestyle. We discuss details of health-promoting "high-vibrational" living at www.heart mdinstitute.com.

Also, emotions are another huge factor, as we mentioned earlier: internalized anger, chronic stress, and even depression. Frankly, I think these are significant risk factors for both men and women.

SOMERS: Internalized anger.

SINATRA: I remember when I was a young cardiologist in psychotherapy training, I had a cardiac patient who was an attorney. A sixteen-year-old boy had keyed his car. The boy had taken a nail and deliberately made a line in this guy's brand-new car. The poor guy was so outraged by the random injustice that he had a heart attack on the spot. Talk about a probable massive cortisol-clotting event!

SOMERS: That feels a little over the top. He blew out his heart from anger?

SINATRA: He was just so enraged. It was like he went on automatic! And another case just came as a flashback. I remember a forty-two-year-old heart attack victim who had brought his car to a mechanic. The mechanic changed the oil filter and drained the oil but forgot to put new oil back in the car. So the guy drives that car a mile away from the service station, and it seizes up, collapses, and stops running. Fuming internally, he aims the car off the road, takes a rope from his trunk, and starts pulling his car in the breakdown lane. Suddenly, he has a massive heart attack.

Hearing his story in the ER, I realized the heart attack was due to internalized anger coupled with intense physical exertion; "double handcuffs," I call it. Exertion while you are angry—especially isometrically straining upper body muscles that literally squeeze your coronary arteries on the inhale—is like the metaphor I gave of driving your car with one foot on the accelerator and one on the brake. In this case, my car metaphor is all too ironic and heartbreaking. I've written about this in *Heartbreak and Heart Disease.*

I also recall another patient who dissected his aorta in a fit of rage in his workplace. He had been ordered to unjustifiably fire his favorite employee and then do a big favor for the superior/boss who'd commanded him to do so. That gentleman had to repress his feelings—and his true self—and betray his heart to keep his job. But his heart told the truth. And it attacked him, metaphorically and literally speaking.

Over the years I've had my fair share of patients who have emotional outbursts and experience cardiac arrhythmias, heart attacks, aortic dissection, and sudden death. I've always felt that emotion is a pivotal factor when it comes to heart disease.

SOMERS: Now I understand your credentialed gift of being a psychotherapist as well as a cardiologist. Do you remember John Ritter? He died from an aortic tear.

SINATRA: Yes, he had aortic dissection.

SOMERS: I've always wondered, Wouldn't you feel anything prior? Doesn't the body "talk"? Aren't there any impending signs that something doesn't feel right?

SINATRA: In most cases, the body gets a warning, even in situations of sudden death, but there's so much denial of symptoms in both men and women. My own father died suddenly of an aortic dissection, right in my arms as I was arriving at home. No warning we recognized. He was a picture of robust health. Devastating.

SOMERS: Particularly men?

SINATRA: Yes, denial is particularly more of an issue for men—but women are not exempt. When it comes to emotion, denial is yet another very serious risk factor. If you deny your symptoms—"Oh, it's only indigestion"; "Oh, it's nothing"; "I just pulled a muscle"; and so on—you could end up in serious trouble.

That's why I always tell people, both men and women, **if you have even the slightest suspicion you may be having a heart attack, then chew on an aspirin, call 911, and get to an emergency room or walk-in medical center for evaluation.**

SOMERS: Do you think we should carry baby aspirin?

SINATRA: No, just be sure you have it in your medicine cabinet. And check the expiration date from time to time to be sure it's active.

SOMERS: Some theories say it should be taken daily as a prophylactic. Do you agree?

SINATRA: I don't believe healthy people need to be taking aspirin as a prophylactic. If you have a history of coronary disease—angina, heart attack, angioplasty, stent, or a coronary artery bypass—then for sure you want to take a baby aspirin a day. Baby aspirin is one-quarter the dose of adult aspirin. But remember, you know, nineteen to twenty thousand people a year die of GI bleeding. So when it comes to aspirin, it, too, has its own baggage in those without heart disease.

SOMERS: What causes thick blood?

SINATRA: Well, thick or sticky blood basically has to do with the toxic chemical and EMF environment. Also, high blood sugar, an indicator of diabetes, contributes to sticky blood. Other medical conditions, like polycythemia, excessive platelet production in the spleen, and more, can cause the blood to clump and clot. Other possible culprits are pharmaceuticals, like some oral contraceptives.

SOMERS: Let's talk about grounding and in particular the positive effects on the heart. You wrote a book with Clint Ober called *Earthing: The Most Important Health Discovery Ever!* You explain why we are increasingly unhealthy. You say it's the missing link.

SINATRA: Even though grounding is a new concept in the health care front, being in close contact to the earth is as old as time. Man used to live, congregate, dance, hunt, eat, birth, and sleep in direct concert with Mother Earth. Modern life and technology have just disconnected many of us, so to speak.

Let's talk about grounding relative to the heart. Each beat of the heart is triggered by an electrical signal from within the heart muscle. This is the activity recorded in twelve different planes by an electrocardiogram [ECG or EKG] in your doctor's office. Each signal is repeated nonstop over the course of a lifetime. The electrical impulse passes through cardiac circuitry, causing the heart to contract and push blood through the chambers and then out into your body. Really, it's a miraculous symphony when you think about it.

Heart disease can disrupt this normal electrical and pumping operation. Problems with the electrical system, known as arrhythmia, make it difficult for the heart to pump blood efficiently.

SOMERS: I would imagine as a cardiologist this would be of great interest.

SINATRA: I am a curious cardiologist, and I was attracted to energy and electrical concepts that might affect the electrically generated cardiovascular system in a beneficial way. When you think about it—our hearts, our muscles, our brains—we are basically electrical beings. There is an electrical charge on the surface of every cell in the body that we can measure!

I met Clint Ober at an electromedicine conference in San Diego. He had this device with him that tested arterial elasticity, so he checked mine. Basically, you want the arteries to be good and elastic. Rigid, constricted blood vessels are symptomatic of high blood pressure and arterial disease. My reading was good, but Clint's was enviously better. He was two years older than I, so I was impressed! He said he believed his results had to do with the fact that he grounded himself all the time; he slept grounded, and he walked barefoot whenever possible.

SOMERS: So are you sleeping grounded and walking barefoot?

SINATRA: Yes. I believe in it. There's just too much scientific evidence to support the power of grounding. My colleagues did research on grounding. They found that grounded rats had lower blood sugars than ungrounded rats. That got me thinking about when I used to walk almost a mile to school as a boy, wearing leather shoes, because that's all we had back then: leather, not man-made soles. Leather conducts the Mother Earth energy of 7.83 hertz (yes, the earth is electrical as well). So when the earth's healing energy is being conducted naturally and gently through your body, you are probably affecting blood sugar dynamics in the body. More research definitely needs to be done on this topic.

But remember the 1960s, Suzanne? The Adidas generation came on board—and the Nike generation—and essentially we switched from leather to rubber and neoprene soles. Seemed exotic and modern at the time. But rubber disconnects you from the earth.

What has happened to all of us is the perfect storm. We discontinued a lot of the physical education offerings in our schools. Then drive-throughs and fast-food diets emerged, with shakes, sweets, carbs, hamburger buns, fried foods, et cetera. So just connect the dots. Now we're walking on rubber. We are eating tons and tons of sugar and fried and highly processed foods. We microwave the nutrients out of our foods, which are already on the lower end due to soil depletion. We are exercising less. We bus or drive most of our kids to school. It's a perfect storm.

Remember when kids began getting bussed to school instead of walking? All of this combined has been, in large part, responsible for the diabetes epidemic. Basically, we started eating more sugar, became less physically active, and gained weight.

Americans are for the most part sugar-holics. In addition to the sugar we add ourselves, our food is already packed with hidden sugars and sugary preservatives like high-fructose corn syrup [HFCS]. You need a PhD to read many food labels. So diabetes has had an exponential rise in the last fifty years. Tragically, we have more diabetics on the planet than ever.

SOMERS: And what does diabetes have to do with grounding?

SINATRA: A lot. Diabetes accounts for about fourteen percent of all health care dollars spent in the United States.[4] The world is losing its battle against diabetes. In fact, the number of people estimated to be living with a predisposition to the disease has hit a new record of one hundred million in the US alone. The vast majority have type 2 diabetes, the kind linked to obesity and lack of exercise. And that epidemic is spreading as more people in the developing world adopt our Western, urban, ungrounded lifestyles. Earthing or grounding has been shown to attenuate blood sugar in the animal model.

Earthing helps to balance the serum cortisol and lowers blood pressure. We did that study with Dr. Howard Elkin in Los Angeles. All twelve people in that study were able to reduce their medications after grounding. Intuitively, I had always felt that earthing would lower blood pressure because it does everything else right for the body. Now we have proof. Grounding lowers what we refer to as sympathetic drive. The sympathetic nervous system [SNS] is the part of the autonomic nervous system [ANS] that sort of revs things up. The parasympathetic nervous system calms things down. When the ANS is in balance, all is well.

But the SNS can go into overdrive—as we see when people are worried, angry, sad, chronically distressed. We mentioned earlier the power of emotions in health, and because I've always believed that emotionality was the key to illness and sickness, it just makes sense that lowering SNS drive leads to optimum health.

If grounding while you sleep, for example, can lower your sympathetic activation by enhancing SNS discharge, it promotes balance of the ANS. It's like recharging your body for free. Maybe that's why all those early Native American warriors liked to sleep directly on the ground after a long day!

Whenever you take grounded energy into the body, you're regulating your hormones, thinning your blood, and regulating the autonomic nervous system. So that's what I mean when I say grounding does everything right for the physiology of the body, and it also alleviates pain as well.

SOMERS: What I like is that it is a drug-free treatment.

SINATRA: It's great. We've heard so many stories from people. Grounding improves functionality. Whenever and wherever I can, I walk barefoot.

As a cardiologist, grounding offers a holy trinity: the perfect trifecta! When you connect to the earth, you lower blood pressure, thin the blood, and improve heart rate variability [HRV is another measure of a healthy heart]—all at the same time. That's my trifecta pick for cardiovascular health. That's what earthing/grounding does!

When early man was walking barefoot, his advantage was his connection to the earth. Humans didn't live as long back then as we do now. They were always foraging for food and had many predators. But now there are invisible, destructive waves in the environment, and because we are disconnected from the earth by walking on rubber footwear that *disconnects* us, we are getting more and more sick as a population. That's why diabetes has had this exponential rise. And more and more people are now becoming hypertensive and depressed, as well as battling cancer.

SOMERS: It seems clear when you connect the dots.

SINATRA: Instead of extending the life of mankind, this perfect storm of technology, EMFs, and pharmaceutical drugs may have the potential to shorten the life of mankind. Short term, and sadly, it's already insidiously causing deterioration of our hearts, brains, and reproductive systems. There's no question about that.

And by the way, when it comes to electromagnetic fields, Wi-Fi, computers, cordless phones, cellular phones, baby monitors, 5G towers—this invisible soup we're living in—the three systems most vulnerable are the heart, the brain, and the reproductive systems. A trinity again! I am deeply concerned that modern man is being knocked out by our own sophisticated technology.

It's tragic; we need our hearts, we need our brains, and we need to propagate for continuation of the next generation and the next. So sad if the three most specialized organ systems are compromised by modern man's technology.

SOMERS: Ever since I started sleeping on a grounding sheet, taking Carditone supplementation, and utilizing EECP, I sleep better, more soundly, no more backaches, and best of all, my blood pressure is normalized.

SINATRA: There are so many benefits of sleeping grounded. In another experiment with nonmedicated subjects, grounding in a single night resulted in significant positive changes in the concentration of minerals and electrolytes in blood serum: iron, ionized calcium, inorganic phosphorus, sodium, potassium, and magnesium.

The grounding perks are also profound for pain and stress, muscle soreness, lowered inflammation and immune response, and stress reduction. The implications for boosting healthy aging are fantastic.

You can easily connect to the earth's healing frequency by simply removing your shoes and socks and walking barefoot on grass, sand, soil, or concrete (asphalt is nonconductive). This is especially important for those living or working in high-rise buildings, many stories up, away from any contact with the earth. When you have the body's ground substance reservoirs saturated with electrons, you can help prevent collateral damage in healthy tissues when grounded. And if the ground surface is wet, even better conduction!

SOMERS: So where does my reader purchase a grounding sheet, pads, patches?

SINATRA: You can resource www.grounded.com or www.earthing.net.

SOMERS: What do you listen for in your body to predict heart attacks?

SINATRA: Women and men are different when it comes to heart disease, especially when it comes to symptoms. One sign I worry about in both women and men—but more in women than men—is dreadful fatigue. Dreadful or profound fatigue where a woman says, "Oh, my gosh, I'm totally exhausted" should never be taken lightly.

Another thing in women is this atypical presentation of jaw pain, neck discomfort. One woman was waiting to see an oral surgeon in our ER. He was not able to come for a few hours. But the patient looked so dreadful that one of our astute nurses made the independent call to do an electrocardiogram. The EKG showed it all: she was having a heart attack. The ER called me immediately. Imagine, her only symptom had been jaw pain.

So "connecting the dots," as you say, between emotions and physical health is very important to mind-body interventions of healing. It is key.

SOMERS: Well, I'm grateful you're on the planet. Thank you for this. Always a pleasure, and . . . because you and I were born a few hours apart on the same day, same year, seventy-three years ago, and that we have each managed to keep ourselves in peak health, I believe we are both going to be around for a long time, so let's celebrate and have a great one hundredth birthday together.

SINATRA: You've got a deal, Suzanne!

CHAPTER 14

ENHANCED EXTERNAL COUNTERPULSATION (EECP)

Looking for an alternative to blood pressure meds and a slew of pharmaceuticals, including dangerous statins? Wait until you read about **enhanced external counterpulsation (EECP)**. This is a nondrug protocol and fast acting. I have seen EECP treatments literally turn people's health around, including mine. I go for treatments regularly to stay in tip-top shape and always will.

EECP enhances blood circulation to the heart and collateral blood flow. People who exercise increase their collateral blood flow. EECP does the same thing but works faster than exercise, so it builds collaterals, increases blood flow to the heart, and decreases the stress on the heart muscle so the heart can pump less vigorously to reduce stress, which is why the blood pressure comes down.

The patient lies on the table and is wrapped in strategically placed blood pressure cuffs. The generator does the inflation and deflation that's underneath. Then the EKG tracks your heart rhythm. During the coronary cardiac cycle, when the arteries dilate, is when blood is propelled into your heart. It's miraculous. Over a period of several weeks, the heart actually makes new blood vessels (angiogenesis), and no drugs are necessary.

How incredible, to regrow new arteries.

No one is ever too old or too frail to be able to withstand the EECP. It actually dilates the vessels, increases circulation, and improves the efficiency of the heart with less effort; ultimately, it decreases blood pressure. It also helps with kidney flow, brain flow, even erectile dysfunction (ED). These are all conditions due to impaired blood flow. I have never been more impressed with a nondrug protocol and have seen it literally perform miracles.

EECP can be used for *all* cardiovascular disease and is becoming a means of prevention and reversal of cardiovascular disease to treat stroke, diabetes, congestive heart failure, hypertension, and renal (kidney) failure as an effective therapy of any cardiovascular disease without side effects or the need for medications. It is also effective for stimulating intestinal tissue, as I recently discovered with great results.

A friend with renal failure who was waiting for a kidney transplant took thirty-five sessions of EECP, flooding his kidneys and arteries with blood pumped from his lower extremities. He regained complete usage of his kidneys and is now healthy. In the beginning, I doubted he would live.

I have witnessed such amazing results with a dear friend of mine. He'd had such high blood pressure that he'd had to curtail all his activities—no more golf, no more tennis—no energy, surely on a fast track to something dark. He had spent two years off and on with EECP treatments. Today he is eighty-nine years young, has energy, plays two hours of tennis daily, loves golf, loves women, and is living a normal and energetic life without drugs.

These are typical of the results you can expect from EECP.

HOW EECP WORKS

EECP improves the flow of blood to the heart, allowing the body to naturally form new small blood vessels called *collaterals*. These collaterals create a natural bypass around blocked arteries. EECP works by squeezing blood from the legs upward to the heart while the heart is at rest. You lie on a padded therapy table outfitted with large blood pressure measurement–like cuffs that wrap around your legs and buttocks. The cuffs inflate and deflate at specific times between your heartbeats; an electrocardiogram (ECG) is used to set the timing of the inflation/

deflation intervals. The painless compression caused by the inflation of the cuffs improves circulation throughout the body.

EECP stands for "enhanced external counterpulsation." It is a safe, noninvasive, nonmedication therapy. It is FDA cleared and Medicare approved for those suffering from ischemic heart diseases such as angina and heart failure when the client's angina diagnosis is class III or IV, whereby the client has chest pain upon minimal exertion, is considered inoperable, and is deemed to be in the end stage of cardiovascular disease.

EECP is available in many communities around the country. I suggest you google it to see if it exists in your area. If not, I highly recommend taking a trip to the nearest place to experience the natural healing properties of EECP.

This is a rather typical testimonial for EECP treatment. I cannot rave enough about this protocol. Read what this man has to say.

My name's Errol Abramson. I'm from Vancouver, British Columbia. I'm a businessman. In 2015, I was diagnosed with congestive heart failure and scheduled for open heart surgery. Because my heart function was so minimal at 17 percent, I was not a candidate for the surgery. They didn't feel I would survive the surgery. So I was sent home basically to die.

I found that there was an alternative for open heart surgery, which was EECP. I came down. I had the sessions that were recommended to me. And I went back and when I had my echo scan in Vancouver, my heart had returned to normal function and I did not need surgery.

When I returned with my results, nobody was excited about learning more about EECP. Everybody seemed to be happy with the results I got and nobody was interested in how I got them. And it's very, very interesting to me where there is so much research on EECP and so little used when it does so much good for so many people. It just seems to be that physicians are only interested in that open-heart surgery.

The interesting thing at the clinic is they take a holistic ap-

proach: diet and nutrition, exercise plus the EECP. Anybody that follows their program is going to get results and be happy. The program's stellar. The results I couldn't be happier with.

When I was diagnosed, I needed two people to help me with medications. I was taking so many. I mean there were probably twenty medications. Interestingly enough, I was able to reduce my medications to zero. I take no heart medications whatsoever now. I had edema. And my edema reduced and my weight reduced. And also, I had diabetic tendencies: high blood sugar, which regulated. My blood sugars are still normal with no medication.

CHAPTER 15

THE HEART AND THE JAW

The joints in your upper neck generate the electrical
power that your brain needs for regulating your heart
and blood pressure, balancing immune response and
hormones, controlling your digestion and sleep, and
coordinating injury repair.

—Dr. Roger Sperry

Have you ever thought the *jaw* could be a factor in heart disease and stroke?

Do you clench your teeth at night? Do you grind your teeth? Do you snore? Do you have sleep apnea? Did you ever have a head or neck injury? Did you get rammed in football as a kid, or did you fall off the monkey bars? Do you experience balance or dizziness episodes? Do you have trouble sleeping? What about atrial fibrillation? How about migraines or headaches? Do you have high blood pressure? Do you live a high-stress lifestyle that could make your jaw tense at night? These seemingly simple and benign issues might be your downfall.

All these issues and more could be your setup for sudden heart attack syndrome or stroke.

How many times have we had friends or relatives drop dead, out of the blue, and then people say, "But he was so healthy!" or "She exercised every day" or "She [or he] ate perfectly."

Listen to what jaw specialist Dr. Leonard Feld has to say. It's a little-known syndrome, and he is one of a very few dentists in the United States and maybe the world who has chosen to specialize in jaw alignment. Because of jaw specialists like Dr. Feld, many NFL and NBA players wear jaw protection appliances during games to protect themselves from misalignment, balance, and strength issues as well as concussions.

This is an area no one has paid attention to until now; read and be fascinated.

Interview with
DR. LEONARD FELD

SOMERS: Thank you for your time, Dr. Feld. I wanted my readership to know why I would put a section in this book about the jaw, as in what does the jaw have to do with going forward in aging this new way?

I really believe God sent me to you, Dr. Feld, because my husband was in such dire straits due to a horrible childhood injury that reared its ugly head decades later. I am not a doctor. I want you to explain to me what you saw when Alan walked into your office that day and what the potential ramifications could have been for him had we not caught it at that time.

FELD: Well, when you, Suzanne, and Alan came to my office, I was taken by surprise at Alan's condition, but the physician that referred you [Dr. Daniel Johnson of Palm Desert, California] was very cognizant of my work and had recognized that many of his patients were suffering from misalignment without realizing it was at the base of their problems. Dr. Johnson examined Alan because sitting in his office, Alan was experiencing severe facial spasms and tics that had become uncontrollable. Upon examination, with his shirt removed it was clear he was, for lack of a better word, "crooked." His shoulders sloped down slightly lower on one side, indicating misalignment, and was most likely causing these vulnerable physical and bodily problems.

Looking at Alan, I saw he was in severe trouble. I had worked with a lot of motor movement disorder patients and worked with their comorbid symptoms. A lot of them have other symptoms besides the motor movement; they have headaches, backaches, neckaches, shoulder pain, migraine headaches, balance issues. But Alan had none of those things; what he had was blepharospasm, uncontrollable blinking of the eye, but his was also not characteristic with usual blepharospasm because his eyes would close and stay closed, and that was my biggest concern. You, Suzanne, had realized Alan could no longer drive as a result. Can't drive if your eyes are closed. It's called functional blindness in the fact that he's not blind, but if your eyes are closed, you can't see.

I had relieved certain motor movement disorders by accident in other patients, not knowing the true connection, because it seemed all these corrections that are done with the jaw are hard to trace and believe.

In the brain, there are twelve cranial nerves, and one hundred percent of the energy of the brain is in those twelve nerves. The trigeminal nerve occupies about thirty-four percent of the energy. It's a big nerve, and it has a lot of functions: it works on the scalp, the muscles, and the ears [external auditory meatus]; it controls the nose, paranasal sinuses, and other things. This nerve also meets with the reticular formation of the brain stem. It then meets with three other nerves: the vagus nerve, the hypoglossal, and the facial. Those four nerves occupy more than fifty percent of the brain's activity. So there's a lot goin' on.

When he came in, I thought I could help him with the blinking but certainly not with the closed eyes.

SOMERS: Alan carries the HLA gene, which makes him more susceptible to chemicals of all kinds, and his lab tests showed that he was severely toxic as a result.

> It is important to note that we are all under a massive environmental assault, perhaps more than ever before. We will all go down if we do nothing about it, but those who carry the HLA gene, identified by Dr. Ritchie Shoemaker, and are susceptible to things like chemicals, will go down faster unless their condition is corrected.

So we were going to Dr. Johnson for chelation [intravenous blood cleaning] because I kept thinking, If we chelate him and get the chemicals out of his system, maybe that would help lower his toxic burden. Alan is like the canary in the coal mine; he reacts first.

That fateful day in Dr. Johnson's office was profound for me. After he examined Alan, he said, "I just went to a lecture at the alternative doctors' conference in Las Vegas to listen to Dr. Leonard Feld, jaw specialist. I had no interest in the jaw, but I had an hour to kill, so I went in and listened to Dr. Feld, and I was blown away. I had never considered it, and it turns out he is a few blocks down the street." This is where I say God intervened, because that day was the worst day of Alan's condition, and when we got to your office, it was so bad, it was like he was in lockjaw. His eyes were closed, and his mouth kept opening uncontrollably, and I started to cry, and you, Dr. Feld, touched my shoulder and looked into my eyes and said compassionately, "I can fix it"—and I believed you. We had been everywhere, all over the United States, for the previous five years, going from one expert to the next, and nobody could figure it out.

FELD: I don't know why, but I felt, I don't know what to call it, maybe it's your ambience or your energy that comes with you, but I felt warm and drawn to both you and Alan, and I said to myself, "I gotta help, I gotta help 'em. I don't know what I gotta do, but I gotta help 'em."

SOMERS: Well, it was that moment that you and I locked eyes that I believed you could do this, and then you went on to the process of educating me, us, about the role the jaw plays in health and, as I would later come to understand, heart health.

I told Dr. Feld that Alan was hung as a child by horrible bullies and left to die hanging in an abandoned barn at eight years old, and most likely, that is how his cranium got moved to the left of his neck.

FELD: Well, I'm convinced of that. There's no doubt in my mind that was major trauma, and after that maybe other traumas, but the fact that all these doctors he had gone to never saw that he had a broken neck surprises me.

SOMERS: He had had MRIs, brain scans, brain SPECTs. That first day, you took all those X-rays of his head, neck, and cranium, and you saw the issue right then. You told me about the vagus nerve, the trigeminal nerve, and the central nervous system and that if the jaw is misaligned, there are serious consequences. Suddenly I realized this is what could be wrong with so many people and why there are so many unexplained heart attacks. That vertigo is something to be very concerned about. I'd like you to talk in that arena.

FELD: Well, a lot of it is misunderstood. I have clinical experience, and the papers I've written are based on other researchers and what has been found. As a clinician I'm in the trenches. I work with patients and keep trying things based on research. I was fortunate to do a residency with Dr. Brendan Stack, who taught me a lot about the brain. Understanding the brain is something that when I studied in dental school I said to myself at that time, "Boy, I'm glad I'm through with this course, because I ain't never gonna do this again."

SOMERS: Why?

FELD: Because there were no answers, just a lot of questions. When Alan came in, I immediately thought about all the nerves in the neck that control muscles and actions. There's fiber stimulation, which causes chronic agitation within. Then you have a crossover of two nerves that are next to each other, the vagus nerve and the trigeminal nerve, and they can affect one another. So—follow me here—there's a bundle of about four millimeters of nerves for the facial, the hypoglossal, the vagus, and the trigeminal nerves that all come together in the neuroelements of the reticular formation, causing reflex actions within the spinal cord, an automatic thing, like knee jerk, so when people are looking for causes for vertigo, for instance, they look inside the ear.

But that's not where the problem is. The auriculotemporal nerve is a branch of the trigeminal nerve that hooks into the jaw, and if the jaw is in the wrong place, then it is misaligned and causes problems, often severe.

A crooked, misaligned jaw could be due to whiplash from a car accident or a blow to the head. Alan had a pretty big blow to his head being hung by the neck, and that's how you displace that ligament structure, because now the jaw is kind of loose, and once you stretch a ligament it doesn't go back to its original tension. It's kind of like a rubber band being out in the sun; it loses its elasticity. With Alan's blinking, he didn't have inappropriate outbursts like some of my patients, so I knew he had none of the signs of Tourette's, and he really had none of the signs of Parkinson's.

SOMERS: Although, by the way, Alan had been diagnosed twice by two other doctors with Parkinson's. I wouldn't accept it. I grabbed him, and we left those offices. I said, "He does not!"

FELD: Well, the only thing that he had that might resemble Parkinson's was his twitching, but he had no bodily shakes and no twitching of his body. He had perfect gait, he could walk fine, he was very coherent, and of course, he's brilliant.

SOMERS: Correct me if I'm wrong, but what I'm understanding is: The central nervous system, along with the vagus nerve and the trigeminal nerve, run from the heart to the brain, behind the jaw. So if the cranium has been pushed to the side of the neck axis from injury and now the jaw is out of line and it's resting on these nerves and arteries, blood vessels, like a kink in a hose, stopping blood flow to some degree, or maybe all the way, this is the pathway to how you get the unexplained heart attacks and stroke?

FELD: That's what we think. There are branches of the carotid artery, which gives oxygen to the brain. If there is a stop in that flow, you are in trouble. If the jaw is misaligned and interfering, you've got trouble.

SOMERS: So if that's the pathway, then that's why these unexplained heart attacks occur—as a result of jaw misalignment?

FELD: Yes, we do know that when you get less blood supply to the brain, you are putting yourself in jeopardy, and we know that's not a good thing. We do know that the brain needs oxygen and blood flow. So if something is obstructing the major arteries that supply circulation to the brain whose function is to provide oxygen to the brain, and you have a condition that creates a kind of "foot stepping on the pathway," you have a dangerous situation.

SOMERS: It's like a kink in the hose.

FELD: Yes, another example: Imagine you're watering the lawn, and your son comes up and he drives over the hose, and the water stops. So you go over to the hose and turn the valve up to get more water out. Same thing with the heart: the heart has to pump harder to get the same amount of oxygen and blood flow through the blood vessels [arteries] to service and support the nerves, so does that increase blood pressure? Yes, people that have jaw misalignment have higher blood pressure and are at risk for heart attack because the heart is trying to push the blood to the brain because the brain's saying "I need more."

This condition is physical. What we're talking about is not a disease, it's not an infection, it's a structural thing that happens when the jaw is out of place. It's now resting somewhere where it shouldn't rest.

This misalignment mechanism is like having a door jam, and the hinge is off, so it doesn't close properly; its main function is impaired. But the jaw is different; it functions in three dimensions. For example: a door hinge is just one dimension, a knee is one dimension, but the jaw moves on all three planes, so people with jaw issues unconsciously compensate and get around their jaw damage by moving their jaw around to try and get it in the right place.

SOMERS: So we compensate for jaw misalignment, just keep adjusting until it feels comfortable, right?

FELD: Yes, when a person gets a clicking or popping noise in their jaw, they unconsciously adjust, but it really has to do with the little "pillow" that sits between the jawbone and the skull. When cartilage or that "pillow" is out of place and not resting in the right place, the jaw goes backward and hits these vessels and nerves.

SOMERS: And that's the danger: stopping the blood flow, that "kink in the hose," putting you in jeopardy because the jaw goes backward and rests on the nerves, stopping blood flow. This is brilliant information. It makes perfect sense.

I had never noticed that Alan's skeletal configuration was crooked. Even knowing it now, without his shirt on, I can barely tell that one shoulder is a little lower than the other, which says to me it's probably been that way all his life and he's been compensating. Unbelievably, it reared its ugly head sixty years later.

Then there's vertigo. I have a friend, a big guy weighs 250 pounds, he was a football player in high school and loved ramming and body slamming into other guys, just loved rough sports, as do so many guys, they are all testosterone. So here he is, sixty years later, with vertigo, this big guy, 250 pounds, falls down in the supermarket from dizziness. Well, of course, his doctor puts him on a bunch of pills, which makes him even dizzier.

FELD: Well, yeah, it's the jaw, it's about hits to the head and neck and concussions he has had. If you want to knock someone out, watch fighters fight. Do they hit 'em in the butt? Do they hit on the shoulder? Do they hit 'em on the head? Or do they hit 'em on the jaw? The nerves that are attached to the head of the jaw with the blood vessels go directly to the brain, and when they are jammed the brain is short-circuited, like a fuse blowout or a dead battery: "Lights out."

SOMERS: So why do fighters go for the jaw?

FELD: They want to hit 'em on the jaw, because it's the most serious blow. Knocks them out most often. Riding a bike and falling, being hit by a snowball, whiplash equals concussion.

SOMERS: Interesting. I remember being with Muhammad Ali a number of years ago at a Vegas event. He was clearly on the downside of his life. He had Parkinson's, and because of it he had a lot of shaking in the face, eye twitching, and a general slowness, clearly from years of boxing and all those hits to the head, neck, and jaw, right?

FELD: Well, it has to be. You just mentioned it, eye twitching, a lot of the effects of these things, have multiple side effects and multiple neurological issues happening.

The vagus nerve is a crucial nerve with a lot of functions, including even effects on the gut. If the vagus nerve is associated with a nerve that's twitching, that means it's sending out the wrong signals, and suddenly the person has issues like restless leg syndrome or they ache all over. Well, why do they ache all over? I don't want to get too technical, but we do know when you injure your body—for instance, if you sprain an ankle—the body sends out fluid to encapsulate that area so you won't injure it anymore. It's all done automatically; the answer is not from the pharmacy with drugs. Our body knows how to take care of itself; we wrap an injury for a football or basketball player right away with Ace bandages and put them on ice, right? That keeps it from swelling because the flow of the protective fluid can cause as much damage as the actual injury. They didn't have Ace bandages or ice fifty thousand years ago, right? So we have developed built-in protective mechanisms; that's part of our evolution.

SOMERS: And think about this: most all kids have fallen off the monkey bars growing up. I did. I also fell out of the car as a kid and got a concussion. So now, hmmm . . . I have had TMJ all my adult life. Is that why? Who knows? I also had a lot of fear as a kid, and I probably clenched my teeth all night long.

Maybe our individual histories of different falls, hits, concussions, accidents, et cetera result in chronic misalignment issues for most of us without realizing it. That means that most all of us are at risk.

The biggest killer of people in our country is heart attacks. I realize there are many reasons—genetics, diet, lifestyle, stress—but the other unknown is the jaw and the little-known and -understood role it plays in blood and air flow. Connect the dots.

FELD: Yes, also think about car accidents—rear-end collisions—and motorcycle accidents as other possibilities for misalignment.

SOMERS: So why are doctors slow to recognize the importance of the jaw relative to heart attacks and stroke? Seems to me jaw examination and taking images are crucial.

When I realize how close Alan was to becoming a victim of an unexplained heart attack, I get shivers down my spine. That day—that fateful day when his eyes slammed shut and his mouth wouldn't close—was the day it could have been his end. Again, I believe God directed us to you and Dr. Johnson. Hopefully this interview will start the necessary change. In all my years of going to the doctor, no one has ever asked me about accidents.

FELD: I believe it should be part of any exam. The medical community takes care of the medical, and the dental takes care of the dental, but there's a crossover; what Alan had could have been construed as a medical problem, and in that context the last thing that would be thought of is bringing in a dentist, yet here is a situation of a medical problem whose solution turned out to be dental/orthopedic.

SOMERS: I believe we, the patients, need to take injuries more seriously and demand jaw examinations as part of our medicals to eliminate the potential of a sudden heart attack from a jaw that has been pushed back compromising the blood flow to the brain.

FELD: Yes. A broken jaw or torn muscles and ligaments need to be thought of on a deeper level. People and doctors need to look at it as a sprained jaw and that it's serious.

It's normal to just chew, but if your bite is not right, it can lead to abnormal tension in these muscles, it can cause tension headaches when the bite is not in the correct position. The trigeminal nerve, which is attached to the back of the jaw, becomes impaired. Brain function activities make up what has been suggested to be a trigeminovascular reflex responsible for migraine pain. Even though you may be feeling your headaches in your sinuses, face, or on top of your head doesn't mean that is where the cause of the problem is located. Many times, when a person has a pinched nerve in their back, they will feel a pain in their leg.

With a jaw that pops, the cartilage slowly wears out and there's grinding and louder popping. Then all of a sudden the popping, grinding stops.

SOMERS: Why?

FELD: Because you've gone through the cartilage. You've worn it out. And now you're bone on bone. It starts impinging on nerves, and you get headaches, migraines. So how does this happen? Because the jaw is out of alignment, and that affects blood flow to the brain.

SOMERS: Let's talk about atrial fibrillation of the heart. So many of my friends suffer from this and often end up in the hospital. How serious is it, and what does this have to do with misalignment?

FELD: Atrial fibrillation, or afib, is a heart rhythm disorder in which the upper heart chambers contract irregularly. Afib ups a person's risk of stroke by a factor of five. Research links afib to sleep apnea, and there is a strong correlation between obstructive [jaw in the way] sleep apnea, where breathing stops while you are sleeping, and atrial fibrillation as leading causes of stroke. The best preventative treatment is to maintain an open airway during sleep.

SOMERS: OSA [obstructive sleep apnea] is noted in forty-nine percent of sleep apnea patients and thirty percent of cardiovascular patients. Why don't people know this? Why are you the only one putting this out there? Is that why so many people are sleeping with those horrible CPAP machines?

FELD: Yes, but in my practice, I make a customized dental appliance like I made for Alan that pushes the jaw forward during the night, prevents snoring, opens the airways, allowing for oxygenation, and, if all goes well, fixes the problem.

SOMERS: The solution you found for Alan was a customized dental appliance to do exactly that. His jaw has become relaxed and calmed down in the two years he has been wearing his appliance. It's been a miracle. He still needs to have Botox injections to calm the nerves that have been damaged, but the jaw is working again and both of us are so grateful. He will wear this appliance forever or until you tell him he can stop.

FELD: It's all about the custom appliance. That's what I do. When someone comes in who grinds their teeth at night or snores badly or stops breathing intermittently or has migraine headaches or dizziness or vertigo, realigning the jaw with a custom appliance is usually the anti-dote.

SOMERS: Well, you have two very happy patients in us.

FELD: Yes, the appliance moves the jaw forward a little bit, takes the tension off the nerves, and the blood flow goes back to normal, the headache disappears. Ninety percent of all headaches are vascular in nature. So all I do is put the blood flow back. It's about getting air and promoting realignment.

The mouthpieces we make for the football players and the basketball players are nothing more than to keep the jaw forward, so they can breathe through their nose.

SOMERS: With Alan, you gave him the appliance because his jaw had moved so far back to such a dangerous place, it was starting to seriously affect the quality of his life. I strongly feel we dodged a bullet, that bullet being a heart attack. You have been moving his jaw forward for the last two years, and I have to say for the reading audience, my husband, who, if we went in on a scale of one to ten—ten being the worst, one being the best—he was at ten. He is now somewhere between one and two. He's able to drive from time to time without any effort. It depends on his stress level. If he has a lot of stress, the central nervous system gets activated. We try to live a very calm life. We are very happy, so we rarely have a cross word with each other. I believe our calm, happy lives that are low stress by design are a big part of his recovery. He wears the appliance religiously, and now we have our life back and we thank you.

FELD: No, thank you, thank you.

PART V

CUTTING-EDGE ADVANCES IN ANTIAGING

CHAPTER 16

NAD+ AND SENOLYTICS

The only constant is change. Learn to love it. As the rate of change accelerates, the result will appear chaotic to the uninitiated. But there is elegant order in chaos. Few so far have learned to recognize and profit from it. This is where the future lies.
—Frank Ogden

I've been waiting to get you to this part of the book. This is the new stuff, the exciting new approach on how to reverse aging naturally. I wanted to prepare you first. So far you are well immersed in the new way to age, but in this part, we move into the mind-blowing new protocols. I can't wait for you to read this chapter with Bill Faloon and also Dr. Galitzer's chapter on energy medicine. Hang on to your hats. This is going to be a great ride.

My friend Bill Faloon has been in the trenches from the start. He is a relentless maverick who doesn't give up, and lucky for us, we are the beneficiaries. I met Bill twenty years ago after a cold call, wanting to speak with him about health and, in particular at that time, bioidentical hormone replacement therapy. I was intrigued by the concept of age reversal or aging "slowdown" that people like myself were experiencing with natural bioidentical hormone replacement therapy.

We clicked and have been friends ever since. It is my great fortune that members of Life Extension's scientific staff have reviewed this book and most of my books from the past. So far, I have never been challenged. He is the founder and editor of *Life Extension* magazine. It was Bill and his group that brought the term *antiaging* to the forefront. He is a dedicated researcher and critical thinker and as of late is focused on longevity, longer life, even indefinite life. He never stops searching. He continually incorporates different interventions into his life extension regimen. Most recently he underwent a series of infusions of a natural cofactor called **nicotinamide adenine dinucleotide (NAD+)**, which David Sinclair, codirector of the Paul F. Glenn Center for the Biology of Aging at Harvard Medical School, says is **"the closest we've gotten to a fountain of youth."** NAD+ helps repair cellular DNA, which is critical for us to remain alive.

Our bodies require NAD+, but its levels decline as we age past forty. When NAD+ levels are boosted in old mice, they look and act younger and live longer.

I will turn seventy-four this year, and I am fascinated by the table on this page showing that the life expectancy when I was born was only around sixty-two years. And the final years of life were often burdened by chronic disease.

AVERAGE AMERICAN LIFE SPAN

Year of Birth	Life Expectancy
1770–1865	A meager 35 years
1866–1900	Gradual increase to 47 years
1900–1940	Gradual increase to 55 years
1940–1960	Gradual increase to 62 years
1960–1980	Gradual increase to 67 years
1980–2000	Gradual increase to 73 years
2000–2012	Gradual increase to 76 years
2012–2015	Gradual increase to 78 years

I credit my being alive and well today to healthy lifestyle practices, bioidentical hormones, dietary supplements, and careful blood testing to ensure that my body stays fine-tuned. In other words, I work at living longer and healthier.

I look at others who also have taken care of themselves who, like me, continue to be mentally and physically active and are often able to sustain their careers. I feel gratified that I chose to go this route. There are, however, upper limits as to how long we can depend on healthy lifestyle choices to keep us youthful. In his interview, Bill Faloon is confident that the medical advances his organization long ago advocated have added ten to fifteen years of healthy longevity to those who have adhered to them.

Imagine: ten to fifteen extra years with great health and quality of life plus the added gift of acquired wisdom that comes only with having lived long enough. Suddenly the concepts of matriarch and patriarch are viable again: elders of the tribe who are cool and hip, healthy and young, both inside and outside.

Today, published scientific studies with lab animals show substantial rejuvenation in response to therapies that are available to people who are turned on by the idea of living longer (much longer) with quality of life, not frail and decrepit.

Maybe the idea of living longer is not your goal but rather living a life rarely experienced today of health, quality, and energy until the end. There are new breakthroughs that will enable you to access this "new way."

I mentioned the remarkable benefits of NAD+ enabling DNA repair, but Bill will go into greater depth in my interview with him later in this chapter. NAD+ will keep your cells healthy. This is significant because our bodies are made up of communicating cells (approximately 37 trillion of them), so caring for the cells is one of the new advances.

If you have healthy young cells, you have
a healthy young body.

The new therapies can be combined in many ways, but the most logical first therapy is to take compounds that selectively remove senescent or "broken" cells from your aging body.

This chapter not only describes the senile cell–removing compounds but explains how to use them. The idea of *removing broken cells* from the body to make it more youthful might not make sense at first; rather, you might think that *adding good cells* would be a better approach. But . . . **senescent ("broken") cells are highly toxic!**

They are often called "zombie cells" because they spew out harmful pro-aging factors. More disturbingly, they act like a contagion throughout our tissues, spreading toxic factors that injure healthy cells. The evidence in laboratory animals, as well as in some initial human research, has shown powerful and consistent health benefits in response to clearance of senescent cells.

These scientific discoveries are the future of medicine, and they are increasingly being recognized by the medical establishment. Here are quotes from two recent publications in *The Journal of the American Medical Association*:

Many human pathologic conditions are associated with the presence of senescent cells. Interventions aimed at eliminating those senescent cells, commonly called senolytic, have also been shown to improve health and extend life in various mouse disease models.[1]

If senolytics are shown to be safe and effective in humans, they could transform care of older adults and patients with multiple chronic diseases.[2]

But it took a 2018 Mayo Clinic report about a study on mice to really open the world's eyes to the potential power of senolytics to *reverse* age-related afflictions in humans. The mice that underwent treatment to have senescent cells selectively removed not only appeared outwardly younger and healthier, but they also lived 36 percent longer than the mice that did not have senescent cells removed.[3]

This is not the first study showing rejuvenation effects. What makes it exceptional is the meticulous way in which it was conducted. An as-yet-unpublished clinical study in osteoarthritis patients showed that when the same senescent cell–removing compounds were tested in a small group of people with severe osteoarthritis, 82 percent had significant relief of pain and improved joint mobility that lasted for at least six months. The study participants want to repeat the study to make their chronic pain disappear again. This certainly seems like a better and safer way to deal with chronic pain rather than prescribing opioid drugs, which has created the opioid crisis that plagues our country and so many other countries around the world. Removal of senescent cells is a critical first step to counteracting the many causes of degenerative aging. But there are other cutting-edge treatments now available to systemically reverse aging.

In January 2019, the results of a small clinical trial using senolytics on people were published by researchers at the Mayo Clinic, Wake Forest, and University of Texas Health Center. They demonstrated safety and partial efficacy against a fatal disease called *pulmonary fibrosis*. This lung disease causes victims to slowly suffocate to death as dysfunctional senescent cells accumulate in the lungs and damage nearby healthy cells.[4]

In a recent study, three pulmonary fibrosis patients treated with senolytics in a clinical trial showed marked improvements, such as being able to walk across a room without wearing an oxygen mask. The trial was to measure the effects of senolytics in osteoarthrosis patients. The three pulmonary fibrosis patients were part of this senolytic study helping to systematically rejuvenate older people. This includes removing senescent ("broken") cells from aging bodies and restoring youthful levels of NAD+, a compound needed to sustain life.

The Age Reversal Network has funded a study to review the compounds that prompt cells to naturally remove waste products that accumulate inside our cells as we age. The name of this cell-cleansing process is **autophagy**, and it can now be naturally "turned on" to remove cellular debris that clogs up critical cellular functions, including natural removal of fat stores. I look at it as similar to cleaning out all the old and broken pipes in your home. Many of us have done that, and afterward the plumbing works like new again; same with our cells.

Interview with

BILL FALOON

SOMERS: Once again, thanks, Bill, for giving me your time. You and your foundation, Life Extension, have been a tremendous source of information and education for me and my readers over the decades. In fact, you actually give away copies of your magazine, a fact that has made my readers very happy.

You began this journey forty-two years ago with the concept of radically extending healthy human life spans. You were a mere twenty-two years old; what on earth got you started at such a young age?

FALOON: There were a number of research projects I felt needed my attention back then. Most shocking were studies published in medical journals that were overlooked by physicians. This meant that proven ways to prevent and treat diseases were being denied to Americans. I needed to get this information out. Most people today forget that in the early 1970s, the medical establishment and FDA claimed that there was no relationship between the types of foods people ate and their risk of heart disease, cancer, and dementia. Yet an abundance of data revealed that groups of people who followed healthy dietary patterns added about seven years to their average life span, and these were often healthy years.

SOMERS: I remember when you were attacked for that. We now know these are the foods that increase heart attack and cancer risk. What was the agenda?

FALOON: The sugar industry led the charge. The sugar industry essentially paid off some prominent scientists to claim sugar was perfectly safe to ingest. This was verified in articles published in 2016 by the American Medical Association. We had been exposing these kinds of industry-funded hoaxes for decades in *Life Extension* magazine. It is analogous to how tobacco companies paid off academia to cast doubt on the dangers of cigarettes. Some of the same scientists essentially bought off by the sugar industry were also harsh critics of dietary supplements.

We know how to reduce degenerative disease risk and slow certain aspects of aging, but at this time, our priority is accelerating research aimed at enabling older people to grow biologically younger.

SOMERS: Please explain.

FALOON: As we age, our bodies accumulate damaged cells that are not fully alive but not dead, either. These are called *senescent cells*, and media sources have picked up on this phenomenon and referred to them as "zombie cells." This name is appropriate, considering the multiple illnesses they cause and the fact that they spread like a contagion inside our bodies to infect healthy cells.

SOMERS: Why are these "zombie cells" so toxic?

FALOON: They release protein-degrading enzymes, along with inflammatory factors that shorten healthy life spans. It's hard to regenerate aging people when they have to battle relentless inflammatory attacks against healthy tissues caused by dysfunctional senescent cells.

SOMERS: How do we eliminate these inflammation-causing senescent ["zombie"] cells?

FALOON: Compounds called **senolytics** can selectively remove senescent cells from the body. By eliminating these toxic cells, a significant source of age-related chronic inflammation can be neutralized. When senolytics are tested in elderly rodents, there are whole-body rejuvenating effects and reversals of multiple age-related pathologies.

SOMERS: What happens when senolytic compounds are tested on people?

FALOON: Well, for instance, we helped support a study that tested senolytics on a group of older people with severe bone-on-bone osteoarthritis. The animal data showed marked improvements in joint function, so we thought we'd put senolytics to the most challenging test to see if we could regenerate cartilage in arthritic joints. After only three weeks, eighty-two percent of the study subjects had almost complete relief of pain and restoration of joint function. Larger studies need to be done to confirm these results, but a number of people have initiated some sort of senolytic therapy with the objective of systemic regeneration.

SOMERS: That's exciting. I know people with bone-on-bone osteoarthritis, and they are in constant chronic pain [inflammation]. How do senolytics regenerate cartilage?

FALOON: Arthritic joints are laden with senescent cells that generate so much destructive inflammation that cartilage is destroyed and natural regenerative factors suppressed. So when we clear senescent ("broken") cells from joint linings, the inflammation ceases and natural cartilage regeneration can rapidly occur.

SOMERS: How do you clear senescent cells? And do you think these same benefits are happening throughout the human body?

FALOON: In the proof-of-concept studies we helped fund, there was evidence of significant clearance of senescent cells using just two doses of a drug called **dasatinib** along with high-dose **quercetin**. We are finding other benefits based on preliminary biomarker data we are collecting now.

SOMERS: Is there another way of removing senescent cells from our aging bodies without using the drug dasatinib?

FALOON: Yes. We looked into how dasatinib eliminates senescent cells and were pleasantly surprised to find that a compound found in black tea called **theaflavins** possesses many of the same senolytic properties as dasatinib. So most readers of *Life Extension* magazine take a nutritional formula comprising black tea theaflavins combined with a highly absorbable quercetin phytosome. The dosage recommendation is just once a week, which is modeled after the dose frequency observed in published studies using senolytics. Another natural substance with senolytic properties is **fisetin**, found in many fruits and vegetables. Researchers at the University of Minnesota Medical School published a paper in September 2018 showing that high doses of a formula designed to dramatically increase the oral bioavailability of fisetin extends the maximum life span of laboratory animals. Other natural senolytics are being investigated, and human trials are already under way.[5]

SOMERS: Is this expensive?

FALOON: Not at all. What I love about senolytic therapy is that it does not require daily dosing, so the cost is quite low. Our readers take a once-weekly dose of a Senolytic Activator formula [theaflavins plus quercetin] that costs less than eight dollars a month. [Go to lifeextension.com /goodhealth to order it.]

SOMERS: So your recipe is to clear the body of senescent cells and then follow up with NAD+ treatments, such as IV NAD+ infusions, or NAD+-boosting supplements?

FALOON: The most popular supplement our readers use to boost their NAD+ levels is an NAD+ precursor combined with resveratrol. It boosts NAD+ blood levels between twenty-six and fifty-eight percent, depending on dose.

NAD+ infusions or patches increase NAD+ much more. People over age fifty usually benefit by first using NAD+ patches or infusions to restore youthful NAD+ blood levels. They then continue with oral NAD+ precursor supplements to maintain youthful ranges. Most, however, start with the oral NAD+ booster because it does not require a doctor's visit. With the emerging widespread availability of NAD+ blood tests, people will know ahead of time if they need an NAD+ infusion or can rely on NAD+ boosting supplements.

SOMERS: It excites me to know that if I can intermittently take short-term steps to clean out the "broken" senescent cells in my body and reduce inflammation and repair DNA breaks that cause so many problems with NAD+, that's pretty powerful.

FALOON: Our Age Reversal Network group is putting together physicians who will prescribe and administer NAD+ infusions or patches, along with senolytics like dasatinib/quercetin and compounds that help clear out accumulated waste products inside our cells via a housekeeping process known as *autophagy*.

These autophagy inducers include metformin, rapamycin, and natural compounds like highly bioavailable curcumin and green tea extract.

Our approach is based on typical people who are aging too fast. I need to emphasize, however, that these rejuvenation therapies should be based on individual needs. What we've done with the Age Reversal Network is create a section on our website where people can receive recommendations via email as to how they may best proceed. Some people need to start on different regenerative techniques, such as boosting their cellular levels of an enzyme called **AMPK**, which can be done with a drug called metformin, or specific AMPK-activating dietary supplements that can be obtained at lifeextension.com/goodhealth.

For your readers who want to find a doctor knowledgeable about prescribing dasatinib or NAD+ infusions or patches, they can visit the Age Reversal Network website. This public benefit group maintains a listing of physicians that prescribe rejuvenating approaches such as restoring NAD+ to youthful ranges.

SOMERS: Has Life Extension developed a blood test to measure NAD+ plasma levels and the senescent cell burden in one's body?

FALOON: Yes, we have developed the testing, but they are not presently available to the public. I am hoping by the time this is published we will be able to provide that service.

Several university labs perform NAD+ blood tests for us to help further clinical trials whereby we boost plasma levels of NAD+ and then assess what degree of age reversal may be occurring. We expect to have several universities offer these tests at affordable prices as part of a larger research initiative we are spearheading. Your readers can check out sources of NAD+ blood tests by visiting our public benefit group's website, www.RescueEldersNow.org. Many of our followers supplement with 250 to 500 milligrams a day of an NAD+ precursor vitamin like nicotinamide riboside. They then have the option of having their blood tested to see if they should go further and have a physician prescribe NAD+ infusions or patches. By trying the oral precursor first, your readers can save money by avoiding baseline NAD+ blood tests. They can do this because we've already established that NAD+ deficiency is epidemic, which corresponds to the loss of vitality people notice after ages forty to fifty. So we suggest that most people first supplement with an NAD+ precursor for thirty to sixty days and have their blood tested for NAD+ later to see if they need infusions or patches to fully restore NAD+ to optimal ranges.

SOMERS: I've read a lot about NAD+ recently where restoring it enables old mice to look and act younger as well as live longer. Why is it so important for aging people to replenish their cellular NAD+?

FALOON: Every day, each one of our cells sustains about ten DNA breaks. NAD+ is essential in repairing single-strand and double-strand DNA breaks.[6]

To put this into perspective, at age fifty, we have about sixty percent of the cellular NAD+ we had at age twenty-one. By the time we reach age eighty, our NAD+ levels are only one to eight percent of what they were in our youth. It may be a coincidence, but average life expectancy is around eighty years, right at the time when NAD+ levels are severely deficient.[7]

SOMERS: What exactly is NAD+?

FALOON: Australian researcher David Sinclair said in *Time* magazine **"[NAD+ is] one of the most important molecules for life to exist, and without it you're dead in 30 seconds."**[8]

NAD stands for **nicotinamide adenine dinucleotide**. NAD+ is a natural and essential coenzyme inside of our cells that diminishes with aging. Each cell in your body suffers about ten DNA breaks every day.

Unrepaired DNA damage is a major degenerative aging factor, and NAD+ depletion turns off DNA repair enzymes. According to Harvard professor David Sinclair, PhD, when cellular NAD+ falls to zero, you are dead.

> NAD+ is the closest we've gotten to a fountain of youth.
>
> —Dr. David Sinclair

SOMERS: How low do NAD+ levels drop as we age?

FALOON: Age eighty happens to be about the average time when Americans [men and women combined] die. Replenishing NAD+ is absolutely essential for healthy longevity.

Until recently, we had to estimate based on one's age: the older a person was, the lower their NAD+ levels. But there are other factors that can cause NAD+ to plummet, such as excess alcohol ingestion and eating unhealthy foods that require extensive liver detoxification.

SOMERS: Oh, no. Does this mean I have to give up my occasional tequila? Haha. What do your human studies show when older people restore NAD+ to youthful ranges?

FALOON: A little alcohol is okay, as long as you also take steps to maintain your NAD+ levels. The good news is that there are ways to immediately increase NAD+ levels now by taking specific vitamin precursors and then follow up with affordable NAD+ blood tests to assess if additional NAD+ restoration is needed. We helped fund two small proof-of-concept studies where generally unhealthy people with an average age of seventy-nine years underwent NAD+ infusion therapy.

We were able to identify multiple improvements in clinical measures such as reduced blood pressure, arthritis pain relief, alleviation of depression, neurological improvements, fewer tremors, improved exercise performance, cognitive enhancement, and improved sleep. We hope to confirm these findings soon in larger clinical trials.

SOMERS: How do we restore youthful NAD+ levels?

FALOON: If you are under age fifty, you can use a natural NAD+ precursor like nicotinamide riboside, which is a dietary supplement. The dose for most people is 250 to 500 milligrams a day.

If you are over age fifty, then you may need to boost your NAD+ to youthful ranges by having a physician administer NAD+ infusions or prescribe patches that deliver NAD+ through your skin into your bloodstream. You can then maintain these higher NAD+ levels with an NAD+ precursor dietary supplement. Most adults over age thirty can benefit by taking an NAD+ precursor that will increase NAD+ levels in their body. To fully restore youthful NAD+ levels in people over age forty to sixty, however, infusions or patches are often needed.

SOMERS: For a great night's sleep alone, it's worth it. Sleep eludes so many, and as we age there's nothing better than waking up in the morning having had a great seven or eight hours of sleep. But most aging people sleep an average of less than five hours and then have great difficulty getting back to sleep. The "lists" begin: all the thoughts going on in the brain. It's extremely frustrating and accelerates aging. What is your personal experience with NAD+ infusions?

FALOON: My systolic blood pressure dropped fifteen to twenty points, and I discontinued my blood pressure medication. There was an eighty percent improvement in my sleep patterns. It was one of the most significant age reversal interventions I've ever experienced.

SOMERS: So what's next? What follows senolytic and NAD+ restoration therapies?

FALOON: As you know, Suzanne, our healthy cells accumulate cellular waste products that interfere with youthful functionality. This is sometimes referred to as "cellular junk" and is a major factor why we suffer degenerative aging. There are now ways to turn on a process called *autophagy* that clears cells of these waste products and improves their functionality.

AUTOPHAGY

Autophagy is a self-degradative process that is important for balancing sources of energy at critical times in development and in response to nutrient stress. It also plays a housekeeping role in removing misfolded or aggregated proteins, clearing damaged organelles, such as mitochondria, endoplasmic reticulum, and peroxisomes, and eliminating intracellular pathogens, giving it a key role in preventing diseases such as cancer, neurodegeneration, cardiomyopathy, diabetes, liver disease, autoimmune diseases, and infections.[9]

SOMERS: So no one likes the idea of "waste" in their cells. How do we clear this cellular debris?

FALOON: An existing drug is being used in a creative way to turn on autophagy, and you only use it once a week. The drug, rapamycin, does its job in about thirty-six to forty-eight hours and then is mostly metabolized out of the body, so side effects typically do not occur.

SOMERS: Is there scientific data that supports the use of rapamycin as an antiaging therapy?

FALOON: In every animal model tested, rapamycin extends life span and reverses markers of pathological aging. This prompted a physician in Great Neck, New York, named Alan Green to start prescribing 5 milligrams a week of rapamycin to his patients, with good results reported so far. But at this stage, we are finding most of our supporters may not need rapamycin because they are achieving similar benefits by taking the antidiabetic drug **metformin** or by using dietary supplements that work via similar pathways as metformin, such as **gynostemma leaf extract** and **hesperidin**, or practicing calorie restriction or intermittent fasting. Any of these approaches beneficially turns down a signaling factor in our cells called **mTOR*** by activating a cellular enzyme called AMPK. This enables cells to remove cellular debris via the process of autophagy. We are funding studies to assess the effects of varying doses of rapamycin on aging persons.

SOMERS: And Life Extension makes an AMPK activator supplement for this purpose. What kind of results are you seeing in human studies?

FALOON: These are ongoing clinical trials with a drug called rapamycin, and one challenge has been that most of the volunteer study subjects are obese. The reason we are attracting overweight people is that when AMPK is activated, it suppresses mTOR, which can enable weight loss to occur. Fat cells replicate faster when mTOR is highly active. Turning down mTOR signaling by activating AMPK can turn down fat cell production in the body. Data on AMPK-activating nutrients that indirectly reduce mTOR as relates to weight loss are compelling.

SOMERS: Now you're talking. Everyone wants to know how to lose weight. Please explain in lay terms how people can lose weight by activating their AMPK?

FALOON: Without getting too technical, when AMPK is activated, it downregulates the cell growth factor called mTOR. We continue to study how effective this rejuvenation approach will be for weight loss. But unless something is done to turn down one's mTOR signaling (which can be accomplished with the drug metformin) it is difficult to shed body fat.

SOMERS: I'd like to add that the natural equivalent of metformin is a supplement called **berberine**.

---

* mTOR (mammalian target of rapamycin) is a protein that helps control several cell functions, including cell division and survival, and binds to rapamycin and other drugs. mTOR may be more active in some types of cancer cells than it is in normal cells. If the body no longer needs to grow in size and mature but mTOR activity remains high, something else can start to grow: cancer. Reducing mTOR signaling has indeed been shown to reduce cancer.

FALOON: Or nutrients such as gynostemma leaf extract/hesperidin and/or calorie restriction. And in case you have not figured this out yet, when you turn down excess cell proliferation, you also reduce cancer risk and the formation of artery-clogging plaque.

A myriad of published studies shows that when AMPK is activated, cancer rates go way down.

Current ways of clearing cellular debris involve severe calorie restriction (which most people cannot do) and boosting AMPK with metformin or a combination of two plant extracts: gynostemma pentaphyllum and hesperidin. Some adventurous people are using rapamycin* today, but some are waiting and using plant extracts to boost AMPK, which has an indirect effect of lowering mTOR, which then induces autophagy [clearing cellular debris]. But with aging or excess calorie intake, most people's mTOR activity remains at dangerously high levels long after we've achieved skeletal maturity, at which the body no longer needs the growth boost that high mTOR levels provide.

SOMERS: Explain how turning down mTOR helps cleanse cells of accumulated debris.

FALOON: When mTOR is turned down, cells sense starvation and start utilizing accumulated fat and begin clearing out accumulated waste products via a process known as autophagy. Studies in elderly people indicate improvements in immune functions in response to mTOR inhibition. Aside from severe calorie restriction, which is impractical for most people, the most efficient way of suppressing excess mTOR is to activate AMPK with metformin.

SOMERS: Okay, so you've removed senescent cells to make room for regenerative therapies to work, you've restored NAD+ levels to repair

---

* The compound was named rapamycin after the native name of the island where it was discovered, Rapa Nui. Sirolimus was initially developed as an antifungal agent. However, this use was abandoned when it was discovered to have potent immunosuppressive and antiproliferative properties due to its ability to inhibit mTOR. It was approved by the US Food and Drug Administration in September 1999 and is marketed under the trade name Rapamune by Pfizer (formerly by Wyeth).

broken DNA and cleared accumulated waste products by turning on "autophagy" and turning down mTOR. What's the final step in your age-reversal research protocol?

FALOON: Until we turn aging into a manageable condition, there is no "final step." What we are seeking to do today is provide people decades of extra time. That being said, the final step in our current protocol is to take advantage of the regenerative effects of very young plasma, umbilical cord stem cells/plasma, mesenchymal stem cells, and/or stem cell–derived exosome factors.

Our philanthropic group has a website where people can learn details about regenerative interventions, communicate with like-minded people including physicians and scientists, transmit their blood test results, and receive periodic updates. Registration on this website at www .RescueEldersNow.org/join costs nothing and is supported solely by those who want to see the science of age reversal accelerated.

SOMERS: My books have always revolved around longer life *with quality*! I had never considered actually reversing aging by using protocols that wipe out the issues that kill us. My husband is ten years older than me; if we could take advantage of these age-reversing protocols, it would allow that much more time together. What a lovely thought.

My dream is that as humans we can revert back to long life, quality of life, and when that time comes die peacefully and *not sick*. The present paradigm of aging is all about sickness. I call it "the long, slow death." What you have laid out in this interview allows all of us to dream big. I know my readers will be very enthusiastic to learn there is another way. Thank you, Bill. Always fascinating to pick your brain. Never stop being curious.

FALOON: And thank you, Suzanne. Your readers can receive a free subscription to *Life Extension* magazine by going to our website or by calling 1-888-884-3666.

CHAPTER 17

TELOMERE LENGTHENING

What is a **telomere**? The word *telomere* (tel-uh-meer) comes from the Greek *telos* (end) and *meros* (part). Telomeres are located in the nucleus of all cells and their shortening is an essential part of the cellular aging process. Telomeres are the caps at the end of each strand of DNA that protect our chromosomes, like the plastic tips at the end of shoelaces. Without those protective tips, shoelaces become frayed until they can no longer do their job. When telomeres get too short, genetic DNA is lost and cells become senescent or die. (Senescent cells are still alive but no longer function as they should. They can no longer divide, are larger than normal cells, and secrete harmful cytokines that affect nearby healthy cells.)

I first met Noel Thomas Patton, the founder and CEO of T.A. Sciences, the provider of the telomere-lengthening supplement TA-65, several years ago. I was fascinated listening to Mr. Patton explain the concept of reversing cellular aging by lengthening the telomeres; for lack of a better description, the telomeres are "tails" on the end of each chromosome in every cell.

Each cell in our body reproduces around fifty times. Each time it reproduces, the "tail" or the telomere gets shorter. By the time a cell has reproduced close to its fiftieth time, the cell stops dividing and either becomes senescent or dies. Telomere lengthening actually "regrows" the tail (Suzanne speak), making the cell young and vital again.

I have been taking telomere supplementation in the form of TA-65 for nine years. I must say, I believe it's working. My skin is not wrinkling much. I have no "sloppy skin," especially considering my age. The skin on my face is minimally wrinkled. However, TA-65 is not promoted as a cosmetic product; the goal of using it is to rejuvenate cells inside our bodies.

Cellular health has taken a front-and-center position in this book. I start a book with no preconceived notion, and eventually a "theme" emerges. So many doctors and professionals in this book refer to cellular health as the fountain of youth, and this theme runs throughout many different forms and explanations of ways to care for the human cell.

The human body is made up of approximately 30 trillion to 40 trillion cells, so the concept of keeping the cells cleaned out and in top form seems to me a no-brainer.

The fact that telomeres protect our DNA was first observed in the 1930s. Scientists made the link between telomeres and cellular aging nearly forty years ago.

In 2009, the Nobel Prize in Physiology or Medicine was awarded to three scientists who discovered how an enzyme called **telomerase** impacts telomere length. TA-65 has been proven to activate telomerase and lengthen telomeres. In fact, TA-65 has the first and only published and peer-reviewed, randomized, double-blind, placebo-controlled study to show telomeres getting longer in humans. Today, there are more than twenty thousand scientific articles published about telomeres. An ever-increasing number of scientists continue to study telomeres and the benefits of stopping or possibly reversing the telomere shortening that happens as we age.

SHORTENED TELOMERES ARE CONNECTED TO PREMATURE CELLULAR AGING

Here is a question you probably can't answer: How old are you biologically? If for some reason you don't know your chronological age, just look at your birth certificate. Depending on your inherited genes and your lifestyle, biologically you are most likely to be younger or older than the number of years since your birth. The accepted way in which scientists calculate biological age is to measure telomere length through blood testing by a qualified doctor. Telomere shortening is involved in all aspects of the aging process. Telomeres cushion the ends of our chromosomes, which is a pretty important job considering that those chromosomes are made up of DNA strands that determine our entire genetic makeup—including the way our skin and hair look and how our liver functions.

Our cells are constantly dying and replenishing themselves throughout our lives, and when that happens, our DNA stays intact while the telomeres shorten slightly each time. So the older we get, the shorter our telomeres become, and eventually our skin, hair, livers, etc., start to feel the wear and tear. Needless to say, keeping telomeres as long as possible for as long as possible is one of the major keys to feeling and looking young.

Through Bill Faloon you have learned about NAD+, which repairs DNA breaks in your cells, and senolytics, which clear our cellular debris, but there is another factor, and that is telomeres and telomere length. What if you could take a "telomere lengthener"? That is the job and purpose of the supplement TA-65 as a means of life extension and optimal health. There are thousands of studies showing that telomere dysfunction is related to poor health, a shorter life, and nearly all forms of disease and aging. Aging and disease are both dependent upon telomere erosion in both normal cells and stem cells, and the rate of erosion determines the rates of mutation, cell dysfunction, and depletion of healthy reserves.

We've talked a lot about the importance of healthy cells, cellular debris, and accelerated aging, when your malfunctioning cells outnumber your functioning cells. If you take away nothing else from this book, take cellular health seriously.

Clearly, healthy cells and a strong immune system are the answers to quality of life and longevity. The best "recipe" for well-functioning cells, as suggested by the doctors in this book:

- Telomere lengthening, with supplements such as TA-65

- The creation of NAD+, as explained by Bill Faloon in chapter 16

- Senolytics, as explained by Bill Faloon in chapter 16

Extremely short telomeres = early cell aging

WHAT DOCTORS SAY ABOUT TA-65

Here is what some prominent antiaging researchers have to say about TA-65.

DR. EDWARD PARK

Dr. Edward Park is an antiaging MD trained at Harvard for undergraduate and residency training and Columbia for his MD and master's in public health. Since 2007, he has personally ingested and prescribed telomerase activators, and the amazing clinical results can be discovered on his YouTube channel, *drpark65*. Dr. Park says:

"Since 2007, I have taken an herbily derived telomerase activator. Based on my own physiological benefits and those of my patients, I believe this will often slow and occasionally reverse changes associated with aging. In my YouTube videos at *drpark65*, I explore conditions ranging from depression, addiction, cancer, sports injuries, diabetes, and high blood pressure. There are thousands of research studies suggesting a relationship between unhealthy telomeres and most diseases, but the good news is that this research also suggests how we can optimize breathing, mind-set, sleep, diet, exercise, and supplements to fight telomere erosion. I explain how to understand and utilize these tools for repairing your telomeres in my book *The Telomere Miracle: Scientific Secrets to Fight Disease, Feel Great, and Turn Back the Clock on Aging*.

"Most people taking a telomerase activator experience improved mood, deeper sleep, fewer colds and flus, and faster recovery from exercise and injury. Back in 2007, I was a forty-year-old with gray hair and reading glasses. Now, eleven years later, I have neither! Although aging also involves other processes like epigenetic gene silencing, stem cell mutation and depletion, and a failure of immune- and apoptosis-mediated senolysis [killing of damaged, old cells], I believe that telomerase activators are a powerful tool in our arsenal and can help to maintain a healthier and longer life."

DR. WALTER PIERPAOLI

"A revolution can only be started by the people themselves, from the ground up. Once the public wakes up to the current medical mafia and understands what is truly possible with alternatives, by which I mean non-orthodox, but nonetheless scientifically proven approaches; then the world of health will become a very different place."[1]

DR. THIERRY HERTOGHE

"The two most important telomere lengtheners I know of are astragalus extracts, and the most well known of these extracts is TA-65. Then there's the one that comes from Russia, a small peptide made by the pineal gland. It is called Epithalon. It may have anticancer properties. I tried TA-65. After six weeks, my eyesight was much better and I felt younger. I didn't need reading glasses. Then I tried Epithalon and had the same effect on my vision after six weeks. What I now do with my patients is to give them 3 milligrams of sublingual Epithalon. It's quite expensive, and then they take TA-65 or another astragalus extract and combine both, and their eyesight really improves. We also have a method of putting injections around the eyes which also improves eyesight along with those two products."

DR. JEFFREY GLADDEN

"TA-65, telomerase activator 65, from the astragalus root is important, but there's a new telomerase activator out. Dr. Bill Andrews from Sierra Sciences has tested thousands and thousands of molecules for activity; they have found one even more potent than TA-65. It's called telomerase activator molecule 818, TAM 818. So we utilize both. They make TAM 818 in a skin cream and also a pill. It's important to have your telomerase measured and depending on your levels, we would either add telomerase supplementation or leave you where you are; it just depends on how you are feeling."

I've been taking TA-65 for six years. I feel a big difference. All you can do is compare yourself to your contemporaries, and I realize I don't have the aches and pains or issues they have, so something's working.

CHAPTER 18

STEM CELLS:
The Future or Now?

It's been said that stem cells are the future, but I say the future is now!

My first experience with advancements in stem cell procedures was with *me*!

The miracle of regrowing my breast, which had been taken by cancer twenty years before, was life changing. I had chosen at the time of surgery not to have reconstruction or implants. I knew deep inside that a better option would come along.

I heard of Dr. Kotaro Yoshimura at the University of Tokyo School of Medicine in Tokyo, Japan, who had successfully regrown the breasts of more than four hundred Japanese women using their own stem cells.

I called Dr. Yoshimura, and to my delight and surprise, he had heard of me and my work. He agreed after several conversations to come to Los Angeles and teach this incredible procedure to my plastic surgeon in Los Angeles, Dr. Joel Aronowitz.

My initial breast cancer surgery required that half my breast be removed to get rid of the tumor and all "evidence." Luckily for me, the surgeon had left the skin and nipple intact, which turned out to be a great advantage. Aesthetically, leaving the nipple and skin not only allowed for the stem cell fat transfer to regrow my breast but also enabled the breast to look as though nothing had ever happened to it. That was my incredible result: whole again, with minimal surgery. The procedure required removing fat from my belly (boo-hoo), then spinning out the stem cells, discarding the weak ones, keeping the strong ones (I am simplifying), and, for lack of a better term, using what looked like a "turkey baster" filled with my fat to inject strong, rich stem cells from my body into my breast. The result was a perfect breast.

You can imagine how pleased I am with the results. After having been disfigured for all those years, I had "me" back again—nothing foreign, full feeling, no implants, just my own fat and my own stem cells. It took three years to obtain permission to open a clinical trial in the United States, and I was the first woman to successfully and legally regrow her own breast. My gratitude to Dr. Yoshimura and Dr. Aronowitz is difficult to express.

This is just one of the many new ways to use stem cells for healing and disfigurement as a simpler way than complex surgeries.

In this part you will meet Dr. Dipnarine Maharaj, the founder and medical director of the South Florida Bone Marrow/Stem Cell Transplant Institute, one of the few completely outpatient bone marrow/stem cell transplant facilities in the United States. This will be like having an appointment with him. I've tried to ask all the questions I thought any of us would want to ask in the examining room. After you read it, you can decide for yourselves if this is the way you want to go.

Also featured in this part is Dr. Marc Darrow, one of the most experienced stem cell doctors in the world. He utilizes stem cell therapy, platelet-rich plasma therapy, and prolotherapy for the treatment of pain in joints, tendons, and ligaments and many other injuries and syndromes all over the body, including back and neck pain.

Stem cell therapy has the potential to revolutionize nearly all aspects of medicine. We may soon see stem cells used to treat everything from heart disease and cancer to spinal cord injuries, Parkinson's disease, and Alzheimer's disease to even baldness and blindness.

As Dr. Michael Galitzer explains, "Stem cells are considered the 'mother cells' of all other cells in the body because they are undifferentiated cells that can differentiate, or turn, into specialized cells, and also divide, through a process known as *mitosis*, to produce additional stem cells.

"Adult stem cells are found in bone marrow and fat, as well as other tissues and organs of the body. The number of stem cells in our body declines drastically with age. At birth, 1 in 10,000 of our cells are stem cells. When we are teenagers, it is 1 in 100,000. In our forties, it is 1 in 400,000. In our eighties, it is 1 in 2 million. Stem cells have three major modes of action: they can reduce inflammation, modulate the immune system, and regenerate tissues."

Autologous stem cell therapy refers to therapy using stem cells harvested from a person's own body. There are three sources of autologous adult stem cells in humans: bone marrow, which involves extracting stem cells from pelvic bone; adipose tissue (fat cells), which involves harvesting stem cells using liposuction (this was the procedure I chose for my breast regrowth); and blood, which involves drawing blood and then harvesting stem cells through a process called **apheresis**.

During apheresis the drawn blood passes through a machine that extracts stem cells and returns the rest of the blood to the donor's body. Stem cells can also be harvested from umbilical cord blood following birth and then banked for future use.

Stem cell therapy is currently becoming popular in the area of orthopedics and sports medicine. Stem cells are extracted from the patient's pelvic bone marrow and immediately injected into a poorly functioning joint such as the knee, hip, or shoulder.

A present area of controversy is collecting placental umbilical cord stem cells from a healthy woman after she gives birth and injecting them either into a joint or intravenously into a person who is looking for a health-enhancing antiaging effect. More research needs to be done as to its safety and effectiveness.

Dr. Galitzer says, "I believe that the body needs to be optimized before one undergoes stem cell therapy. Optimal nutrition, exercise, proper supplements, drainage and detoxification, and hormonal balance will result in a more beneficial outcome when using stem cell therapy."

And no small thing: clinical researcher Dr. Jonathan M. Fishbein has very interesting things (and science) to say about non-THC CBD for managing pain. With the opioid crisis being epidemic, it's time to look for natural pain management. We have CBD receptors all throughout our body, as though our bodies have been waiting for this. You will be interested in what he has to say.

Interview with
DR. DIPNARINE MAHARAJ

Dr. Maharaj is a friend and a doctor "most admired" by his peers. It's his background, passion, and caring that have put him at the top of his field.

He studied hematology/oncology and stem cell transplantation because that was where he felt he could make a real difference in the advancement of health care. He also has advanced degrees from some of the most respected medical schools in the world, including University of Glasgow Medical School in Glasgow, Scotland.

As part of his extensive work in cancer care and research, Dr. Maharaj focused on the healing power of the human immune system and dedicated his career to the concentrated study of the immune system, specifically the vital stem cells that give it its unique regenerative qualities. He has been handling highly complex clinical cases and performing outpatient bone marrow stem cell transplant procedures for more than ten years. His research and clinical work have led to evidence of true advancements in the treatment—and even the prevention—of life-threatening diseases that have historically been difficult to manage.

Dr. Maharaj is the founder and medical director of the Maharaj Institute of Immune Regenerative Medicine and its affiliates, the Stem Cell Cryobank and the Advanced Stem Cell Education Program (ASTEP).

> I chose to study hematology/oncology/stem cell transplantation to make a real difference in the quality of care and to help change people's lives for the better. My education helped shape me as a doctor and as a person. But for me, learning never ends. My patients are far too important.
>
> —Dr. Dipnarine Maharaj

SOMERS: Thank you for your time, Dr. Maharaj. You have been actively involved in stem cell research for quite some time. My husband and I had the pleasure of visiting your clinic in Boynton Beach, Florida, and we were both impressed with the advances in stem cell application right now and also for our health going forward in the future. Tell me how you are using stem cell therapy in your clinic, and how can my readers access it today?

MAHARAJ: Thank you, Suzanne. What is very encouraging is that more and more people are becoming aware that there are stem cells and that there are different types of stem cells with a better understanding of what each of these different types do.

Stem cells are the key cells providing the opportunity to regenerate aging cells and tissues—helping us to stay young. However, as we age, our stem cells begin to lose their function.

SOMERS: Can patients use stem cells only from their own body?

MAHARAJ: There are potential risks to using somebody else's stem cells. It can be more effective and safer to use your own.

SOMERS: I understand. Today so many of our babies, sadly, are born toxic. Do we have to rethink cord blood stem cells?

MAHARAJ: That's a very important point, and most people aren't aware of the risks. You would assume that stem cells from a newborn baby are pristine. When they are pristine, they can be used for many different indications.

What many people do not understand is that stem cells form the immune system of the body—that's one of the main functions of our stem cells. In a baby, these stem cells have not matured enough to form a fully functional immune system.

SOMERS: Meaning the immune system of a baby is immature?

MAHARAJ: Correct. Secondly, there are different types of stem cells, and the numbers in cord blood are low because the actual volume we normally collect and keep is low when compared to the volume we collect from an adult to be used for a transplant. So the important points to notice are the amount of toxicity, the immaturity of the immune system, and the numbers of stem cells.

A fourth important point is that the stem cells in that baby will form a particular tissue type when they differentiate—a tissue type specific to that baby. If those stem cells are taken and given to somebody else and they differentiate, they will actually form the tissue type of the baby from whom they originated. So injecting stem cells from a baby could be harmful to somebody if it's not the right "fit" or tissue type.

SOMERS: So I assume that the safest thing is to bank your own stem cells for future use from birth and beyond. I did this fifteen years ago.

But what if you haven't done this? What if you get leukemia? Where does this person get stem cells?

MAHARAJ: If somebody comes to our clinic with leukemia and we consider them for a transplant, there are two options. One is that stem cells from the individual with leukemia could be considered, depending on the age of the individual. The alternative source of stem cells would be from a donor, and that donor has to be tissue-typed to the person who is requesting the treatment.

I have had a lot of experience utilizing an individual's own stem cells. I was part of a group in Scotland where we pioneered this treatment, even in patients with advanced leukemia. Once we were able to get these patients into remission, we collected some of their stem cells which were not affected by the disease. That allowed us to do a bone marrow transplant using their own stem cells. The reason is because leukemia arises from particular lines of stem cells but not all lines of stem cells in the bone marrow are affected by the leukemia. So it is possible to get rid of or to destroy the lines that are affected by the leukemia and then use the normal stem cells to recover the immune system, which is basically what results in long-term survival.

SOMERS: Is this now your standard of care?

MAHARAJ: Yes, It's called an autologous stem cell transplant. It's a standard of care not only for leukemia but also for patients who have other types of blood or immune disorders. These disorders include multiple myeloma, lymphomas, and other immune dysfunctional or deficiency disorders. So we can do an autologous stem cell transplant. Or the other option is an allogeneic transplant (basically using a donor), but that donor has to be a match to the patient.

SOMERS: What is the best match?

MAHARAJ: The best match is actually getting it from a relative, preferably a sibling. Usually we ask for a six-out-of-six HLA match. That's a full match, and then, if there are varying degrees of that, we would go for a mismatch or partial mismatch.

SOMERS: I'm getting confused.

MAHARAJ: Meaning we can still use those cells but there is a bigger risk of complications, including an autoimmune disease called graft-versus-host disease. Death associated with the transplant procedure is also greater because of that.

SOMERS: Aging is about worn-out parts. Do you think the immune system is the first to go because of the enormous environmental assault and toxicity?

MAHARAJ: Yes. To answer that question fully, one has to consider how the immune system is formed. Babies have lots of stem cells, but their immune system is immature. As the person grows, the immune system matures and the stem cells in the bone marrow increase. When we're between the ages of eighteen and forty, our immune system is at its peak. After forty it begins to decline, and that's directly related to dysfunction, which occurs in particular types of stem cells called **lymphoid stem cells**.

Normal aging is caused by a decrease in the function of lymphoid stem cells, which causes the immune system to decline.

Most people are not aware of this because they go to their doctors and have a complete blood count [CBC], the cells of which are formed by the myeloid stem cells. Myeloid stem cells are most plentiful and don't decline to the same extent as the lymphoid stem cells.

Aging creates an imbalance of these two types of stem cells—myeloid versus lymphoid—which form different components of the blood.

The key components of the blood that maintain our immune system are B cells, T cells, and natural killer cells. This is what we call the functional immune system. In the aging process, the functional immune system declines.

At our institute we are able to measure a patient's immune system. They might have a normal blood count, but when we look at their immune system, we can tell the level at which their immune system is functioning.

So to come back to your question about people being exposed to environmental toxins. If we consider normal aging of the immune system, which is a decline of the lymphoid stem cells and their precursor stem cells, which are the pluripotent stem cells, then we can attribute twenty-five percent to genetics, but the other seventy-five percent is related to the environmental toxin exposure and lifestyle factors.

If we use this as a guide for "normal aging," then after age forty, people's immune systems begin to decline, and by age sixty-five it takes a nosedive. That's the reason why older people experience the onset of at least one chronic disease, including cancer, by age sixty-five, which can increase to as many as eight chronic diseases by age eighty.

SOMERS: So it appears paramount that in order to prolong life with optimal health, we have to keep our immune systems strong and firing. What do you do about this?

MAHARAJ: This is why the area of stem cells and regenerative medicine is so exciting, because we have and are developing new strategies to improve the function of "worn-out" stem cells to strengthen the immune system.

But first it's important to educate individuals of the need to take responsibility for their health and to learn the type of lifestyles and diets that improve and preserve their immune systems, and this is a big part of whether you age well or not: they need to avoid the habits such as smoking, excessive alcohol, and exposure to all the other toxins that are driving accelerated aging.

SOMERS: The immune system degrading is clearly evident by the startling amount of people with cancer today, which feels like an epidemic. What kinds of cancer respond to stem cell therapy?

MAHARAJ: Individuals who have blood cancers such as leukemias, lymphomas, and multiple myelomas. Blood cancers and other cancers are caused by driver mutations within the stem cells, and this, together with the decline of the immune system, causes rapid growth of the cancers.

We used to think that leukemia was the only cancer that arose from a stem cell. But now we realize that all different types of cancers arise from mutations within the DNA of stem cells.

If you look at the cells within a particular tumor, they are very different in the types of mutations they have: some of them are slow growing, some of them are fast growing. It's the fast-growing cells that have the driver mutations, and this makes the disease more aggressive.

SOMERS: What about metastases? How do you treat cancer that spreads through the body? Normally it's a death sentence.

MAHARAJ: Metastases have different types of cells caused by different mutations. Right now, immunotherapy with stem cells is being used in an experimental way to treat metastatic cancer, with stem cell harvests that contain not only stem cells but also B cells, T cells, and natural killer cells. Some of the T cells are being used as treatments, which can kill the cancer, because the T cells can be modified genetically to cause activation so that they target the cancer cells. This is a new form of treatment called CAR-T cells.

SOMERS: That's exciting news. Blood cancers usually have ominous outcomes, but now if you have a blood cancer, there's the promise of maintaining or curing. Can I use the word *cure*?

MAHARAJ: Yes.

SOMERS: I have read that there is increased risk of multiple myeloma when exposed to glyphosate. Have you heard that?

MAHARAJ: Yes. There isn't any doubt that toxins, for example in pesticides, cause cancer. In Florida around Lake Okeechobee, where there are a lot of toxins, there are clusters of people with multiple myeloma compared to other parts of Florida. People often go fishing and eat the foods from that contaminated water. Also, I think that water is draining out and affecting other parts of the state as well.

SOMERS: I appreciate my great health; I eat healthy and take care of myself. Would I come to you to get an immune system boost with stem cells? Could I do that proactively to reactivate my immune system? You said there was a test that one could take to determine the health of your immune system. What's it called?

MAHARAJ: Yes, there is a blood test that allows us to evaluate your immune system, called an immune profile.

SOMERS: So if I wanted to come to your clinic to make sure going forward that I have a strong immune system, I could have that therapy in your clinic?

MAHARAJ: Yes. You would have a blood sample taken, an immune blood profile. It's an extensive analysis of the cells that form the **functional immune system** (a combination of the **innate immune system** and the **adaptive immune system**), and then from those results we can identify a pattern allowing us to determine if an abnormality exists.

From these tests we can characterize someone as having evidence of immune dysfunction if it isn't normal. There's a decline of the immune system with normal aging, but there are groups of people who actually have a normal immune system right up until the time when they die. And that's the goal.

SOMERS: What if I have a torn meniscus or a frozen shoulder? Would I come to your clinic for that?

MAHARAJ: Yes, we have platelet-rich plasma [PRP] for that use. It is a series of injections.

SOMERS: Is this what you're calling supra-PRP?

MAHARAJ: Correct, yes.

SOMERS: You've been involved in this for a long time, in fact, you were one of the first ones. It was Ray Kurzweil, called one of the smartest men on the planet by Bill Gates, who told me to contact you years ago, that you were at the forefront of stem cell science and protocols. That's a big endorsement. It's clearly the way of the future.

If this is "the way," then should we all start thinking early on, while we're still healthy, of banking our own stem cells?

MAHARAJ: Yes. When we consider the fact that our bone marrow stem cells, which form our immune system, are being exposed to environmental toxins and lifestyle factors which accelerate aging, then it makes perfect sense to have healthy stem cells banked for future use. They will be invaluable.

It's called planning for our future to have a good quality of life and to know that our health is determined by our immune system. Taking our stem cells when they're healthy can afford us a future where we extend our health span with quality.

SOMERS: Then we have our stem cells stored and keep them for a later date.

MAHARAJ: Yes, the work we pioneered in Scotland showed that even if somebody had developed leukemia, there were still normal stem cells in the bone marrow, so we could take those normal stem cells and give them back to the patient. It's almost like "rebooting" their immune system, and these patients were cured or have long-term survival. We know for a fact it works for blood disorders and immune disorders. Now we are exploring how it would work for other diseases caused by aging of the immune system, which is called **immunosenescence**, meaning aging of the immune system.

SOMERS: What does aging of the immune system correlate to in terms of diseases?

MAHARAJ: Diseases associated with immunosenescence include chronic inflammatory diseases like Alzheimer's, Parkinson's, and other neurological disorders associated with neuroinflammation, chronic heart disease, chronic lung disease. Also, autoimmune diseases, cancer, recurrent infections, and frailty occur with immunosenescence.

As people begin to get older, they suddenly realize they can't do what they used to do before. That's the beginning of frailty. The five categories I've just described are all caused by this immunosenescence, which is the aging of the immune system. So when somebody has their blood test done, I can usually tell if they've got evidence of immunosenescence and if it's likely they are going to get one of these diseases.

SOMERS: I'm a proponent of bioidentical hormone replacement, and myself and the people that I know who have gone on replacement just seem healthier to me. Are hormones part of your protocol?

MAHARAJ: It's a very important category. When we consider immunosenescence and we find immune dysfunction in someone's blood test, we look at their hormones as a root cause of the immune system dysfunction. The brain, the immune system, and our hormonal system are key organs affected by aging. Maintaining our hormones is a key component of our immune systems working well.

SOMERS: Life is wonderful only if you have health.

MAHARAJ: Yes, and our health care system is based upon disease care. So I agree with you: let's look at our health proactively, let's prevent the onset of diseases. The key component is to maintain a healthy immune system. That's what centenarians and supercentenarians show when tested, and they maintain it right up to the time when it suddenly declines and then they die. But along the way they're living a good quality of life.

SOMERS: Isn't that what we all want? Live healthy until the final day.

MAHARAJ: Yes, and what we've learned from them is they have found a way. If we, as insurance, bank our stem cells, then we will have them to be used at a later date, when our immune system begins to decline. You can be in control of a strong immune system.

HOW TO MAINTAIN A STRONG IMMUNE SYSTEM

1. **Get enough sleep.** On average, we need about seven to nine hours of sleep each night.

2. **Get regular exercise,** the right amount but not too much. Superathletes who overexercise have a shorter life span because their immune systems are weakened.

3. **Eat well.**

4. **Control your stress.** We can measure and see the effects of stress on the immune system.

SOMERS: Well, I do know I'm aging differently than my contemporaries who are not doing these same things.

MAHARAJ: Absolutely.

A huge problem we have in the United States is Alzheimer's disease. In the state of Florida there are 750,000 people sitting in nursing homes with no hope that they will ever be able to leave, all because their immune systems went down twenty years before the onset of Alzheimer's.

Their neuroinflammation caused damage to the point where it's very difficult to do anything to be able to get them back.

The real way to deal with that epidemic is actually to prevent it. One of the main ways of prevention and preserving our immune system is by banking our stem cells for the future.

SOMERS: Well, that makes me want to run to your clinic and bank my stem cells right now. It almost seems ridiculous that we have the ability and knowledge to renew our immune systems using our own stem cells—that we cannot reject, since you can't reject yourself—thus guarding us against the worst diseases, and yet we do not bank our stem cells.

My theory: toxins are entering our bodies through our skin, the food we eat, and the air we breathe, and they will eventually end up in the GI tract, where the toxins will eat through the lining, allowing for "leaky gut." To me, that's where all the trouble begins. It seems to me a big part of prevention is to protect yourself from the environment by the choices we make. Right?

MAHARAJ: Yes, absolutely. We know that seventy percent of the immune system of the body is in the gut. The immune system is there for a reason: to prevent toxins, bacteria, viruses, and fungi that cause infections and death.

For example, Candida are organisms which, if they are working well, are supposed to help keep our immune system working. But if the gut is populated by abnormal viruses, abnormal bacteria, abnormal fungi, then they cause damage to the immune system and create what's called a leaky gut.

So yes, it's exposure to toxins, but also exposure to these abnormal pathogenic bacteria, viruses, and fungi, that causes our immune systems to weaken and causes inflammation in the lining in the cells of the gut. When that happens, the gut is vulnerable and allows food or any other toxins to go straight into the bloodstream. People who have a leaky gut have a high risk of fatty liver.

Toxins also go to the fat normally protecting our organs and cause inflammation, and that causes obesity. You can link obesity to the abnormal gut microbiome. An abnormal gut microbiome leads to an abnormal immune system, and this leads to chronic diseases like diabetes, metabolic syndrome, obesity, and fatty liver.

SOMERS: So if I'm a patient and I come to you with all those issues— obesity, diabetes, leaky gut—what could you do for that patient?

MAHARAJ: The first thing is the immune test. I want to look at markers of inflammation. We expect abnormalities, but we want to see baselines. As we correct the baselines, our goal is to get the gut back to normal.

Then we identify root causes. We measure the toxins that person is exposed to—for example, do they have high levels of cadmium, lead, or high levels of arsenic? Many patients have heavy metals, and we know this has been associated with chronic diseases like heart disease. Inflammation causes different diseases. We want to see specific foods that person is eating that's driving their B cells to produce antibodies against the food in much the same way you would see with a viral or bacterial infection. We also measure their nutrients and micronutrients. If their micronutrients (vitamins and trace metals) are abnormal, we want to correct it.

We look at their gut's microbiome to see if they're populated with abnormal bacteria so we can correct it. We also look at viruses, bacterial fungi, to identify the ones that normally cause disease. For example, some people are exposed to Epstein-Barr, which causes glandular fever. Or a virus called cytomegalovirus, which is a member of the herpes family of viruses. If those remain activated, we are concerned because they have been associated with certain inflammatory disorders of the brain. More frequently, they are associated with accelerated aging of the immune system.

We look at sleep levels, stress, exercise, measure their vitamin D levels, and look at alcohol consumption or other things they might be doing to affect their immune system.

That's a simplified profile of how I treat my patients.

SOMERS: I think what you're doing is detective work. Down the road, do you see that pancreatic cancer patients could utilize stem cell treatments, or is that still the worst cancer of all?

MAHARAJ: Pancreatic cancer patients respond sometimes to immuno-therapy; utilizing and improving the immune system ultimately causes the paradigm shift, so treating these patients with immunotherapy is gradually moving toward a cure.

We are talking about cure because it is possible to treat patients with cancer and cure them. We have to have that mind-set when we look at these diseases. If we don't, we are undervaluing the potential of what we could be providing to our patients. When we look at the immune system, we can find specific cells that are responsible for killing cancer in patients, and we can also find the specific cells that block the immune system from killing these cancers. By readjusting and coming up with new treatment protocols, we can make a difference in the lives of our patients.

I can describe a patient with leukemia who received the "standard of care" with chemotherapy, radiation, bone marrow transplantation, and donor lymphocyte infusion, but this "standard of care" failed.

I measured the immune system and the mutations driving the cancer. We used a targeted therapy to block the mutations driving the cancer and boosted the immune system. We've seen many successes like this. These are patients who basically had exhausted everything. Many of the patients I treat are in that situation, and we've been able to help them.

SOMERS: I'm sure you'd prefer these patients come to you before they have chemical poisoning.

MAHARAJ: Yes. Absolutely. I think that's the point I'd like to emphasize, because as soon as somebody gets cancer or even before they get cancer—often five, ten years before they get cancer—their immune system is breaking down. If cancer occurs as a result of a breakdown of the immune system, it doesn't happen overnight, it happens over a period of time.

If we can catch that person early at the onset of the cancer and correct their immune system and target the cancer cells, with **genomic analysis** we can actually identify the specific genes driving the cancer cells.

Chemotherapy is like a cluster bomb: you give it to the patient, and it destroys not only the cancer but everything else. Instead, we target the immune system to correct it and target only the cancer cells driving the cancer. The patient has less toxicity that way and better outcomes.

SOMERS: What are naive T cells as compared to memory T cells? What's the difference?

MAHARAJ: *Naive* means they have never been exposed to cancer or other antigens like viruses before; *memory* means having been exposed to cancer, and now the onset of the response is a lot faster. Our stem cells are within the bone marrow and called pluripotent stem cells. They divide into myeloid and lymphoid stem cells. The lymphoid stem cells can be divided further into naive T cells and memory T cells. A naive cell is basically a cell which is early in terms of differentiation and has never been exposed to an antigen before.

Let's say, for example, we get a viral infection and we've never been exposed to that viral infection before. The naive cell will actually recognize that virus as being abnormal and it will then produce memory cells so that the next time we are exposed to that virus, our memory T cells are there to be able to kill it.

One of the problems older people encounter is herpes zoster, which is shingles. You would think people exposed to that virus (which is really the chicken pox virus) should be able to respond to it, but the problem with aging of the immune system is that the naive T cell numbers go down, along with their memory cells not functioning well. As a result, they will get a reactivation of that herpes virus, which had caused chicken pox in childhood but now causes herpes zoster [shingles].

SOMERS: You mentioned people who were far more resistant to cancer. Are those the people you were just talking about who have those extraordinary immune systems?

MAHARAJ: Yes.

SOMERS: How do you get to be one of those people?

MAHARAJ: Well, I'm sure you are.

SOMERS: No, I've had cancer twice. Frankly, having had cancer twice has benefits; I no longer fear it. I know how to deal with this demon. Every choice I make of every moment of every day, I look at food and I think, "Am I choosing great health down the road or the nursing home?" It's as simple as that.

MAHARAJ: We all have to have that same mind-set. Your question earlier about how can we prevent cancer? We can measure it. There are certain subsets of cells within the immune system called natural killer cells. Individuals who maintain their natural killer cell function have a lower incidence of cancer.

Natural killer cells are cells of the innate immune system, and they're able to recognize cancer cells because they're different from normal cells. **The way to prevent cancer is to make sure all of our natural killer cell numbers are high and functioning well.** People with high natural killer cell numbers, who are functioning well, live to be one hundred and healthy.

SOMERS: You must go home at night pleased with yourself and the work you have chosen to do, right?

MAHARAJ: When I have patients who I am able to help get better when nothing else has worked, I feel a great sense of accomplishment. I attribute that to the gift that we're given. God gives us all gifts, and we have to use those gifts to their fullest extent to help others; otherwise we are not fulfilling our lives.

As a transplant physician helping patients with critical illnesses after they were told that nothing else could be done, it has given me the courage and desire to change this paradigm. We need to educate people so they don't get chronic diseases, and then we will be able to provide true health care rather than disease care.

SOMERS: Thank you for this incredible information, Dr. Maharaj.

In alternative medicine I always try to find nondrug therapies for all conditions, in particular to manage pain or tissue damage. If you go to a sports surgeon, he or she is going to want to do surgery to try to fix your problem, but today we have the marvel of stem cell therapies as the first option, including the therapies you will read about in the following interview.

Interview with

DR. MARC DARROW

Dr. Marc Darrow, a leading sports doctor located in Santa Monica, California, is one of the most experienced stem cell doctors in the world. He is "in the trenches" daily. He utilizes stem cell therapy, platelet-rich plasma (PRP) therapy, and prolotherapy for the treatment of joints, tendons, ligaments, and many other injuries and syndromes all over the body, including back and neck pain.

Sports medicine is a natural for stem cell therapy, but very few sports doctors or pain management doctors utilize stem cells. Dr. Darrow's practice differs from Dr. Maharaj's practice, which focuses mainly on cancer, oncology, and rebuilding the immune system. Dr. Darrow is the go-to doctor for injuries, pain, and regenerative medicine, which is done by way of a natural injection series.

Prolotherapy is an early form of regenerative medicine that has progressed throughout the years to include platelet-rich plasma (PRP) and stem cell therapy.

Regenerative medicine involves injecting a dextrose solution, platelets from the blood, stem cells and platelets from bone marrow, or stem cells from fat into places where soft tissue is injured, such as the joints, muscles, tendons, or ligaments. Most recently, stem cells have been used from umbilical cord blood and other perinatal products from live births.

I have been Dr. Darrow's patient for "writer's back," a condition created by sitting too long at my computer while writing a book. He has also been able to successfully treat my son, Bruce Somers, who as a cyclist has had more accidents than a mother wants to know about. I find out by casually asking Dr. Darrow from time to time, "Have you seen Bruce lately?" to which he answers, "Oh, yes, he's here all the time." Sigh. He's a grown man. What's a mother to do? All I know is that he has no issues at present and I can thank Dr. Darrow for that.

SOMERS: Hello, Marc, so nice to speak with you. Stem cells: they are all the buzz, but you've been treating with stem cells in your Los Angeles clinic for quite some time. Stem cells and stem cell treatments seem to me a much better option than surgery in most cases. I feel there are a lot of unnecessary surgeries. Tell me what goes on in your office in a typical day. What did you do today?

DARROW: Thanks, Suzanne. Okay, I normally see about fifteen to twenty people a day, and we average about seventy bone marrow stem cell treatments per month for orthopedics. Also, in addition to that, we do maybe ten to fifteen platelet-rich plasma [PRP] injections for orthopedics per day. In the last few months, we started offering cord blood stem cells to our healing menu. We mix those with PRP.

SOMERS: Let's break that down so my reading audience knows what these treatments are. Let's start with the bone marrow.

DARROW: Okay. Bone marrow is a substance inside our bones that produces blood, stem cells, and things like exosomes and cytokines, things I am able to use to stimulate tissue growth.

The growth of the tissue I work with has to do with the musculoskeletal system, or orthopedics, as it's called. This goes from the top of the head, for instance with people getting headaches, to having a back or neck problem that causes headaches. It can also be injected into the C [cervical] spine or the neck and shoulders down the entire spine into the low back and, along the way, into the periphery of the shoulders and different muscles, elbows, wrists and fingers, plus hands, hips, knees, and the ankles and feet and toes. We typically heal muscle tears and all of these different conditions that get aggravated with arthritis and issues all the way down to the bottom of the feet, like plantar fasciitis, ankle arthritis—you name it.

Also, a big issue is meniscal tears in the knee and rotator cuff tears in the shoulders. Additionally, labral tears in the hip and the shoulders generally heal well using regenerative medicine.

Most areas of the body can be repaired without surgery, and most important for your readers to know about, Suzanne, is that we can no longer trust imaging to tell us where pain is being generated.

So if you have an MRI that shows that you have a meniscal tear, obviously a surgeon is the one that wants to get that image, because that shows him where he can cut.

But I always tell my patients, if you go to a barber, you get a haircut. If you go to a surgeon, you get a surgery. But that doesn't mean that the surgery ever should have been done. Research tells us that images do not necessarily correlate with pain. In other words, experiments are done doing imaging on people who have no pain. Guess what? Much of the time, pathology is seen that would normally be operated on if the patient had pain. And for the wrong reason. Conversely, patients with severe pain often have no imaging pathology at all.

SOMERS: I know that from my own experience. I tore my meniscus in my knee doing my one-woman Broadway show. It was a constant pain that was low, deliberate, steady, and throbbing. I went to a surgeon who said, "Well, we've got to cut out that tear." I told him I'd think about it, and then I thought, Cut out what? As in, you cut out the tear, then what do you leave? A scar, another tear?

Instead I went to you, where you injected prolotherapy using sugar water into my knee several times. Injections, not my favorite, haha, but today my knee is perfectly fine.

DARROW: And we now have studies. I just wrote a book that you were so delightful in writing the foreword to, called *Stem Cell and Platelet Therapy: Regenerate, Don't Operate.*

The book features 256 studies showing that surgery is no longer the way to go. It never really was, but now it's researched and shown that it usually doesn't work long term and that regenerative medicine using platelets and stem cells is safe and reliable.

We must be careful not to look at the imaging to decide where the pain generator is, because we could have someone that shows herniated disks in their back, facet arthropathy, or spinal stenosis, and the surgeon looks at the images and says that this patient should need surgery. And the person says, "But I don't have pain, Doc. Why do I need surgery?"

Now there are other ways to heal, and they are as simple as an injection.

I've been doing this work for over twenty years with amazing success. Eighty to ninety percent of our patients get better. No surgery. Just platelets or stem cells.

SOMERS: This all began because you had serious wrist and shoulder problems, right?

DARROW: Yes, it started with my wrist and shoulder, and those both healed, in fact, overnight.

SOMERS: One injection of PRP?

DARROW: No, this was back a long time ago before we knew about PRP. This was just the old prolotherapy using sugar water, like I used on your knee.

SOMERS: I'm grateful, but it wasn't the most pleasant experience, Marc.

DARROW: It's more pleasant today, because we now use an ultrasound, and we inject in the suprapatellar pouch, where it doesn't hurt. We can also numb the area for injection, or we can freeze it with a spray. There are a lot of ways to make it comfortable. Ask your son, Bruce. I mean, my God, I've treated him so many times.

SOMERS: He's Humpty Dumpty, and you've put him back together more times than I want to know.

DARROW: He is active.

SOMERS: Great (says the mother). It's exciting you're doing this work, because I believe there's no surgery that doesn't have consequences. Any time we can avoid it, I feel we are better off. When you need it, it's a godsend, but surgery is presented like it's a magic bullet, and it's not.

DARROW: Same with medications.

SOMERS: They may fix it, but now you've got something new that you never had before.

DARROW: That's right, and with the orthopedic procedures, Suzanne, those doctors are simply taking out tissue for the most part. Which poses the question: Why would someone want to take tissue out of the body and destabilize the area when we can grow the tissue back and make it stronger?

SOMERS: And you can regrow tissue with stem cells?

DARROW: Yes, that's what's so exciting about this work.

SOMERS: Where do you get stem cells themselves?

DARROW: There are many places to get them. Originally, we had two ways for years, but now there are three.

The first is from fat, adipose derived. I used to utilize fat, but I found it to be very abrasive on the patient; you've got to make an incision on the tummy or butt or thigh or somewhere else where you can grab some fat, depending on the patient's body habitus.

And then you've got to beat up the tissue in order to remove it. It's a liposuction, a miniliposuction, because, believe it or not, fat is very dense and firm. And once it's beat up and you aspirate it [suck it out], it is centrifuged to remove unwanted fluid. Then the bad part: you've got to use a very thick needle to inject the viscous fat. Some areas that I inject twenty or thirty times to cover the entire area could not tolerate a thick needle. Shoulders are like this. Not only is the joint and subdeltoid bursa injected but also the labrum and many points on the rotator cuff tendons.

With bone marrow–derived stem cells, it literally takes me, on average, ten to fifteen seconds with a drill to put a needle into the back of the pelvis—not into the spine but the back of the pelvis into a spot called the PSIS, or the posterior superior iliac spine. It's a very safe thing to do. I've done more than three thousand bone marrow aspirations. As a bonus, bone marrow contains stem cells, PRP, exosomes, and cytokines, which all assist in the tissue growth process.

SOMERS: Is the patient out while this is happening?

DARROW: No, it's not necessary. We use a local anesthetic injection, lidocaine, to numb the area.

SOMERS: That's good. I believe anesthetic kills brain cells. So many people taking anesthesia are cavalier about its long-term effects. You don't want to have lots of surgeries and lose valuable brain cells in the process. We're trying to hang on to the brain cells that we have.

DARROW: Sure, it's dangerous to put people out. I mean, let's face it, some people don't wake up from anesthesia.

SOMERS: Six or seven years ago I had my breast regrown from cancer surgery using my own stem cells. It's a remarkable success.

DARROW: At a stem cell seminar, I saw the case of a man whose jaw was partially destroyed by cancer. His surgeon inserted a scaffold and put stem cells around it. The last photos showed the jaw regrown and normal looking. This is an amazing result. The future of medicine is in the stem cell arena.

To recap, we have adipose-derived, bone marrow–derived. Obviously, we do not want to obtain **embryonic stem cells** from aborted fetuses. In eastern Europe, where abortion is a method of birth control, embryonic stem cells flourish. And today, we're testing the efficacy of **umbilical cord stem cells** from live births. There are many labs selling umbilical cord blood, placental tissue, and other perinatal cells to inject.

- The healing mechanisms of perinatal material can be shown in research as a repair activator through growth factors, immune system enhancer, and as an anti-inflammatory agent.

- The components of the perinatal cells help change the joint environment from degenerative to regenerative. There is research on that.

- There is controversy as to whether or not the stem cells in cord blood are alive at the time of injection, and it may be that the other healing elements in the solution are tissue productive.

- In addition, there is research showing that the healing mechanism of stem cells may be to awaken the nascent stem cells already in the patient's body.

SOMERS: Do you generally obtain stem cells from the patient you're working on at that time?

DARROW: In the past I was convinced that the best way to obtain stem cells was from the patient's bone marrow.

SOMERS: You can't reject yourself.

DARROW: That's right. But the new cells we are testing are not from the patient.

SOMERS: You are referring to umbilical cord blood, right?

DARROW: Yes.

SOMERS: Taking stem cells from the patient makes sense because you can't reject yourself. But my concern relative to cord blood is this: Are there any clean babies born anymore? With the present environmental assault, are there any clean wombs remaining where babies are grown? Mothers are innocent, never thinking their imbalanced microbiome, their leaky gut issues, and degraded immune systems as a result could negatively affect their babies' lives. So how do we know the cord blood is clean and safe?

DARROW: The umbilical cords are only taken from live births of healthy moms and healthy babies. Each mother is medically tested prior to her donation of the umbilical cord, and then the perinatal product is again tested by a lab—much as one would test blood prior to transfusion.

The fun part in the office is that when I offer bone marrow (with drilling the pelvis), patients laugh and tell me they'd rather have the cord blood cells.

I would also like to start administrating IV stem cells once I know that the FDA has no issues with it.

One of the experts in this area is Ahvie Herskowitz, MD, in San Francisco. Under clinical research protocols, he studies the efficacy of stem cells for autoimmune, cardiopulmonary, metabolic, and neuro-degenerative conditions.

SOMERS: Aging people have issues like arthritis requiring new hips, new knees, and my husband, Alan, now has titanium in his hip. (He didn't fall, he jumped.) Wouldn't it be wonderful if we could count on our joints and other body parts to work optimally throughout our entire life? So my question is: Are stem cells the answer?

DARROW: Well, it's one of the answers, but with something like a traumatic issue like hip fracture, it has to be operated on and replaced immediately to avoid a potential thrombus to the lungs or brain.

SOMERS: Let's talk practically. Someone like my eighty-two-year-old husband, Alan Hamel, comes in—because he was showing off for his wife and jumped off a six-foot wall—dislocated his hip, and the residual from that is a knee that's bothering him.

DARROW: Yeah, that's common, by the way.

SOMERS: Jumping off a wall? Haha! He doesn't have crushing pain but is aware of it, especially if it's cold. What would you do for him?

DARROW: Well, the first thing is an examination. See how the knee moves. See how it feels, then find out if there are any spots in the area that are red hot for him. I could use PRP [platelets from his blood]. That would be the easiest procedure in this scenario. If appropriate, I'd draw his blood, spin it in a centrifuge, and then inject it under ultrasound guidance. Please, never have a knee, shoulder, or hip injected without ultrasound guidance. The chances of the healing cells missing the joint are about one-third of the time unless the needle is visualized.

Or I could use cord blood stem cells or his bone marrow which contains platelets, exosomes, stem cells, cytokines, and several other growth factors in the solution. If it's advanced arthritis, then I'm going to go straight to the bone marrow or umbilical cord cells. If it's a good knee that was just sprained, then I'm going to just use the PRP.

SOMERS: Is this all done in your office in a day?

DARROW: Yes. It is so simple. You walk in, and you get the treatment. You walk out.

SOMERS: What do you do for shoulders?

DARROW: It is the same treatment I use in the shoulders. The entire body is treated in the same fashion. Since collagen is the structural protein of the body, regenerative medicine works all over. And collagen is the major constituent of cartilage.

SOMERS: I hear about frozen shoulders.

DARROW: My shoulder was frozen about a year and a half ago. It's perfect now. I have no pain. And by the way, I have a labral tear and two rotator cuff tendon tears.

SOMERS: What did you do?

DARROW: I self-injected my shoulder with amazing success.

SOMERS: With what?

DARROW: Well, I can't get stem cells from my bone marrow because I can't reach back there, so I just used PRP and umbilical cord blood cells.

SOMERS: Why do people's hips wear out as they get older?

DARROW: Typically, it's from osteoarthritis. Often it is traumatically in-duced from a fall or years of sports or yoga, but when a hip fractures, it's generally from osteoporosis, which you and I both know is from a decrease in hormones. If you can treat a person with bioidentical hormones, they can actually regrow the density of their bones. I've had women with severe osteoporosis who have grown back most of their bone structure in one year with hormone supplementation. But if you let it go for years and allow the bones to become fragile, it's more difficult later to strengthen the bones.

Studies have shown that a person's hip can fracture and cause a fall. You would think the fall caused the fracture, but it could be that osteoporosis was a precondition to the fracture and then the person falls. It could fracture either way.

SOMERS: Those are the skinny older ladies with protruding bellies. The belly is actually from vertebral fractures causing kyphosis of the spine pushing out the abdomen, and it's not really fat in the belly.

DARROW: Men have the same issue.

SOMERS: Can bone or cartilage be rebuilt? It has long been thought that once these tissues are gone, they are gone, and there's not been much you could do about it.

DARROW: Stem cells have changed this. With stem cells we can regrow cartilage in the joint, and now there are studies showing that bone can be regrown. The goal is avoiding surgery and eliminating pain.

SOMERS: When someone comes in with pain, do you want to see their X-ray or MRI?

DARROW: I always want to see imaging because it gives me an idea of the condition of the area, and I wouldn't want to miss something really important like a cancer.

SOMERS: Does it mean much to you when you see it?

DARROW: No, it doesn't mean much. There is a diagnostic code called "failed back surgery." What does that tell you? It means there are so many people that have failed surgeries that an insurance company must recognize it as a syndrome. My toughest job with patients is convincing them that they should not have surgery.

SOMERS: Belief is a big part of healing. If you believe you will heal, you will heal; conversely, if you don't believe it, most likely it won't work.

DARROW: Correct; if you don't believe in the treatment, you will resist on some level. I hope I'm wrong, but I see it over and over; that patient will most likely have shoulder replacements, and I have seen far too many of those that failed. One man came in for his right shoulder pain after a failed left shoulder replacement. He couldn't even move his left arm. The prosthesis didn't even fit into the shoulder joint, and his arm was useless.

SOMERS: So your clinic offers stem cell therapy along with PRP and prolotherapy. And you take the stem cells from the patient themselves?

DARROW: My practice is mostly PRP and stem cells at this point. I find that prolotherapy is a weaker healing agent than PRP or stem cells.

SOMERS: A friend of mine had a torn labrum.

DARROW: Yes. Shoulder or hip?

SOMERS: Hip. It became bone on bone from repeated surgeries and never got better. All I heard was there's nothing you can do about labrum. How do you react to that?

DARROW: I treat labral tears every single day and have even treated my own. *Labrum* means "lip" in Latin, and the labrum is like a lip around the bone that holds it in the joint. I've injected endless hip labra with amazing success. I've self-injected my shoulder labrum with one hundred percent success. We don't know when we look at an MRI or an X-ray or a CT if what we see is the pain generator. You can have a labral tear and not have any pain, so I imagine what this doctor said to this gentleman: "You have a labral tear. I have to fix it, or I have to cut it out." By cutting, I can assure you he caused more problems; in fact, the surgery probably caused the arthritis or the bone on bone. When you take out tissue, what is left?

And even bone on bone is not typically an issue in healing. I hear the term all day long, and when I do the exam, I often laugh and tell the patient that they really don't have bone on bone, or the joint would not even move.

SOMERS: This person is in show business. As a result, he has a doctor waiting who shoots him up with painkillers midshow so he can get through the second half.

DARROW: Does he give him cortisone shots?

SOMERS: Yes.

DARROW: Yeah, well, guess what cortisone does to the cartilage? It disintegrates it. Yes, the patient feels better for a while, but it's a long-term catastrophe. You win the battle and lose the war.

SOMERS: So it's this ongoing, never-going-to-get-better situation. There's no changing him. He believes he's with the best doctors. I've gone to more funerals lately for the people who had the "best doctors."

And what can you do for back pain?

DARROW: Most low back and neck pain is from sprained ligaments. Another word is *enthesis*. Most of people's neck and back pain, and I don't care what the MRI shows, is from an enthesopathy. An enthesis is the connection of muscle, tendon, or ligament to bone. So if someone has low back pain and they have a herniated disk and some other wild diagnosis, when I touch their back, instantly I can tell them if I can help them, because I reach for the spot of the enthesis, and when that's inflamed, it hurts. You touch it, and they say, "Ouch." That can't be a herniated disk, which is deep inside the body. The ligaments are fairly superficial in comparison. And studies have shown that with regenerative injections, the ligaments can thicken and be strengthened with resolution of the pain.

SOMERS: I also hear a lot about sciatic issues. Is that something stem cells can help?

DARROW: It depends. I hear the word *sciatica* every day. If it truly is an impinged sciatic nerve, that's a problem that may need surgical intervention. The good news is studies show that ninety-four percent of them go away by themselves. We don't know how long it'll take, but ninety-four percent go away without a doctor's help.

SOMERS: Does sciatic damage cause nerve damage?

DARROW: If it is true sciatica, it can be impingement on a nerve, which can cause permanent damage in the form of leg pain or weakness. It can also be bone overgrowth, as in spinal stenosis. It could be a herniated disk that's popping out and sitting on it. Those are the two main reasons for nerve damage.

It could be facet arthropathy. The facets are the joints between the vertebrae, and if they become arthritic, they start to overgrow and hypertrophy, and then you get what are called osteophytes. *Osteo* is bone, and *phyte* is the overgrowth that can press on a nerve. The foramen, which are the holes between the vertebrae where the nerves from the spinal cord exit and go down the arms and legs, can be impinged upon and then cause pain or weakness down the arm or leg.

PRP and my other treatments may not work for this; oftentimes that person needs to see a chiropractor. Randy Weinzoff, DC, in Santa Monica is where I send all my sciatica patients, and he fixes them. How does he do it? He realigns the body. The first time I heard about him, I referred a patient with sciatica. He was a middle-aged gentleman with what I'm going to call a dead left leg. I said, "I can't help you. Let me send you to my friend down the street." He went, and in one treatment the guy's leg came back to life.

SOMERS: That is generous of you. He'll be happy to be in this book.

Going forward, I see myself living a long time. I can easily wrap around 110 years with the way I take care of myself. I'm against all drugs unless absolutely necessary. I want to see how few drugs I ever have to take for the rest of my life. It's been ten years since I've had an antibiotic or, frankly, anything.

What I like about your approach to pain and regenerating broken parts and rebuilding bone is that yours is a nondrug therapy. Limiting foreign molecules in the body can only be good. I believe this gives the edge, allowing for the new long, extended life that we can take advantage of starting right now.

You must feel good at the end of each day that you're doing this work.

DARROW: I feel good every minute. I truly want to see the world happy. I know we all have that in us. My part in the puzzle is to regenerate people's bodies. I love helping people, and I feel upbeat and excited about life, the love in my life, and my work.

I teach patients about meditation as a possibility for healing; that their pain could be a manifestation of some hidden emotional issues, and to ask in meditation what really is going on that brought them to this point. It often resonates.

SOMERS: People will do anything to get rid of pain. The most sound-minded person in extreme pain will take any drug to just stop it. What you are doing is exciting, especially given the opioid crisis, which sadly is leading to suicides and unhappiness. Your work in alleviating pain without surgery and drugs is a true gift to humanity.

DARROW: Thank you. As to opioids, the first thing I do with a person on opioids is to wean them off. Opioids upregulate pain receptors and make patients more sensitive to their pain. Then they need more medicine, and then they're addicted. I always tell people, don't be seduced by a surgery, by a quick fix, or by drugs; that route will take you down a slippery slope.

SOMERS: You genuinely seem to enjoy your work and love your patients. You have a kindness about you.

DARROW: I like taking care of people. It gives me the greatest joy.

SOMERS: It's a beautiful thing and a beautiful way to live. I always say if you live in gratitude, it leaves room for little else.

CHAPTER 19

NON-THC CANNABIS FOR PAIN

The new epidemic in the United States and most other parts of the world is the **opioid crisis**. In most cases, normal people who are riddled with pain have no means of relief except for strong pharmaceuticals. Eventually they become reliant on them and develop a need for stronger and stronger drugs—all with side effects—requiring yet more drugs to address the problem.

Cannabis users are familiar with the well-known cannabinoids THC and CBD, the therapeutic compounds that have provided an abundance of medicinal relief for various medical conditions, including nausea, inflammation, and pain.

Cannabinoids and their terpenoid cousins are chemicals that provide relief by acting on special receptors that are found in the cells and tissue of the human body. They are among the more than 480 natural components that make up the cannabis plant.

These special receptors form part of what is known as the **endocannabinoid system (ECS)**. This system helps modulate many bodily functions, including anxiety level, appetite, and cognition; it is intimately connected to the immune system and nervous system. Interestingly, certain cannabinoids produced by the cannabis plant target particular types of receptors found on the surface of the cells in various areas of the body.

If substances originating in the cannabis plant can have similar ac-

tivity as molecules that exist in the human body, is there reason to believe that they can have therapeutic effects as well? Is there a better way,
a natural way, to eliminate the need for strong addictive pharmaceuticals? Many individuals suffering from pain could find significant relief
without undertaking serious risk to their lives, and the opioid epidemic
could be curtailed.

Interview with
DR. JONATHAN M. FISHBEIN

I asked Dr. Jonathan M. Fishbein, a physician with thirty-two years of professional experience in clinical research and the executive director of the Kavana Research Initiative, whether cannabinoids, particularly the nonpsychoactive ones such as CBD, can be an antidote for pain.

SOMERS: Thanks, Dr. Fishbein, for your time. We all know humans will do anything to get rid of pain; even those who normally would never abuse drugs are susceptible. I have friends in the entertainment business who won't have a glass of wine, but they are all loaded up on oxycontin due to pain. Can CBD shut off the pain signal?

FISHBEIN: A substantial impact on the opioid crisis can be made if it can be definitively demonstrated that CBD alleviates pain. Anecdotally, there is plenty of evidence that it does, and published research suggests it's very promising. But not all CBD is created equal, and the quality and quantity of CBD can vary significantly from supplier to supplier. There have been studies published that show a lot of the products on the market don't contain the quantity of CBD they state on the label. Fraudulent products can be cut with coconut oil and contain very little CBD. Furthermore, some have detectable levels of heavy metals, toxins, and pesticides, so they actually can be hazardous to your health. A reputable manufacturer will not make health claims. That is patently illegal. Health claims require approval from the FDA and are substantiated by multiple clinical studies. Because there is so much interest in CBD's therapeutic potential, it is not surprising that unscrupulous manufacturers have emerged to take advantage of consumers. But legitimate suppliers do indeed exist, and they have recommended the FDA adapt stringent regulations to protect the public.

SOMERS: I guess that's why you talk to some people and one person will say, "I had great results," and the next person says it did nothing.

FISHBEIN: I'm a physician, and I've been working with the pharmaceutical and biotech industry for a long time. Again, much of what the public believes about CBD and pain relief is based upon anecdotal evidence. We are very committed to finding out whether CBD has a lot of therapeutic value, and so far, the research shows a great deal of promise.

CBD is produced from the two major species of cannabis plants, hemp and marijuana, but marijuana also contains THC, the psychoactive intoxicating substance that makes marijuana a federally controlled substance. Some of the suppliers who sell CBD have a product that contains more THC than is legally allowed. The THC content is not to exceed 0.3 percent by dry weight, by law. But aside from the quality of the product, individual variability in people's response to CBD could be a function of genetics, age, gender, type of pain or injury, even the use of concomitant medication.

SOMERS: So that's what we should be looking for with pain management?

FISHBEIN: The first thing one should look for is a high-quality CBD product that does not include THC. Then the product's use must be supported by research. For a manufacturer to receive approval for their CBD product, rigorous clinical trials to prove its safety and efficacy must be conducted. As we speak today, CBD has been approved by the FDA for only the narrowest of indications: two rare forms of childhood seizures. I should also note: CBD has not been approved as a food additive.

SOMERS: What's the difference between CBD, CBG, and CBN?

FISHBEIN: Actually, there are 144 different cannabinoids identified by their molecular structures. THC and CBD are the major cannabinoids. THC has the psychoactive intoxicating properties, and it remains a federally controlled substance. CBD makes up forty percent of the extract of a single hemp flower. That amount may vary depending on the particular strain. The precursor molecule by which the cannabis plant produces all the other cannabinoids is cannabigerol, or CBG, one of the earliest cannabinoids identified. Along with another related substance, cannabinol [CBN], CBG is undergoing extensive preclinical testing to determine whether it may have therapeutic potential.

SOMERS: That's a bit confusing.

FISHBEIN: Aside from the potential usefulness of any one particular cannabinoid, the really big story here is the emerging understanding of the endocannabinoid system, as scientists are learning more about how it regulates many different functions in our body. The discovery of cannabinoids in the 1960s by Dr. Raphael Mechoulam opened our eyes to the existence of the ECS [endocannabinoid system], a previously unknown system within the human body which profoundly effects our physiology. To find out definitively whether administering a single plant-derived cannabinoid or a combination of these exogenous substances can evoke a therapeutic effect is a huge scientific undertaking, and many established researchers are taking up the challenge.

SOMERS: Could CBD unlock brain receptors? I'm asking because I've read there are powerful endocannabinoid pain receptors in the brain and I'm wondering: Could this be a key to understanding Alzheimer's?

FISHBEIN: Perhaps, but it is a very complicated answer; we have to find out. CBD can do many things, but we need to do the clinical work to really understand in great detail. We know there are receptors in certain parts of the brain that control pain and the endocannabinoid system is part of that pain control system. We've talked about its role in pain, but it also regulates appetite, mood, memory, and immune function. It appears to have neuroprotective properties, which means that there are implications in the treatment of stroke and traumatic brain injury. Many researchers have postulated that manipulating the ECS could have benefits in slowing the progression of Parkinsonism, ALS, and Huntington's disease.

SOMERS: The possibilities seem endless, considering how many different functions the endocannabinoid system serves.

FISHBEIN: The fascinating thing about the human body is its redundancy. There are many systems that work in harmony to regulate our bodily functions. Just where cannabinoids like CBD work best, or even work at all, is what scientists are actively trying to learn. There is so much ahead of us to study, but that's what makes this such an exciting field right now.

SOMERS: If there are endocannabinoid receptors throughout your body, then it sounds like this is something the human body wants or craves; that nature provided this substance and we've been ignoring it all these years because we got sidetracked by the rock 'n' rollers who were stoned all the time and it got labeled bad. You were saying it affects mood, so does it affect your serotonin levels?

FISHBEIN: Yes, it affects dopamine.

SOMERS: Dopamine.

DOPAMINE

In the brain, **dopamine** functions as a neurotransmitter, a chemical released by neurons (nerve cells) to send signals to other nerve cells. The brain includes several distinct dopamine pathways, one of which plays a major role in the motivational component of reward-motivated behavior.

FISHBEIN: Maybe the rock 'n' rollers were onto something the rest of us didn't know! What we do know is that cannabis is one of the oldest medicinal plants known to man. And it was commonly used in this country as such into the twentieth century. But once cannabis was designated as an illegal substance, it created a stigma and the medical community shunned it for decades.

SOMERS: I write so much about hormones and dopamine receptors in the brain, and I know firsthand that women truly suffer until they get their hormones balanced. CBD sounds like it could be an antidote for perimenopausal and menopausal moodiness, right?

FISHBEIN: Actually, speaking of women's health, one of the places where the cannabinoid receptors are very concentrated is in the uterus. Extensive research is under way in Israel in regard to the role of the ECS in fertility and fetal development, as well as endometriosis and its associated pain.

SOMERS: As a clinical trialist, you straddle the natural versus the pharmaceutical worlds. How do you bring these two worlds together?

FISHBEIN: They overlap considerably, so it isn't hard to reconcile. Whether a product is considered "natural" or a drug, we look for the same things: safety and efficacy. And there are many natural substances that have been evaluated thoroughly as drugs and are a major part of our therapeutic armamentarium: cyclosporin, digitalis, taxol, penicillin, and quinine, to name just a few. The advantage for a natural product to be designated a drug is that extensive research must be conducted so it can earn its labeling claim. With the drug designation, CBD can now be subjected to rigorous clinical trials to demonstrate safety and effectiveness in a wide variety of disorders. But what is particularly exciting to me about cannabis is the sheer number of substances that can be tested and the broad spectrum of disorders where they may possibly have a therapeutic effect.

SOMERS: Off the top of your head, can you list the potential for conditions people are suffering today that could be helped by cannabinoids?

FISHBEIN: Let's see . . . spinal cord injury, PTSD, mood disorders, anxiety, obesity and other eating disorders, insomnia, autism, osteoporosis, glaucoma, myocardial infarction, drug addiction, nausea. These are all disorders that appear to have an endocannabinoid component, and preclinical and clinical research is under way.

SOMERS: We've already talked about epilepsy and Alzheimer's.

FISHBEIN: Responsible growers and manufacturers produce product that is consistent and of the highest quality. The product in every lot, every bottle, every pill or oil is always the same. Companies devoted to excellence do things according to good manufacturing practices.

SOMERS: What I'm getting from you is CBD could possibly be nature's remedy because we have endocannabinoid receptor sites all throughout our body, almost as if the body has been waiting for this. You just mentioned the possibilities and potential. Could this be the most explosive thing that's happened to medicine in our lifetimes?

FISHBEIN: Perhaps you are right. We may have found a class of natural products, the cannabinoids, that can have a major impact on public health and improve the quality of life for so many.

SOMERS: I know when something hits my passion button. I feel emotional when you are saying this because it sounds like this could be so very important. Thank you, Dr. Fishbein.

CHAPTER 20

ENERGY MEDICINE

Your body is this orchestra in which these organs and glands are instruments in that orchestra. Some are sluggish and out of tune. Some are strong and in tune. My goal is to find out what is sluggish and out of tune and get it strong and in tune so the orchestra plays better music.

—Dr. Michael Galitzer

The above quote encapsulates the work of energy medicine. When I first started working with Dr. Galitzer, I was intrigued by the fact that he could test for energy in my various glands and organs. What a spectacular idea. What ages us? The answer is: worn-out parts (organs and glands). Therefore, if along the way we could constantly be checking for optimal output of each organ and gland, we could catch aging, disease, or breakdown before it has a chance to get a stronghold.

I feel it puts me ahead of the game. I feel as though I'm onto something. There will be no surprises for me of a kidney that fails or a liver that betrays; rather the testing will tell me long before the possibility of a catastrophic event that there is a problem, and then I can get to work to fix it.

This is why I felt it so important to include Dr. Galitzer in the "cutting-edge" section of this book. This is advanced medicine; it works to alert me when something is amiss. Dr. Galitzer is my primary care physician. I rely on him to be the "alpha" doc overseeing my health. He's helped me though all my health challenges, including cancer. I trust him implicitly and he is always learning, going to conferences, to be "in the know." His work is part of my regular check on my health, my aging progress, and my desire to remain in optimal health.

Interview with

DR. MICHAEL GALITZER

Dr. Michael Galitzer is my antiaging doctor. He's the guy I go to for aches, pains, mineral IVs, and chelation, but most of all to keep a check on the energy of my internal parts, such as organs and glands. Aging is about a loss of energy, so his specialty is especially pertinent to those of us who want to stay vital and energetic. His clinic is in Santa Monica, California. He treats without drugs for the most part, using them only when absolutely necessary. He is also an expert in bioidentical hormones and homeopathic medicine.

SOMERS: You spent fifteen years as an emergency room doctor until you needed to move on. So many ER docs I've interviewed all say the same thing: at some point the emergency room is so stressful that you must make a major change. But how can you go back to normal doctoring?

GALITZER: I found the integrative and alternative world a natural transition, as it is a business that is constantly changing and growing exponentially, with cutting-edge breakthroughs happening at a pace that's difficult to keep up with and that provide the passion and excitement. There are three ways medicine can assess the body: *physical*, *chemical*, and *electrical* or *energetic*. When I was a board-certified ER doctor, most traditional medicine was physical or chemical.

SOMERS: Please explain *physical* and *chemical*.

GALITZER: *Physical* are X-rays, CT scans, MRIs, biopsies, mammograms—they look for structural changes. *Chemical* are blood tests, but those really look for diseases and traditional medicine believes that health is the absence of disease. I believe physical and chemical are exact opposites: health is on one end, and disease is on the other.

SOMERS: Most people don't know what antiaging doctors do, and certainly most patients have never heard of "electrical" testing.

GALITZER: In order to analyze health, you have got to go beyond the physical and the chemical and look at the *electrical*. A cardiologist looks at the electrical heart because the electrical impulse of the heart precedes the physical heartbeat. A neurologist looks at the electrical brain. There are also the electrical liver, kidneys, pancreas, adrenals, and thyroid.

Your body is this orchestra in which these organs and glands are instruments in that orchestra. Some are sluggish and out of tune. Some are strong and in tune. My goal is to find out what is sluggish and out of tune and get it strong and in tune so the orchestra plays better music.

SOMERS: Lovely metaphor.

GALITZER: Part two is toxins. In the ER we were concerned about life-threatening toxins—overdose of sleeping pills, carbon monoxide poisoning, oil spills—but in this new medicine we are looking at chronic low-level toxicity. Pesticides, heavy metals, chemicals, viruses, bacteria, yeast, over-the-counter medications, prescription medicines, these are all chemicals also. The goal is to reduce toxicity, because when toxins accumulate in the body, the body doesn't work as well as it should. That's the overall assessment of a patient, in addition to blood tests and X-ray studies that people frequently bring in to me.

SOMERS: You often mention **bioimpedance**; can you explain?

GALITZER: Bioimpedance looks at body fat, body water, but more importantly, something called the *phase angle*, which is a measure of regeneration. Our bodies are always destroying old cells and strengthening or creating new cells. The phase angle tells us how well we are regenerating and how well we are creating new cells.

The last thing I do in addition to a physical examination is look at heart rate variability. The autonomic nervous system is the subconscious nervous system, where all your old emotions are stored. The autonomic nervous system has two parts: the *sympathetic*, which is *energy producing*, and the *parasympathetic*, which is *energy recovery*. The healthier the autonomic nervous system, the healthier the heart.

SOMERS: Would I be correct in calling this energy medicine?

GALITZER: Yes, because health is energy. The energetic level of the body correlates to how people feel. I have people come in with normal blood tests and X-rays but they are fatigued or they can't sleep or they have allergies or their joints hurt. Their doctors tell them, "Hey, you look okay to me." Well, that's on the physical and chemical level, but on the electrical level they don't look okay. They are toxic, their liver is overloaded, their adrenals are tired. Being able to assess that overload and help people is a great thing for people.

SOMERS: Nice. At less expense and no poking with needles.

GALITZER: Yes. So I thought if this protocol could figure out which are the energy-drained organs and glands found noninvasively without blood, I wanted to learn. I went to see the physician from Europe who was conducting his first seminar—December of 1986—and after listening to his seminar I realized the tremendous value of this protocol and I have been doing it ever since.

SOMERS: You use a screening called electrodermal, and I used to make you annoyed by calling it hocus-pocus and I never meant to do that, especially since I find the readings from this machine so accurate. I have great respect for electrodermal screenings. Explain what it actually does.

GALITZER: The real value in electrodermal testing is to find out specifically what food, nutrient, herb, homeopathic, and even medication—sometimes it's needed, as in high blood pressure or antidepressant medications—works for that person.

SOMERS: It's an individualized assessment which allows you to exactly give the right thing to the right person?

GALITZER: Yes, eventually what you are trying to find, Suzanne, is if it's effective and if it's tolerated. That means does it work, is it effective, are there no side effects, and is it tolerated?

An example of something that's effective and probably tolerated is cancer chemotherapy; it kills cancer cells but has a whole lot of side effects. But if we can find out what's effective and what's tolerated and what works for that individual person and what supplement can work for one person and not work for the other, we are ahead of the game.

We are all different, but you know about the person who drinks a cup of coffee in the morning who can't sleep at night, and then there is another person who can drink coffee right before they go to sleep and sleep fine? We are all different in our ability to break down and metabolize substances, so the real value of electrodermal testing is to find out exactly what will work for that person, which is a huge breakthrough.

SOMERS: It was interesting in rereading your book about fascia [fascia are the connective tissues below the skin and around muscles]. My understanding of fascia is similar to when you peel an orange and you get rid of the skin but there is always this sort of white web that's around the orange itself that you peel off called the fascia. I know in yoga I have fascia right under the skin between the skin and the muscles, and we are always trying to break that down and soften that to eliminate cellulite. Not that I have any! Haha. How does that work in your approach to health?

GALITZER: This connective tissue is called mesenchyme and is the interface between the blood vessels and the cells.

SOMERS: Why do I care?

GALITZER: You're funny. So the heart pumps the blood and the blood goes into the aorta and then to the arteries and arterioles and finally down to the capillary. The capillary then delivers oxygen and sugar (or glucose) to the cells to create energy. The connective tissue is important because that interface between the cell and the capillary is where nutrients are delivered and toxins are removed.

SOMERS: The magnificence of the human body—what a journey.

GALITZER: Connective tissue is vitally important, and the health of that connective tissue can be helped with all sorts of procedures I do in my office like liver drainage, lymph drainage, and kidney drainage. When we get these organs to work optimally, the connective tissue is able to function at its highest level.

There are only a few people in this country who practice this kind of medicine and certainly not many physicians.

SOMERS: You've found a very unique niche, and that's why people come from all over the world. I have seen people in your office from Indonesia, Europe, and Asia, and I'm always impressed that somehow the word has gotten out. People spend years trying to figure out what's wrong with them and keep hitting allopathic walls where finally pills don't work; then they hear about you. When they sit down for the first time, what are the usual complaints?

GALITZER: They don't have enough energy. Their body's ability to handle stress in their lives has been severely compromised, their toxicity level is very high. People feel if they eat organic, meditate, or exercise, that's all they have to do. Exercise is key, but people are toxic and have low energy, and the symptoms are a result of that combination.

SOMERS: Do you start with hormones?

GALITZER: Absolutely. But it's more than that. The initial complaints are usually "I don't have enough 'juice,' I don't have the energy I used to have, I can't focus, I can't concentrate like I used to, my memory is a problem, my sleep is a problem."

Sleep is a game changer. They also complain their digestion is off, that they bloat after meals or they bloat all the time. Women complain about this more often than guys. They also say they can't lose weight no matter what they do.

My approach is first do bioimpedance, then after the physical I take a look at their blood tests and X-rays and everything else that they bring in. The bioimpedance tells me their regeneration potential, and if the regeneration potential is good, then I am quite confident they are going to get better pretty quickly.

The second part is the heart rate variability, that gives me information about the heart and the parasympathetic nervous system. The sympathetic is "How fast did you run the hundred-yard dash?," whereas the parasympathetic is "How long did it take for you to get your breath back?" The parasympathetic is most important because most people are sympathetically driven and can't relax and can't recover as well as they should.

THE PARASYMPATHETIC NERVOUS SYSTEM

The **parasympathetic nervous system**, organwise, corresponds to the liver and the adrenals. The liver is the major organ that removes toxins from the body. It is also an organ that has to process all the foods we eat and absorb, whereas the adrenals are glands that are more affected by stress. Stress can be in the form of mental stress, emotional stress, nutritional stress, or eating food you are allergic to, such as gluten or dairy products. Environmental stress means you are exposed to pesticides. Electromagnetic stress is when you are talking to your friend, holding your cell phone to your ear for an hour.

SOMERS: Is physical stress damaging to the adrenals?

GALITZER: Yes. Imagine you have had surgery or you are hurt at the gym or you contract infectious bacteria or viruses. Whenever there is a stressor, the adrenals create the stress hormones, noticeably cortisol, which is the major stress hormone. If the stress recurs for too long a period of time or if there are multiple stresses occurring at the same time, the adrenals get tired, the cortisol goes down, and with that your ability to handle stress goes down. Your body can't differentiate big stress from little stress, so you overreact to little things, and ultimately you are going to get anxious.

Imagine if you wake up in the morning and your brain is having a conversation with your adrenals and your brain says, "Look, I got a lot on my plate today. I have got to do this, this, this, and that, and I know you can secrete hormones to get me through the day." The adrenals say, "I have got nothing to give you. You are going to be anxious, because you don't have the reserves to deal with the stressors of the day."

SOMERS: Interesting: adrenal fatigue, inability to sleep, is because your cortisol is off. It's a cascade. A meltdown.

GALITZER: Correct. I find adrenals to be weak and tired in just about everybody, and there is the thinking that you can't sleep because your cortisol levels are high at night. But what I see is the exact opposite: most people's cortisol and adrenal function are too low. Basically, they need adrenal support. The key nutrient for the adrenals is vitamin C.

I utilize a lot of vitamin C intravenously. Ninety-five percent of the people I see have suboptimal adrenal gland functioning.

SOMERS: The major and minor hormones work in concert with one another, and when the minors are off, the majors—insulin, thyroid, adrenals, and cortisol—are off, producing either not enough or too much, depending.

GALITZER: The body wants balance with thyroid and adrenal hormones. I liken it to running your Ferrari around the racetrack, and of course you would put high-octane fuel into this car; I see the thyroid as the fuel injection system and the adrenals as the gas pedal. If you have low insulin but optimal thyroid and adrenals, the Ferrari is going to take off as long as you are feeding it high-octane fuel. The adrenals are paramount, and in women adrenals represent survival and the stress response. The ovaries represent reproduction.

The body always wants to maintain the "stress and survival" response and frequently at the expense of reproduction. Here's how it works: If the adrenals are tired—and this most often will happen with women in their forties and early fifties—the body will start shunting progesterone to the ovaries and cortisol to the adrenals. Then estrogen goes to the ovaries, which in turn shunts DHEA to the adrenals, all in order to maintain survival at the expense of reproduction. In this scenario a woman gets depleted in progesterone and estrogen and consequently goes into perimenopause and menopause.

The adrenals affect the ovaries more often than the other way around. When people come in with premenopause or menopausal symptoms, you not only have to replace the progesterone and estrogen, but you also have to strengthen the adrenals so you are not shunting those hormones that put a woman back to maintaining survival.

SOMERS: So it's nature perpetuating the species. And it's also alchemy. This is all each individual's complex chemistry, right?

GALITZER: Right. Absolutely.

SOMERS: This "new way to age" requires detective work, a new approach. I don't remember the last time you ordered a blood test on me; you seem to get more out of bioenergetics.

I've started taking my 20 milligrams of cortisol all in the morning, rather than spreading it out throughout the day, and I have so much more energy. Why is that?

GALITZER: Normally your cortisol is highest in the morning. Your own adrenal glands produce about 20 milligrams daily and in some people 30 milligrams a day. So giving you 20 milligrams cortisol is still physiological, and if you get sick, that is when you double the dose.

SOMERS: Do you treat the heart?

GALITZER: I see heart patients, cancer patients. I see cancer as a tug-of-war: the energy of the cancer person and the energy of the body.

Traditional medicine tries to win the tug-of-war by killing the bad guys. Unfortunately, then the good guys are weakened. My approach has always been to strengthen the body, and I thoroughly believe that people with cancer can get better with chemotherapy or with immunotherapy as long as somebody is paying attention to the body. This thing about chemo only working five percent of the time, and maybe that's true, but my experience has been that if you give intravenous vitamin C on the weeks between chemo, and if you strengthen the liver, the adrenals, and work at controlling the stress and worry of having cancer, you've got a good shot at winning. **Everybody with cancer has weak adrenals, and you need to know that chemo kills cancer cells but all that chemical debris has to be cleared by the liver, so supporting the liver is crucial for survival.** So if you are supporting the adrenals and supporting the rest of the organs in the body, people seem to do better.

You have got to win the tug-of-war, and the only way to win the tug-of-war is to make a concerted effort to support the body. My approach has always been to honor the belief system of the patient but tell the patient that you have to go both ways.

SOMERS: Any patient that has cancer and is on chemotherapy must understand the concept that if you are breaking down, you've got to build it up.

GALITZER: The real mandate for us as we get older is a continual need to optimize our cardiovascular system. Exercise is key, and that's one of the hard things to do when you are sick. Traditional medicine has two weaknesses: an inability to motivate patients to change and an inability to show people how to change. Motivation is key; people need to exercise. I put my patients on the Sonix vibrational machine just to get their body moving. They seem to like that a lot. Then I use the EECP [enhanced external counter pulsation], which improves blood flow throughout the body. It's a great technology for a lot of people. CoQ10 is also a great nutrient for the heart, as is the herb hawthorn.

SOMERS: One of the nicest things that happened to me this year was being in your office when you asked me how I was feeling and I said, "I think I am the happiest I have ever been in my life." And then you used your bioimpedance testing and went "Whoa!" and said my oxytocin [the "love and sex" hormone] was off the charts.

I thought about that because for years I've practiced gratitude in my daily meditations. It's the first thing I do every morning. I wake up and thank God for the life I live and the life that I was able to create. How important is happiness relative to health?

GALITZER: It's critical. The Beatles said it so well: "All you need is love." I can measure oxytocin or oxytocin energy, so to speak, and I find it so important in treating my patients. I think guys don't have nearly as much oxytocin as women because women are mothers. They deliver babies and as a rule are more intuitive and more connected to the world than men. There are, of course, exceptions. Interestingly, I find cancer patients don't have enough oxytocin. I actually believe that cancer fills in the space that love is supposed to fill in, as in: Were you loved as a kid? Do you deserve love? Are you loving in your relationship with your wife or husband? Do you love your kids? Do your kids love you? How do you express love?

All of that is reflected in oxytocin levels, and you, obviously, are extremely loving and have high levels. Women with cancer, I can tell you, don't have enough love in their life. Men would actually benefit from taking a little bit of oxytocin, especially the hard-driving men that aren't too concerned about other people's feelings. They could probably use a little oxytocin.

SOMERS: Am I loving because I make high levels of oxytocin, or do I have high oxytocin, which then makes me a more loving being?

GALITZER: Don't know, but it's something I prescribe when it feels called for. I actually take it from time to time, especially when I am seeing patients at the office. In the kind of work I do I am always holding hands with people, and you pick up a lot of energy that way, frequently good energy but not always good energy, and so while I am a little flustered and a little irritable, I find oxytocin sublingually is wonderful.

SOMERS: One of the things I find so enjoyable about writing a book is when things manifest that I don't plan. I love free form. Throughout this book the importance of our thoughts and that *thoughts create* keeps arising as a theme; that we are in charge of our health and happiness by the thoughts we think and that if we grew up in an environment that wasn't emotionally healthy, our job as adults is to recognize who we are—or aren't—and do the work that we can to change it. Do you concur that thoughts are that important?

GALITZER: Absolutely. I used to have this thing that was on the wall in the office that said, "Thoughts that make you happy make you well." The three key things in life are purpose, passion, and gratitude. You talked about gratitude earlier. But your purpose: Why are you here? What's your vision? What's your goal? What's your dream? If you find your purpose and let your purpose drive you, they are very important elements to happiness. The people that don't do well are the people that focus on what they don't have or what they don't control.

Then the hormones that really make people feel good, as you have written about so extensively, Suzanne: estrogen, progesterone, testosterone for women, and testosterone for men. These are important.

If you are a big guy and your blood test for testosterone is a range of 300 to 1,000 [nanograms per deciliter] and you are at 400, well, you didn't get to be a big guy by having a testosterone level of 400 when you were twenty years old. So as you age, men and women need more testosterone.

Natural bioidentical hormones, when used in a program that addresses toxicity and hormonal balance, exercise, and optimal nutrition all together, have an antiaging effect. This keeps your brain sharp and your heart strong.

SOMERS: I don't know who I would be without my bioidentical hormones.

GALITZER: I agree, they do keep one happy and upbeat.

SOMERS: There is a myth out there that you take hormones for a while and then you don't need them. That is not true; once you drain out, you are never going to rev up again, so once you start hormone replacement, it's a commitment for life.

GALITZER: Yes, and you will feel so good you will want to be committed to this for life.

SOMERS: It's a simple thing to do, rubbing on some cream every day.

You started talking about NuCalm. What is it, and why have you been so very enthusiastic about it? Is this because our stress levels are so off the charts that here is a nondrug protocol that allows you to calm yourself down and destress?

GALITZER: To be healthy, you need energy coherence; that means the cells need to talk to one another and have proper signaling. The autonomic nervous system is part of the signaling process, sending impulses to the sympathetic and parasympathetic nervous system.

Most people have an imbalance. If their sympathetic nervous system is too strong and their parasympathetic nervous system is too weak, it's not good; a great example is a heart attack.

The new research seems to indicate that people who get heart attacks have an underlying weak parasympathetic nervous system and then they get a sympathetic stress. That stress can be an emotional outburst, anger outburst, or physically exercising too much can throw these systems out of balance and cause the heart to get acidic. Then the heart swells, the coronary artery gets smaller, clots form, and you have a heart attack.

But if you have a strong parasympathetic nervous system, you could handle any sympathetic stress, and we have sympathetic stresses every day. NuCalm has been proven through heart rate variability to strengthen the parasympathetic or relaxation or energy recovery nervous system. With NuCalm you put on headphones and listen to music, but underneath the music there are brain frequencies that put you into what's called alpha and theta states. When you and I are talking, we are in beta; that means our brains are beating twelve to twenty times a second. Alpha is the meditation state, so the brain slows down to eight to twelve beats per second, and theta is a deep kind of dreamlike creative state where the brain goes between four and seven beats per second.

NuCalm takes you from your heightened thinking state into a calm or relaxed alpha and theta state. Doing it for thirty minutes relieves stress. Sleep is enhanced, and people feel so much better.

SOMERS: Where can my reader get NuCalm?

GALITZER: Well, there is a website, nucalm.com.

SOMERS: You are the new version of the old country doctor, just in a much more sophisticated way. I come to you because I want you to figure out my "body language": my aches and pains, bloating, constipation, moods, dry skin, and the things that go wrong as we age. All issues of "body language" are actually your body telling you something is wrong or "off." This, I believe, is the kind of care people are looking for, this is what people want; we don't want a prescription pad anymore.

GALITZER: Yes, people want to feel great. That's why I titled my book *Outstanding Health*.

SOMERS: It's exciting as a patient. I am as happy as you said that I tested. I feel it every day. Thank you for your pearls of wisdom.

GALITZER: It is my privilege to assist in the journey.

CHAPTER 21

ELECTRONS AND
THE HEALING POWER OF TOUCH

And one last thought: the healing power of touch . . .

We've covered a lot of ground in this book, so many of the newest nondrug advances, opportunities for relief of pain without drugs, balancing hormones, stem cell advancements, and the new way and the new kind of doctors to approach your health.

Sometimes it's the simplest things in life that can make a difference and have a positive effect on your quality of life. This is one last thing to add to all you've already learned from the brilliant doctors, scientists, and professionals presented in this book. I'm speaking of the healing power (physically and emotionally) of touch.

Why does it feel so good to hug your loved ones? It's a simple process of sharing electrons. What are electrons? When electrons are running through a conductor such as copper wire, either they are there or not. If the switch is on, there is an electron donor. If the switch is off, there are no electrons. There are electron donors and electron stealers. An electron stealer is having an acidic body, as opposed to an alkaline body. An electron stealer is a free radical; an electron donor is an anti-oxidant. Electron stealers cause damage.

You will hear statements such as "All disease occurs when you are acidic." What this is really saying is that all disease occurs when your voltage (or energy) is low or in an elecron-stealer state. *Alkalize or Die* by Theodore Baroody said you must have electrons available to do their work, or your cells will die.

A free radical is a molecule that is missing electrons. It's like a mugger looking for a purse to steal. When a free radical steals electrons from the cell, it damages the cell. We maintain our health and heal primarily by making new cells.

So how does the power of touch fit into this scenario?

Try this tonight: when you get into bed with your loved one, hold each other very close. What you are doing and why it feels so good is that you are sharing positive electrons. It's the same thing that happens when you pet your cat or your dog. They stay put because it feels good, because from being to being you are sharing electrons. Electrons are healing.

We all need to be touched. As babies, we thrived on it; as adults, it's also what puts us back together. We forget in today's high-stress world that it's the little things that count: a dance together, a hug for nothing, holding each other until we sleep, a morning kiss. It's part of the human experience and has so much to do with antiaging. When you are touched frequently, you feel happy and fulfilled. It's a running theme with me and my husband, Alan; he'll say, "Give me some electrons." What happens next is always good.

The information throughout this book is meant to be provocative in order to stimulate interest in the newest possibilities. These amazing professionals gave me their best so I could pass it on to you.

There is clearly A NEW WAY TO AGE. It's exciting, and it makes the present paradigm of aging appear to be a dinosaur.

All of us are watching what I call the "slow death" of so many of our friends: first the knees go, then the back goes out, then the brain stops firing, diseases come, the pills mount up, more and more drugs turn a once vibrant person into a zombie: no energy, no vitality, no highs, no lows, just a medicated semi-even stream of nonconsciousness.

If you have stayed with me throughout this entire book, I know you don't want to end up that way.

Start now, today. Call one of these doctors, and make an appointment. Fly there, go there. You really need to go only once. After that it's phone calls and lab work.

Imagine the possibilities: renewed energy with senolytics clearing out your old dysfunctional immune cells, bone marrow stem cell treatments to strengthen your immune system. Dr. Maharaj says a failed immune system is what ultimately does us in.

Put back all your declining hormones to get your "juice" back. Life without hormonal balance is not living. Take telomere-lengthening supplements such as TA-65 to renew cell strength, take NAD+ precursors to help repair DNA breaks, try EECP to lower your blood pressure. I've done this and cannot believe the results: a nondrug protocol that strengthens the heart and has even shown to grow new blood vessels in the heart. Why wouldn't you do that instead of taking blood pressure medicine, which is known to have such harmful side effects?

As explained by Dr. Hertoghe, peptide protocols that rejuvenate and target every body part—muscles, organs, glands, brain, skin, hair, sex organs, and more—are a very exciting development, and understanding the life-lengthening importance of the hormones cortisol and adrenals functioning at optimum as explained by Dr. Hertoghe is crucial not only for internal health and brain health but for rejuvenation of the skin (good-bye, wrinkles, without cosmetic treatments). Again, how exciting!

This new life is yours. It's a new way to age: without drugs, with "juice," sexuality, energy, beautiful hair and nails, happiness, vitality, and, best of all, an intact memory.

You did it right; you raised your kids, loved them, and educated them, but the new way is not to sit in the corner as the old grandmother; no more of that! Now we are vibrant, contributing members of society.

The NEW WAY TO AGE opens the possibilities to experience another life chapter. All those regrets—what you didn't do because life was in the way, the education you didn't have access to—are things you can change now.

Your brain is working at optimum because of bioidentical hormone replacement, and in spite of our kids making fun of us, we have learned to operate our computers, enabling us to earn an online college degree. How exciting to learn something new, focused on what you are interested in, and then use that new knowledge and/or skill to make money for now and the next chapter of life.

Social media, when used productively, is the new way to make acquaintances, rendering loneliness unnecessary.

You can make this time of life anything you want, dream your biggest dream, see before you what it is you want, and then go for it.

At the top of my list is optimal health. With health, everything is possible.

I wish you great health, long life without illness, and vibrant great energy. I look forward to seeing those who have chosen A NEW WAY TO AGE grab their spot on the planet and soar.

ACKNOWLEDGMENTS

So many people make a book: the publisher, the editor, the doctors, the scientists, my staff, my family, and MORE.

First to my new editor, Lauren McKenna. This is my twenty-seventh book, and starting with a new editor can be daunting; I have my way, and she has hers. But from the start Lauren and I clicked. Her insights into and understanding of what I am trying to present to you were enhanced by her thoughtful, wise overview. She has definitely made this a better book.

To Jen Bergstrom, my publisher, thank you for providing a wonderful new home for me at Simon & Schuster!

Thanks to the Gallery team:

John Vairo, art director

Christine Masters, senior production editor

Jennifer Robinson, publicity director

Abby Zidle, marketing director

Maggie Loughran, editorial assistant

A heartfelt thank-you to Life Extension, a scientific group, and in particular to Bill Faloon, founder and editor of Life Extension. Along with the scientific advisory board they have provided invaluable assistance in the writing of all my books, this one being no exception. I have been working with this team of professionals for many years and I deeply appreciate their contributions. In this book they specifically helped to verify the facts presented related to the biology of aging. I'm not a doctor so I rely on interviews and research for my information. The interviews with the medical doctors represent the opinions of the doctors, which sometimes differ from those of other doctors and Life Extension.

Thank you to the whole Life Extension team, in particular:

William Faloon, cofounder, Life Extension group, Age Reversal Network

Hernando Latorre, MD, MSc, medical editor, *Life Extension* magazine

Scott Fogle, ND, executive director of clinical information and laboratory services, Life Extension

Blake Gossard, ELS, MWC, chief editor, *Disease Prevention and Treatment*

And to Dr. Mike aka Michael Smith, MD, director of education, who gives my readers and customers the luxury of an "office visit" online when he participates on my live social media shows. My readers love it because he takes the time to answer their questions with such expertise and charm.

Having the right PR is paramount to making a successful book launch and I'm pleased to partner with Couri Hay and his team for the first time.

My literary lawyer, Marc Chamlin, has been with me for almost all my books. He is always protecting, negotiating, making sure all legalities are perfectly lined up. I deeply appreciate his excellence.

Thank you to Caroline Somers, president of SOMERS Companies. She is the perfect person for the job. She not only brings so much to this company, but she brings so much to me as my facilitator, respecting and appreciating my message and the importance of bringing it correctly to my constituency. In addition to running the businesses, she produces our IGTV and Facebook LIVE shows, which have turned out to be an incredible way to speak directly with my readers and customers on a regular basis. She is a powerhouse, super smart, incredibly organized and in touch with all aspects of our various companies. And, no small thing, she's also an amazing and loving wife to my son, Bruce, and mother to my granddaughters.

Thank you to Danielle Shapero, my longtime graphic designer, who keeps me on brand in all facets of my businesses. She and Caroline work with all the companies with whom we partner to make sure my collaborations visually represent me.

Thank you to my office staff, who are invaluable to me, in particular Julie Turkel, my assistant, who does everything for me with such heart, kindness, and professionalism.

Thank you to the unflappable Jill Schugart, who heads our operations, wearing many hats with grace and ease.

Thank you to Jason Latshaw for his skillful job in running my website and digital marketing.

Thank you to Samuel Harwitt for handling my social media.

Thank you to Jon Edison, who is my daily go-to and an absolute joy.

Thank you Dave Henson, my IT who makes sure I don't lose my work!

Thank you to Herb Schmidt and Silke Boersch for making all the numbers line up!

Thank you to Cindy Gold and her team, Paul, John, and Bonnie for the beautiful cover photograph. I love working with all of you again and again.

My husband, Alan Hamel, is my everything. He runs the businesses oversees all departments. I call him "Mr. Idea" because he is very creative! Ours is an incredible love, allowing me the confidence to achieve my best work. He's got my back, appreciates me and US, and supports me completely. I love him fiercely and deeply.

Finally, thank you to the doctors in this book, all of whom gave me their best knowledge to pass on to you, my dear readers.

I profoundly and deeply appreciate everyone involved in helping me to put out this book, which, for me, was life-changing.

BLOOD TESTING

As promised throughout the book, here is a comprehensive list of all the tests you might want to do. To inquire about these tests or order them directly, you can call Life Extension at 888-671-8127 twenty-four hours a day or log on to www.labprevent.com.

THE NEED FOR BLOOD TESTS

Ever since I started writing health books, readers have asked me what should be their first step in youth restoration.

My response is that there is no "one-size-fits-all" approach to reversing what can be several underlying factors that rob our vitality as we age past thirty to forty years.

Readers often tell me they have been to multiple doctors and none has been able to diagnose the underlying cause of their chronic conditions. I am amazed that most people have never had a comprehensive blood test. This means that something as simple as balancing one's hormones is sadly overlooked.

In many cases, those who cannot shed body fat have an underactive thyroid, excess levels of insulin, and deficiencies in sex hormones such as DHEA. Not only do these hormone imbalances make weight loss difficult or impossible, but they contribute to the loss of a youthful sense of well-being that affects so many beginning in their middle years.

My suggestion is that before you visit another doctor or try some new weight loss program, you first have a comprehensive blood test panel done. The results of the tests can help you and your doctor identify correctable factors that are causing chronic problems and accelerating your rate of biological aging.

The good news is that as more efficient laboratory methods evolve, the cost to the consumer of comprehensive blood testing has plummeted.

Below I describe a comprehensive blood test panel that can identify risk factors before a serious age-related illness manifests itself. If the results of these blood tests show that your markers are out of the optimal range, there are easy steps you can take to help resolve chronic conditions. These corrective steps can also help to rejuvenate you from within.

For those who suffer health issues related to environmental hazards, such as mold or pollutants, there are tests that can pinpoint your individual susceptibilities. This will enable you to neutralize what may be a simmering underlying cause of your health problems.

The first step for most of you will be a comprehensive female or male blood test panel.

THE FEMALE BLOOD TEST PANEL

Age-related problems such as weight gain, clogged arteries, and cancer don't manifest themselves suddenly. They are the result of decades of underlying abnormalities, many of which are detectable via comprehensive blood testing. My favorite is the Female Panel, which evaluates a large number of common irregularities that typically affect women as they age past thirty to forty years. The tests include:

- **Chemistry Panel.** The chemistry part of the Female Panel provides an array of markers to help assess cardiovascular risk such as glucose, LDL cholesterol, metabolic function, and minerals important for bone health, plus liver and kidney function.

- **Complete blood count (CBC).** This part of the Female Panel evaluates three types of cells that circulate in the blood: red blood cells, white blood cells, and platelets. These markers can help provide information regarding your immune system, your possibility of getting an infection, whether you have anemia, any nutritional deficiencies you may have, and more.

- **Free and total testosterone.** Known as the "feel-good hormone," testosterone helps maintain a woman's libido, bone and muscle mass, cardiovascular health, mood, and sense of well-being. Testosterone in conjunction with estrogen is crucial in minimizing hot flashes, sleep disturbances, night sweats, and vaginal dryness. The Female Panel includes tests for both total and free testosterone.

- **DHEA-S.** Produced primarily by the adrenal glands, DHEA is the most abundant steroid hormone in the human body. DHEA plays a fundamental role in hormone balance, as well as supporting one's immune function, energy, mood, regulation of body fat, and maintenance of muscle and bone mass. This test is often overlooked by doctors but is included in the Female Panel.

- **Progesterone.** Progesterone is instrumental in balancing the powerful effects of estrogen; an imbalance between the two is linked to weight gain, insomnia, anxiety, depression, migraine, cancer, uterine fibroids, ovarian cysts, and osteoporosis.

- **Estradiol.** The primary female sex hormone, estradiol is a form of estrogen responsible for regulating mood, skin elasticity, bone strength, and bladder and vaginal health. This part of the Female Panel, along with the progesterone test, enables a woman to balance her primary sex hormones optimally.

- **Homocysteine.** Elevated homocysteine can damage the delicate cells that line the inside of the arteries, resulting in vascular inflammation, arterial plaque rupture, and blood clot formation. What's more, elevated homocysteine can contribute to mental depression, mood disorders, and increased risk of dementia. Easy steps can be taken to lower your homocysteine level, but you won't know whether this is necessary unless your blood is tested. That's why it's included in the Female Panel.

- **C-reactive protein (high sensitivity).** CRP measures the general level of inflammation in your body. Uncontrolled, systemic inflammation puts you at risk of developing many degenerative diseases, including heart disease, cancer, dementia, and a host of age-related disorders. Like many tests included in the Female Panel, the C-reactive protein marker is unfortunately omitted from conventional blood tests.

- **Thyroid-stimulating hormone (TSH).** TSH, which is produced by the pituitary gland, stimulates your thyroid to produce thyroid hormones T_3 and T_4. The TSH test can be used to screen for thyroid imbalances, which can be an underlying cause of mental fatigue and unwanted weight gain that does not come off no matter how little you eat. Testing for TSH should be routine, but so often it's omitted, which is why it's included in the Female Panel.

- **Vitamin D.** Known as the "sunshine vitamin," vitamin D is important to every cell and tissue throughout the body. From proper immune function and bone density to heart health and mood disorders, vitamin D is critical for optimal health. If your Female Panel test shows you are deficient, just take more of this low-cost vitamin supplement.

- **Hemoglobin A1c (HbA1c).** This part of the Female Panel shows your average level of blood sugar (glucose) over the past three months. HbA1c is a useful indicator of how well your blood glucose is being controlled and is also used to monitor the effects of diet, exercise, and drug therapy in diabetic patients.

- **Apolipoprotein B (ApoB).** ApoB is a more sensitive marker of your future risk of heart attack and stroke than is LDL cholesterol. If your ApoB level is elevated, there are steps you can take to bring it into a safer range. This test was expensive initially but is now included in both the Female and Male Panels.

- **Insulin.** As people age and accumulate surplus body fat, their fasting insulin level often surges upward and contributes to more weight gain. This happens because excess insulin acts like a growth factor to drive glucose into fat cells, which can make the cells "fatter." Weight loss can be challenging for those with high fasting insulin levels. Excess insulin can also increase the risk of developing certain cancers. This one test alone, which is included in the Female Panel, can provide information to help protect against a range of age-related disorders, including obesity.

The results you get back from the blood tests in the Female Panel can form the cornerstone of your antiaging program while identifying underlying causes of chronic conditions you may be confronting, such as loss of the feeling of youthful well-being and unwanted weight gain.

The cost of all these tests done in a doctor's office can be prohibitively high, but through Life Extension you can obtain them for a fraction of what commercial laboratories charge. What's nice about this service is that you can call in your order twenty-four hours a day, be sent a list of blood-draw stations in your neighborhood, and have your blood drawn at your convenience.

With modern technology, you'll get your results back quickly. If you have questions about your results, you'll have free access to people who can help provide guidance as to the best way of counteracting any abnormal result.

With the results of the Female Panel in hand, the next appointment you have with a doctor can be more meaningful. That's because it provides information your doctor can use to help you feel better.

The Female Panel is the best value I've ever seen. It provides a broad spectrum of blood tests that are cost prohibitive if purchased separately. Not only will you save around 70 percent compared to normal pricing, but you will have free access to knowledgeable people who can help you understand the results and possibly refer you to the proper medical doctor.

The Female Panel can be ordered twenty-four hours a day by calling 1-888-671-8127 or logging on to www.LabPrevent.com.

THE MALE PANEL

As men age past forty to fifty years, they start experiencing urinary issues, while the incidence of prostate cancer surges. A prostate-specific antigen (PSA) blood test can identify a reversible cause of prostate enlargement and early changes in prostate cells that can be corrected before clinically relevant prostate cancer manifests itself.

The Male Panel contains all the tests included in the Female Panel minus progesterone and plus prostate-specific antigen (PSA).

For aging men, testing for testosterone and estrogen can provide a basis to optimize these hormones to help reduce abdominal fat mass, improve mood, and reduce the risk of developing a number of degenerative disorders.

Perhaps most important is the ability of the tests in the Male Panel to identify cardiovascular risk factors that, if corrected, can dramatically reduce the risk of stroke, heart attack, kidney failure, and dementia.

You'll be sent a listing of blood-draw stations in your neighborhood so you can have a blood draw at your convenience. With the rapid turnaround, you'll know your results fast and have free access to knowledgeable people to answer any questions you might have.

The cost is the same as that of the Female Panel, which is considerably lower than what commercial laboratories charge. You can order the Male Panel twenty-four hours a day; call 888-671-8127 or visit www.labprevent.com.

TESTING FOR TOXINS

To assess your individual response to chemicals, toxins, and immune susceptibility, consider a combination of the following two tests.

HLA-DR Mold Genetic Testing

The HLA-DR genetic test provides information on genetic susceptibility to an overactive immune response to environmental toxins, chemicals, and mold. This is based on the work of Dr. Ritchie Shoemaker. Unfortunately, mold exposure is often misdiagnosed, and some doctors will even tell you that mold illness cannot be diagnosed or there is no such thing! The HLA-DR Mold Genetic Testing blood test measures the specific genes involved in increased susceptibility to biotoxic mold illness, chemicals, and toxins. It reveals why some people can be exposed to molds and chemicals and seemingly suffer no ill effects, while others who are exposed to the same levels of molds and toxins suffer significantly. The difference is in the genetic makeup of the immune system.

Biotoxin Mold Illness Panel

The biotoxin mold illness panel, developed with input from Dr. Ritchie Shoemaker, measures some of the various markers associated with the immune response to mold exposure. The symptoms of biotoxin mold illness can be similar to those of fibromyalgia, chronic sinus infections, or chronic fatigue syndrome. These include allergies, headaches, coughing, GI problems, body aches, burning or watery eyes, fever, anxiety, mood swings, and more.

TESTING FOR HARMFUL METALS

Two more tests evaluate the presence of harmful metals in your body.

Toxic Metals Panel (Fecal)

This at-home test assesses your environmental and dietary exposure to toxic metals. This test is best combined with a heavy metals blood test for a more complete picture of the body's detoxification process.

Heavy metals cannot be readily metabolized by our body, meaning they have the potential to be highly toxic. Toxic metals can bind to tissues and enzymes, causing systemic dysregulation of multiple systems in the body. The results of this test will provide a direct measurement of your environmental exposure to thirteen toxic metals.

Heavy Metals Panel (Mercury, Arsenic, Aluminum)

Since heavy metals tend to accumulate in our body tissues, it is important to evaluate circulating levels. This test evaluates circulating levels of mercury, arsenic, and aluminum, three key toxic metals. Blood testing for metals indicates recent exposure. Metals move out of the blood into other tissues and will no longer show up in the blood after a few weeks or months. When combined with the fecal toxic metals test, this test provides a complete picture of toxic metal exposure and detoxification.

ADRENAL AND SLEEP HORMONE TESTING

For adrenal function concerns, salivary cortisol testing is the preferred method of assessing cortisol levels throughout the day. Life Extension offers the following two salivary cortisol at-home testing kits.

Adrenal Stress Profile

Stress and disrupted adrenal function may be associated with fatigue, sleep issues, hormone imbalances, impaired cognition, and more. This panel was designed to evaluate four crucial stress biomarkers that may be compromising your health. The adrenal stress profile includes a four-point cortisol test (four cortisol measurements), along with measurement of the adrenal hormone DHEA and secretory IgA, an important marker of immune function.

Sleep Hormones Profile

Disrupted or inadequate sleep is closely associated with stress and irregular adrenal function. Cortisol and melatonin help regulate our sleep-wake cycles, but when disrupted result in poor sleep and daytime fatigue. This panel includes a four-point cortisol test (four cortisol measurements) to assess adrenal function during the day and a melatonin test to evaluate melatonin secretion at night.

COGNITIVE/MOOD URINARY TESTING

A great starting point for cognitive and mood concerns is the at-home urinary Neurotransmitter Panel (Basic), which provides a comprehensive overview of the major neurotransmitters that regulate important cognitive and mood-related processes.

Neurotransmitter Panel (Basic)

Urinary neurotransmitter testing provides an overall assessment of your body's ability to produce and metabolize neurotransmitters. Whole-body neurotransmitter levels correlate well with various symptoms and provide a valuable tool for achieving a sense of wellbeing. This panel includes measurements of nine neurotransmitters, including:

- Serotonin

- Gamma-aminobutyric acid (GABA)

- Dopamine

- Norepinephrine

- Epinephrine

- Glutamate

- Glycine

- Histamine

- Phenylethylamine (PEA))

Neurotransmitter Panel (Comprehensive)

This tests for the same neurotransmitters as the basic panel but adds nine neurotransmitters and metabolites:

- Taurine

- Tyrosine

- Tyramine

- 3,4-dihydroxyphelnylacetic acid (DOPAC)

- 3-methoxytyramine (3-MT)

- Normetanephrine

- Metanephrine

- Tryptamine

- 5-hydroxyindoleacetic acid (5-HIAA)

This is the best test, especially for more complicated situations. It provides a tremendous level of detail to help get your neurotransmitters balanced.

AUTOIMMUNE CONCERNS

Researchers have identified eighty to one hundred different auto-immune diseases and suspect at least another forty diseases to have an autoimmune basis. These diseases are often chronic and can be life threatening. Life Extension's Autoimmune Disease Screen is a starting point for those who suspect an autoimmune concern or who may want to monitor their immune balance over time.

Autoimmune Disease Screen

This test includes an expansive list of inflammatory markers, including TNF-alpha and antinuclear antibodies, as well as an immunoglobulin profile (IgA, IgG, and IgM).

- **Antinuclear antibodies (ANA) Screen.** This is a primary test to help evaluate a person for autoimmune diseases.

- **C-Reactive Protein (CRP).** Elevated CRP is a primary marker of inflammation throughout the body.

- **Tumor Necrosis Factor Alpha (TNFα).** This is a cytokine involved in the inflammatory process that helps regulate immune cells.

- **Immunoglobulins IgA, IgG, and IgM.** These tests provide a differential analysis of various antibodies produced by the immune system. The various patterns in these antibodies can help differentiate one autoimmune condition from another as well as help monitor the progression and severity of overall immune response (in other words, "How badly has your immune system regressed?").

DIGESTIVE, INFLAMMATORY BOWEL, AND GASTROINTESTINAL COMPLAINTS

Gastrointestinal complaints are among the most common in medical care. This comprehensive profile helps pinpoint the causes of gastrointestinal symptoms and chronic systemic conditions and measures key markers of digestion, absorption, and inflammation. Using a growth-based culture, the standard of practice in clinical microbiology, as well as sensitive biochemical assays and microscopy, this thorough profile evaluates the status of beneficial and pathogenic microorganisms, including aerobic and anaerobic bacteria, yeast, and parasites. Antimicrobial susceptibility testing to prescriptive and natural agents for appropriate bacterial and fungal species is also included. This is an at-home stool test.

SIBO Home Breath Kit (Lactulose)

Small intestinal bacterial overgrowth is an underrecognized cause of bloating, discomfort, digestive inflammation, and more. This at-home breath test can determine if bacterial overgrowth may be a factor in digestive problems.

Lactulose-based SIBO breath testing can detect bacterial overgrowth throughout the small intestine, including the lower end, where it most commonly occurs. The fermentation of lactulose by intestinal bacteria results in the production of hydrogen and/or methane gas, which can be measured with this breath test collection kit.

FOOD SENSITIVITIES

Another factor associated with digestive complaints and unexplained overactive immune response is unknown food sensitivities. This fingerstick test assesses IgG immune sensitivities to more than 190 different foods and spices.

Food Safe Allergy Test—Combo

IgG-mediated food sensitivities tend to be "masked" or hidden, since IgG-antibody-related symptoms tend to occur hours to days after food exposure, making it hard to pinpoint a cause of the symptoms without IgG testing. The Food Safe Allergy Test—Combo measures sensitivity to a vast array of foods and spices based on an IgG-mediated immune response. Food categories tested include dairy products, meats, nuts, fish, vegetables, fruits, grains, spices, and more.

FATTY ACID STATUS

Dietary fatty acid balance is critical in various health concerns and inflammatory response throughout the body. This at-home test assesses the blood levels of twenty-five different fatty acids, including the important omega-6 to omega-3 ratio and more.

Omega-3 Index Complete

Dietary fat imbalances are often the culprit behind compromised health. Many Western diets do not contain adequate omega-3 fatty acids yet contain an abundance of pro-inflammatory omega-6 fatty acids and saturated fats. Even diets rich in sources of healthy fats do not guarantee adequate absorption, metabolism, and balance. This makes it essential to test the overall balance of circulating fatty acids with the Omega-3 Index.

The Omega-3 Index Complete can give you an unbiased view of your dietary intake of omega-3s as well as your overall cardiovascular risk. An optimal omega-3 index in the range of 8 to 12 percent is an indicator of better overall health and can help support and maintain heart, brain, eye, and joint health.

FOR VEGETARIANS AND VEGANS

People following a vegan or vegetarian diet garner significant health benefits from it but can face deficiencies of critical nutrients, such as iron, vitamin B_{12}, and vitamin D. This panel also includes TSH, a marker of thyroid function and possible iodine deficiency.

Vegan/Vegetarian Panel

This panel contains the following blood tests, which are important for those following a plant-based diet:

- **Complete Blood Count with Differential and Platelets.** This group of tests helps assess concerns related to anemia and immune function.

- **Comprehensive Metabolic Panel and Lipid Profile.** These two tests assess kidney and liver function, as well as glucose management, and provide a cholesterol profile to assess cardiovascular risk. Some vegetarians/vegans can have low cholesterol levels that may not provide adequate support for hormone production.

- **Ferritin, Iron, and TIBC [total iron-binding capacity].** This comprehensive iron panel helps assess circulating iron and long-term iron storage (ferritin), as well as the body's ability to transport iron. This set of tests is the best way to establish your iron status.

• **Vitamin B$_{12}$ and Folate.** Many plant-based diets do not contain B$_{12}$, meaning that B$_{12}$ deficiency is more common in the vegetarian/vegan diet. If left untreated, B$_{12}$ deficiency will ultimately lead to irreversible nerve damage. Though folate is often abundant in plant-based diets, excess folate intake can mask an underlying B$_{12}$ deficiency.

• **Vitamin D, 25-hydroxy.** Vitamin D testing is important for all individuals; however, as it is a fat-soluble vitamin, low-fat, plant-based diets often do not provide adequate vitamin D to create an optimal level in the body.

• **TSH.** This tests thyroid-stimulating hormone (TSH), a marker of thyroid function that may also help indirectly reveal an iodine deficiency.

HOW TO PAY FOR THESE TESTS

Some people have great health insurance that may cover some of the costs of these tests. Most of us, however, face denials by insurance companies of even critical diagnostic procedures. Thankfully, consumers can gain access to these tests at affordable prices compared to what commercial labs charge.

As I stated at the beginning of this appendix, I think diagnostic testing is a critical first step for aging individuals to identify their points of vulnerability. Most of you can benefit from the Male or Female Panel, which provides a comprehensive overall picture of your physical condition. The results of this test provide a convenient road map of what you should do to restore youthful health and well-being, while identifying "correctable" blood factors that predispose you to degenerative illnesses and accelerated aging. To inquire about these tests or to order them, call 888-671-8127 twenty-four hours a day or visit www.labprevent.com.

TESTOSTERONE THERAPY IN MEN WITH PROSTATE CANCER

Which men with prostate cancer can take testosterone therapy safely?

In the interview with Dr. Abraham Morgentaler in chapter 10, he described his revolutionary research regarding the use of testosterone (T) therapy in men with prostate cancer. Whereas it had been believed for decades that T therapy in men with prostate cancer was like "feeding a hungry tumor" and no man with prostate cancer should ever receive T therapy, Dr. Morgentaler has shown this to be incorrect. Dr. Morgentaler's experience in several hundred men has been reported in medical journals, and he has shown that in many cases T therapy provides much-needed health benefits and is not associated with any greater risk of prostate cancer recurrence or progression. But T therapy is not for everyone, and some men should definitely not take testosterone. Here is a brief overview of which men Dr. Morgentaler believes can reasonably take T therapy and which should not. Note that Dr. Morgentaler offers T therapy only to men with symptoms from low testosterone levels and not to men with normal levels.

PROSTATE CANCER TREATED WITH SURGERY OR RADIATION WITH APPARENT CURE

This is the safest group of men to receive T therapy. Numerous studies now show that cancer recurrence rates appear to be no greater in men treated with T therapy than men who did not receive T therapy. Based on the work by Dr. Morgentaler over the last two decades, some health care providers now will also offer T therapy to men who appear cured of their prostate cancer after surgery or radiation treatment. If your PSA is undetectable or less and 0.1 nanogram per milliliter after radical prostatectomy or has stayed low after radiation treatment, you may be a reasonable candidate for T therapy.

MEN ON ACTIVE SURVEILLANCE

Men on active surveillance have been identified with prostate cancer by biopsy and have deferred treatment because their cancer has been deemed low risk. Some men on active surveillance later go on to undergo surgery or radiation if follow-up biopsies show their cancer has become more worrisome.

Testosterone therapy in these men is highly controversial, since the long-standing belief has been that raising testosterone will cause these cancers to grow more rapidly or become more aggressive. In 2011, Dr. Morgentaler and his colleagues at Baylor Medical College reported on results of T therapy in thirteen men on active surveillance. None of the cancers progressed during the study, and no cancer at all was found in 54 percent of the follow-up biopsies.[1] PSA levels did not rise over two years. More recently, Dr. Morgentaler compared rates of cancer progression (more of it or of higher grade) in twenty-eight men who received T therapy for three years and ninety-six similar men who did not receive T therapy. Stunningly, the rate of cancer progression was nearly identical between the two groups, indicating that T therapy did not appear to influence the growth or aggressiveness of the cancers in these men.

Few health care providers currently offer T therapy to men on active surveillance. As many as 15 to 25 percent of men will have progression of their prostate cancer over time without T therapy, so there is the fear that if cancer progression occurs, the automatic response will be to blame the T therapy. Though Dr. Morgentaler tells me he routinely offers T therapy to these men and has not observed increased risk, he cautions that it is far too soon to conclude that T therapy is safe for men on active surveillance.

BIOCHEMICAL RECURRENCE AND METASTATIC DISEASE

The standard treatment for men with recurrence of prostate cancer, called biochemical recurrence, or with metastases is treatment with medications that lower testosterone or block its effects, called androgen deprivation therapy (ADT). New forms of ADT, such as with enzalutamide and abiraterone, have been shown to reduce mortality. In chapter 10, Dr. Morgentaler described his experiences with small numbers of men in this situation whom he treated with T therapy, actually raising their testosterone instead of lowering it. The men were miserable from the effects of low testosterone and were willing to accept the risk of a shortened life span in order to feel better while they were still alive. Interestingly, new reports of alternating high-dose testosterone with ADT, called bipolar androgen therapy (BAT) suggests a therapeutic cancer effect using testosterone in this way.

Treatment in men with biochemical recurrence or metastatic disease should be considered investigational and cannot be recommended at this point in time, as there is a risk that it may cause rapid disease progression and even death.

THE BOTTOM LINE

Though we still lack large prospective studies, a large amount of evidence indicates that there is little, if any, increased cancer risk with T therapy in men after successful surgery or radiation. However, the use of T therapy in men with more advanced disease has not been adequately studied and may cause serious complications. Treatment with T therapy in these men must be considered investigational.

DOCTOR CONTACT INFORMATION

These are the doctors interviewed or referenced in this book. If you can't find a doctor near you, go to www.foreverhealth.com (a free service) to find a qualified, vetted doctor who specializes in this new kind of medicine.

DR. RUSSELL BLAYLOCK
The Blaylock Wellness Report
www.blaylockreport.com

JULIE CARMEN
https://yogatalks.com

DR. MARC DARROW
Stem Cell Institute
11645 Wilshire Boulevard,
Suite 120
Los Angeles, CA 90025
800-734-2210
www.prolotherapyinstitute.com
www.stemcellinstitute.com

DR. LEONARD FELD, DDS
Southeast Dental Group
4332 East Slauson Avenue
Maywood, CA 90270
323-771-7777
or
74-976 Highway 111
Indian Wells, CA 92210
760-341-7920
www.southeastdentalgroup.com

DR. MICHAEL GALITZER
The American Health Institute
12381 Wilshire Boulevard, Suite 102
Los Angeles, CA 90025
800-392-2623
www.drgalitzer.com

DR. JEFFREY GLADDEN
Apex Health, Human Performance
& Longevity Optimization
2301 Cedar Springs Road,
Suite 405
Dallas, TX 75201
855-861-3820
www.apexhhplo.com

DR. THIERRY HERTOGHE
Dr. Hertoghe Clinic
7 Avenue Van Bever 7–9
B-1189 Uccle—Brussels I, Belgium
+32-2-736-68-68
www.hertoghe.com

DR. JOY KONG
Chara Biologics, Inc.
www.charabiologics.com
888-906-4550

DR. KENT MACLEOD
NutriChem Compounding
Pharmacy & Retail Store
2599 Carling Avenue
Ottawa, ON, Canada K2B 7H7
613-820-4200
www.nutrichem.com

DR. ALLAN MAGAZINER
Magaziner Center for Wellness
1907 Greentree Road
Cherry Hill, NJ 08003
856-424-8222
www.drmagaziner.com

DR. DIPNARINE MAHARAJ
Maharaj Institute of Immune
Regenerative Medicine
10301 Hagen Ranch Road
Entrance C, Suite 600
Boynton Beach, FL 33437
561-752-5522
www.stemcellimmuneregenerative
.com

DR. ABRAHAM MORGENTALER
If a reader wants to set up a
consultation, they can do so
by emailing him at pmh@
menshealthboston.com.
www.menshealthboston.com

DR. ED PARK
Recharge Biomedical
600 Anton Boulevard, Suite 1138
Costa Mesa, CA 92626
714-369-8633
www.rechargebiomedical.com
YouTube channel: *drpark65*

DR. WALTER PIERPAOLI
www.drpierpaoli.ch/eng

DR. STEPHEN SINATRA
Dr. Sinatra is no longer doing
active patient consultation. His
office number is 800-228-1507
if someone needs to leave a
message for him.
www.dr.sinatra.com

DR. JONATHAN V. WRIGHT
Tahoma Clinic
6839 Fort Dent Way, Suite 134
Tukwila, WA 98188
206-812-9988
www.tahomaclinic.com

SUZANNESOMERS.COM SUPPLEMENTS!

For your convenience, my dear readers, I am including information obtainable from www.suzannesomers.com about supplementation as discussed in this book. Our formulators are excellent, and whatever I cannot offer you, Life Extension has available, as you have read earlier. Those who are interested in the natural senolytic approach can read more about it by visiting www.lifeextension.com/goodhealth. Senolytic supplements available there include:

- Senolytic Activator

- Theaflavins

- AMPK Metabolic Activator

- NAD+ Cell Regenerator

Other supplements can be ordered from *Aging Matters* magazine (aging-matters.com), an international publication that highlights the developments being made in preventive and regenerative medicine. They include:

- Thyrotropin-releasing hormone (TRH)

- Melatonin with Zinc and Selenium (MZS)

Supplements available at www.suzannesomers.com include the following.

ADVANCED PROBIOTIC INTESTINAL RENEW

A comprehensive probiotic blend to support good gut health

Have you got a little gas or bloating? This has become a problem for so many people.

Let's talk about the digestive tract. First of all, we all have "good" and "bad" bacteria in our gut. It's pretty simple: a healthy gut has a ratio with more good than bad. Stress is one of the factors that can increase the bad bacteria.

One of the ways to improve that ratio is by taking a probiotic. RestoreLife Formulas Advanced Probiotic Intestinal Renew is a great one because it has two ways to help increase the good bacteria in your gut.

First of all, it uses a blend of four bacteriophages. What are bacteriophages? you ask. They are the "warriors" that help fight the bad bacteria in your gut. So that's step one. Second, this blend contains multiple strains of probiotics that can repopulate the gut with healthy bacteria; it's like bringing in the "good guys."

You can see the full list of warriors here: the bacteriophage to help fight the bad guys and the probiotics to bring in the good guys. This is how we help turn around that ratio.

I want you to see what the doctors and scientists at RestoreLife Formulas came up with to help these incredible probiotics last longer in your digestive system. Look how cool this is: the dual encapsulation technology means that the probiotic doesn't immediately disintegrate in the acidic environment of the stomach and the live bacteria are protected for longer. I always say, if you are going to take only one product, take a good-quality probiotic—and this is a really great one.

Potential Benefits at a Glance

- Helps relieve gas and bloating

- Can improve the ratio of good bacteria to bad bacteria

- Helps fight the unwanted bacteria in your gut

- Helps repopulate the gut with good bacteria

- Doesn't immediately disintegrate in the acidic environment of your stomach, thereby protecting the live bacteria longer

CURCUMIN

Supports the brain and cardiovascular system and can help ward off inflammation

When I talk to the experts on the medical and scientific advisory board at RestoreLife about curcumin, you know what they say: Just take it!

Seriously, curcumin, an extract of the spice turmeric, benefits several systems in the body. It can help improve parameters related to brain, cardiovascular, and inflammatory health.

Now, you may be thinking, I'll just use turmeric in cooking and get the benefits that way. But you won't likely be using turmeric routinely in your cooking, and that's why you want to supplement with a high-quality curcumin product.

Curcumin can be hard to absorb, so RestoreLife curcumin uses a special form called BCM-95 BioCurcumin because of its excellent absorption.

This is one of my foundational supplements. I take it every day to help improve parameters related to brain, cardiovascular, and inflammatory health.

GENTLE COLON RENEW

A potent mineral formula for occasional constipation

We all know how important our digestive tract is to our overall health. In fact, many experts say we are only as healthy as our digestive system. In the normal process of digestion, we digest our food, extract the nutrients, and eliminate regularly. But many things can disrupt the normal process.

One of the biggest issues many people face is occasional constipation. Staying regular can be a problem, especially for aging women. How can we improve gastrointestinal function when we aren't as regular as we want? Here's a great approach. Gentle Colon Renew uses the basic nutrients of vitamin C and magnesium; both help with gastrointestinal functions for gentle relief.

Key Ingredients

- Vitamin C (as ascorbic acid), 4,500 milligrams (7,500% of the RDA)

- Vitamin B_6 (as pyridoxine HCl), 4 milligrams (200% of the RDA)

- Magnesium (as magnesium carbonate), 250 milligrams (63% of the RDA)

Gentle Colon Renew includes 4,500 milligrams of vitamin C and 250 milligrams of magnesium in a great-tasting fizzy drink. I take this every night with hot water as a soothing cup of tea.

Vitamin C and magnesium are both antioxidants and help protect the lining of the gut and also to promote overall health of the digestive system.

Magnesium is known for helping move things out! You might be aware of products that use fiber for this purpose. Fiber is great; however, it can create more volume, which can be uncomfortable for some people.

Gentle Colon Renew uses magnesium, which is an easy, calming way to work with the muscles to help with gastrointestinal functions. Magnesium is also known for its calming effects, which is why I like to take this before bed.

By morning, you should have your gentle colon renew!

Potential Benefits at a Glance

- Helps with gastrointestinal functions

- Provides antioxidants

- Supports cardiovascular health

LIVER RENEW

Helps ensure healthy liver and prostate function

Your liver is the organ responsible for detoxing your body of the nearly nine hundred chemicals a day it encounters! Silymarin, a compound found in milk thistle, has long been used to support liver health.

European milk thistle with advanced phospholipid delivery is a potent weapon to support liver health. Milk thistle helps optimize liver function and support the body's natural detoxification pathways and is safe for daily use.

Potential Benefits at a Glance

- Promotes liver health

- Supports liver function and the body's natural detoxification pathways

- Increases active compounds in the liver

- Provides standardized concentrations of silybin and isosilybin A and B not found in other milk thistle extracts

SEXY LEG RENEW

Supports youthful appearance of the legs

This is one of my most popular products because many of us, as we age, develop problems with our legs. In fact, some studies suggest that as many as 50 percent of American women will probably develop unsightly leg veins. It can happen to men, too. When we lose elasticity in our veins, it may also lead to swelling in the legs, ankles, and feet.

One way to support elasticity in your veins is Sexy Leg Renew, which contains diosmin-95, an extract of sweet orange. European women have had access to diosmin for thirty years. In RestoreLife Sexy Leg Renew, we use a standardized form of diosmin to help with absorption and effectiveness.

This product helps support healthy veins by helping to maintain the elasticity of the veins. Having healthy veins can help with leg, ankle, and feet swelling. Plus, Sexy Leg Renew helps improve the appearance of unsightly leg veins. The recommended dosage is one tablet daily for three months and then repeat as needed.

Potential Benefits at a Glance

- Helps support healthy veins
- Helps maintain the elasticity of the veins
- Helps improve the appearance of unsightly leg veins

VITAMIN D$_3$, 5,000 IU

Helps maintain bone health

Evidence suggests that Americans, even those who live in sunny regions, have insufficient vitamin D in their bodies. Vitamin D supplementation helps support overall health in the following areas:

- Cardiovascular system

- Endocrine system

- Immune system

- Cognition

Vitamin D helps protect against:

- Osteoporosis

- Fractures

Vitamin D may help reduce the risk of falls in older individuals. It can also help support muscle strength and postural stability.

BONE RENEW

Comprehensive bone support

Bones! We all want to maintain healthy bones, right? First let's do a little review, so we'll go back to science class in middle school, when we learned how bones are made.

Bones are constantly being made and broken down throughout our lives. Calcium, which is a mineral, is transported into bones, and then it's removed from bones. This process of breaking down and building up bone is called *remodeling*—and the building part requires calcium. That's why it's important to make sure we are getting enough calcium to continue healthy remodeling throughout our lives.

Now, you can get calcium from food, including milk, cheese, yogurt, and even vegetables such as kale and broccoli, but many of us don't eat enough of these foods. So supplementation is important.

But we need more than just calcium. In combination with a healthy diet, we need to get enough calcium plus vitamin D_3, which may reduce the risk of developing osteoporosis and help maintain good bone health. And we all know how important it is to stay strong.

With Bone Renew, you are getting an excellent source of calcium and vitamin D_3.

Plus, when we discuss bone health, we also want to look at bone density to make sure our bones are strong enough to support our bodies, especially as we age. Loss of bone density is associated not just with calcium deficiency but with insufficient intake of vitamin D_3 and magnesium.

So again, with Bone Renew, you have the calcium and vitamin D_3, *plus* additional minerals such as magnesium, zinc, manganese, and boron. With Bone Renew, when combined with a healthy diet, you should have the proper dosage of calcium, vitamin D, and other minerals to help reduce the risk of developing osteoporosis, help maintain good bone health, and support healthy bone density. It's a strong choice!

Potential Benefits at a Glance

- May help reduce the risk of developing osteoporosis

- As part of a healthful diet, can help build and maintain good bone health

- Contributes to good bone health

DIGESTIVE RENEW

Promotes healthy digestion

Time to talk about my favorite topic: the gut! No wonder I talk about it so much—so many people are struggling with gas, bloating, and digestive issues. Let's start with a basic understanding of the digestive process.

When we eat, our bodies break down food with digestive enzymes. These are the proteins that dissect food into its "building blocks," so our bodies can absorb macronutrients—proteins, fats, and carbohydrates—and micronutrients—vitamins, minerals, and antioxidants. That's the healthy, normal digestive process.

As we age, we may secrete fewer digestive enzymes, which means we can't break down food as well. That can lead to a horrible feeling of gas, bloating, and discomfort. Plus, if the food isn't properly broken down, we aren't getting full use of the macro- and micronutrients.

That's where it makes great sense to supplement with digestive enzymes, such as those in RestoreLife Formulas Digestive Renew.

Digestive enzymes help break food into its building blocks, help improve digestive function, and may help relieve bloating. I take this every day, one capsule in the morning and one in the evening with meals. This helps promote optimal digestion for better absorption of nutrients and can help get on top of that horrible bloated feeling.

Potential Benefits at a Glance

- Helps break down food

- Helps relieve gas, bloating, and discomfort

- Helps absorb macro- and micronutrients

- Helps improve digestive function

HAIR, SKIN, AND NAIL RENEW

Promotes collagen and keratin health to support healthy hair, skin, and nails.

Your hair, skin, and nails are constantly renewing and growing, so you need to make sure your body has the nutrients needed to support this growing process. This supplement is like a multivitamin specifically for your hair, skin, and nails.

Hair, skin, and nails all need the same nutrients to be strong and healthy. Putting things on top of your hair, skin, and nails can also help strengthen and support them, but this formula is specifically designed to support them from the inside. It contains four key ingredients:

- Biotin
    Everyone in the beauty business is talking about biotin as a beauty nutrient. I'm sure you've heard your facialist, manicurist,

and hairdresser talking about it. This product contains 2,500 micrograms, so you can get an optimal amount.

- Bioactive Collagen Peptides

- Soluble keratin complex

- Silicon

Potential Benefits at a Glance

- Helps support healthy nails

- Helps support skin's elasticity

- Helps improve the appearance of the skin

- Helps support the top layer of the skin

- Helps improve hair brightness and luster

NATURAL CALM RENEW

Provides relief from stress

Got a lot on your plate? Feeling a little stressed? I can't think of anyone who would say "No." If daily life has you stressed and makes it hard for you to relax and wind down, I want to tell you about Natural Calm Renew. It is one of my bestselling supplements because it can provide a natural way to help you relax.

The primary ingredient is L-theanine, an amino acid derived from green tea, which can help bring a calming effect without making you drowsy. L-theanine increases the natural production of gamma-aminobutyric acid (GABA), which is a neurotransmitter that helps us feel calm. In addition, Natural Calm Renew contains lemon balm, an herb in the mint family, which can help promote calmness and relaxation.

So if you are looking for a natural alternative to deal with occasional stress, this is a wonderful product to have in your cabinet to help you relax, and I'm sure that's why it's one of my top-selling supplements.

Potential Benefits at a Glance

- Helps you relax naturally

- Creates a calming effect without drowsiness

JOINT EASE

Supports joint health and eases range of motion

We all know that exercise is important. But we can come up with a lot of excuses to skip it! Joint discomfort is a really good excuse, and many of us struggle with joint issues. If you have some joint discomfort, you may not exercise as much as you'd like to or as much as you should.

The problem is, one of the ways to help support joint health is to exercise, but when we feel achy, the last thing we feel like doing is exercising. Then the problem can get even worse, because the less active we are, the more joint discomfort we have! So how can we reverse this cycle?

One of the reasons Joint Ease can help with discomfort is that its blend of herbs helps ease inflammation in the joint space.

These herbs can also help to maintain healthy cartilage. Cartilage protects our joints at the connecting point of our bones. When healthy cartilage deteriorates, that can be where the discomfort comes from.

Just one tablet per day of Joint Ease can help ease joint discomfort, so you can enjoy your life and stay active!

Potential Benefits at a Glance

- Helps support healthy joints

- Helps support and maintain healthy cartilage levels

Introduction: The New Way to Age

1. Richard J. Johnson, Mark S. Segal, Yuri Sautin, et al., "Potential Role of Sugar (Fructose) in the Epidemic of Hypertension, Obesity and the Metabolic Syndrome, Diabetes, Kidney Disease, and Cardiovascular Diseases," *The American Journal of Clinical Nutrition* 86, no. 4 (October 2007): 899–906. Boyd A. Swinburn, Gary Sacks, Sing Kai Lo, et al., "Estimating the Changes in Energy Flux That Characterize the Rise in Obesity Prevalence," *The American Journal of Clinical Nutrition* 89, no. 6 (June 2009): 1723–28. David S. Ludwig, Karen E. Peterson, and Steven L. Gortmaker, "Relation Between Consumption of Sugar-Sweetened Drinks and Childhood Obesity: A Prospective, Observational Analysis," *The Lancet* 357, no. 9255 (February 17, 2001): 505–08. Kevin D. Hall and Carson C. Chow, "Estimating the Quantitative Relation Between Food Energy Intake and Changes in Body Weight," *The American Journal of Clinical Nutrition* 91, no. 3 (March 2010): 816. Tanya L. Blasbalg, Joseph R. Hibbeln, Christopher E. Ramsden, et al., "Changes in Consumption of Omega-3 and Omega-6 Fatty Acids in the United States During the 20th Century," *The American Journal of Clinical Nutrition* 93, no. 5 (May 2011): 950–62. Urmila Nair, Helmut Bartsch, and Jagadeesan Nair, "Lipid Peroxidation–Induced DNA Damage in Cancer-Prone Inflammatory Diseases: A Review of Published Adduct Types and Levels in Humans," *Free Radical Biology and Medicine* 43, no. 8 (October 15, 2007): 1109–20.

Chapter 1: Can We Reverse Aging?

1. Donald W. Light, "New Prescription Drugs: A Major Health Risk with Few Offsetting Advantages," Edmond J. Safra Center for Ethics, Harvard University, June 27, 2014, https://ethics.harvard.edu/blog/new-prescription-drugs-major-health-risk-few -offsetting-advantages.

2. Enzo Nisoli and Michele O. Carruba, "Nitric Oxide and Mitochondrial Biogenesis," *Journal of Cell Science* 119, no. 14 (July 15, 2006): 2855–62.

3. "Attention-Deficit/Hyperactivity Disorder (ADHD)," Centers for Disease Control and Prevention, September 21, 2018, https://www.cdc.gov/ncbddd/adhd/data.html.

Chapter 2: What Do You Fear Most About Aging?

1. M. F. McCarty and A. L. Russell, "Niacinamide Therapy for Osteoarthritis—Does It Inhibit Nitric Oxide Synthase Induction by Interleukin-1 in Chondrocytes?," *Medical Hypotheses* 53, no. 4 (October 1999): 350–60.
2. Allan E. Smith and Diane M. Secoy, "A Compendium of Inorganic Substances Used in European Pest Control Before 1850," *Journal of Agricultural and Food Chemistry* 24, no. 6 (November 1, 1976): 1180–86.

Chapter 3: Stress: The Real Killer—and the Part You Play in It

1. Matthias Blüher, M. Dodson Michael, Odile D. Peroni, et al., "Adipose Tissue Se-lective Insulin Receptor Knockout Protects Against Obesity and Obesity-Related Glucose Intolerance," *Developmental Cell* 3, no. 1 (July 2002): 25–38. Matthias Blüher, Barbara B. Kahn, and C. Ronald Kahn, "Extended Longevity in Mice Lacking the Insulin Receptor in Adipose Tissue," *Science* 299, no. 506 (January 24, 2003): 572–74.
2. "Women and Heart Disease," Centers for Disease Control and Prevention, May 14, 2019, https://www.cdc.gov/heartdisease/women.htm.
3. "Lifetime Risk of Developing or Dying from Cancer," American Cancer Society, Jan-uary 4, 2018, https://www.cancer.org/cancer/cancer-basics/lifetime-probability-of -developing-or-dying-from-cancer.html.
4. Kyle J. Foreman, Neal Marquez, Andrew Dolgert, et al., "Forecasting Life Expec-tancy, Years of Life Lost, and All-Cause and Cause-Specific Mortality for 250 Causes of Death: Reference and Alternative Scenario for 2016–40 for 195 Countries and Territories," *The Lancet* 392, no. 10159 (November 10, 2018): 2052–90.

Chapter 4: Supplementation

1. Sohair A. Moustafa, "Effect of Glutathione (GSH) Depletion on the Serum Levels of Triiodothyronine (T_3), Thyroxine (T_4), and T_3/T_4 Ratio in Allyl Alcohol–Treated Male Rats and Possible Protection with Zinc," *International Journal of Toxicology* 20, no. 1 (January 1, 2001): 15–20.
2. N. Veronese, S. Watatantrige-Fernando, C. Luchini, et al., "Effect of Magnesium Sup-plementation on Glucose Metabolism in People with or at Risk of Diabetes: A Sys-tematic Review and Meta-analysis of Double-Blind Randomized Controlled Trials," *European Journal of Clinical Nutrition* 70, no. 12 (December 2016): 1354–59.
3. Jonathan Stoddard, "Shilajit Boosts CoQ10 Efficiency," *Life Extension*, February 2016, https://www.lifeextension.com/Magazine/2016/2/Shilajit-Boosts-CoQ10-Efficiency /Page-01.

Chapter 9: The Hormone System: The Juice of Youth

1. Joseph Mercola, "Skyrocketing Male Infertility May Threaten Mankind's Survival," *Templeton Times*, August 9, 2017.

Chapter 11: The Devastating Effects of Toxicity on Aging

1. "Salad Dressing, Home Recipe, Vinegar and Oil: Nutrition Facts & Calories," *Self*, https://nutritiondata.self.com/facts/fats-and-oils/562/2.
2. "Chicken, Broilers or Fryers, Leg, Meat and Skin, Cooked, Roasted: Nutrition Facts & Calories," Self, https://nutritiondata.self.com/facts/poultry-products/717/2.
3. Robert C. Block, William S. Harris, Kimberly J. Reid, and John A. Spertus, "Omega-6 and Trans Fatty Acids in Blood Cell Membranes: A Risk Factor for Acute Coronary Syndromes?," *American Heart Journal* 156, no. 6 (December 2008): 1117–23.
4. Vicki Batts, "Homes Are Laden with Chemicals That Are Increasing Your Risk of CANCER," Natural News, March 3, 2019, https://www.naturalnews.com/2019 -03-03-homes-are-laden-with-chemicals-increasing-your-risk-of-cancer.html.
5. Alexis Temkin, "Breakfast with a Dose of Roundup?: Weed Killer in $289 Million Cancer Verdict Found in Oat Cereal and Granola Bars," EWG's Children's Health Foundation, August 15, 2018, https://www.ewg.org/childrenshealth/glyphosateince real/.

Chapter 12: The Gut

1. Avandish K. Nehra, Jeffrey A. Alexander, Conor G. Loftus, and Vandana Nehra, "Proton Pump Inhibitors: Review of Emerging Concerns," *Mayo Clinic Proceedings* 93, no. 2 (February 2018): 240–46.
2. Victoria J. Drake, "Cognitive Function in Depth," Micronutrient Information Center, Linus Pauling Institute, Oregon State University, February 2011, https://lpi.oregon state.edu/mic/health-disease/cognitive-function.

Chapter 13: Dispelling Myths About Heart Health

1. "How Common Is Breast Cancer?," American Cancer Society, January 8, 2019, https:// www.cancer.org/cancer/breast-cancer/about/how-common-is-breast-cancer.html.
2. "Women and Heart Disease," Centers for Disease Control and Prevention, May 14, 2019, https://www.cdc.gov/heartdisease/women.htm.
3. Terry Young, "Menopause, Hormone Replacement Therapy, and Sleep-Disordered Breathing: Are We Ready for the Heat?," *American Journal of Respiratory and Critical Care Medicine* 163, no. 3, part 1 (March 2001): 597–98.
4. American Diabetes Association, "The Economic Costs of Diabetes in the U.S. in 2017," *Diabetes Care* 41, no. 5 (May 2018): 917–28.

Chapter 16: NAD+ and Senolytics

1. Nir Barzilai, Ana Maria Cuervo, and Steve Austad, "Aging as a Biological Target for Prevention and Therapy," *The Journal of the American Medical Association* 320, no. 13 (October 2, 2018): 1321–22.
2. Tamara Tchkonia and James L. Kirkland, "Aging, Cell Senescence, and Chronic Disease: Emerging Therapeutic Strategies," *The Journal of the American Medical Association* 320, no. 13 (October 2, 2018): 1319–20.
3. Ming Xu, Tamar Pirtskhalava, Joshua N. Farr, et al., "Senolytics Improve Physical Function and Increase Lifespan in Old Age," *Nature Medicine* 24, no. 8 (August 2018): 1246–56.

4. Jamie M. Justice, Anoop M. Namblar, Tamar Tchkonia, et al., "Senolytics in Idiopathic Pulmonary Fibrosis: Results from a First-in-Human, Open-Label, Pilot Study," *EBioMedicine* 40 (February 2019): 554–63.
5. Matthew J. Yousefzadeh, Yi Zhu, Sara J. McGowan, et al., "Fisetin Is a Senotherapeutic That Extends Health and Lifespan," *EBioMedicine* 36 (October 2018): 18–28.
6. Michael R. Lieber, "The Mechanism of Double-Strand DNA Break Repair by the Nonhomologous DNA End-Joining Pathway," *Annual Review of Biochemistry* 79 (January 7, 2010): 181–211.
7. James Clement, Matthew Wong, Anne Poljak, et al., "The Plasma NAD+ Metabolome Is Dysregulated in 'Normal' Aging," *Rejuvenation Research* 22, no. 2 (April 2019): 121–30.
8. Alexandra Sifferlin, "Is an Anti-aging Pill on the Horizon?," *Time*, February 15, 2018.
9. Danielle Glick, Sandra Barth, and Kay F. Macleod, "Autophagy: Cellular and Molecular Mechanisms," *The Journal of Pathology* 221, no. 1 (May 2010): 3–12.

Chapter 17: Telomere Lengthening

1. Phil Micans, "The Rotational Theory of Aging: An Interview with Walter Pierpaoli, M.D., PhD.," *Aging Matters*, https://aging-matters.com/the-rotational-theory-of-aging/.

Appendix B: Testosterone Therapy in Men with Prostate Cancer

1. Abraham Morgentaler, Larry I. Lipschult, Richard Bennett, et al., "Testosterone Therapy in Men with Untreated Prostate Cancer," *Journal of Urology* 185, no. 4 (April 2011): 1256–61.

GLOSSARY

adenosine triphosphate (ATP): a molecule that supplies energy for many biochemical cellular processes.

adrenaline: the hormone responsible for feelings of heightened energy, excitement, strength, and alertness that occur when someone is in a dangerous, frightening, or highly competitive situation.

AMPK: an enzyme that helps maintain cellular energy equilibrium by activating glucose and fatty acid uptake and oxidation when cellular energy is low.

androstenedione: a steroid sex hormone that is a precursor of testosterone and estrogen and is secreted by the testes, ovaries, and adrenal cortex.

apheresis: the process through which blood is withdrawn from a donor's body, one or more components, such as stem cells, is removed from the blood, and the remaining blood is transfused back into the donor.

autologous stem cell therapy: therapy using stem cells harvested from a person's own body.

autophagy: a process in which cellular components are digested by enzymes of the same cell, clearing out "waste products" that accumulate in a person's cells as a result of aging.

berberine: obtained from the roots of various plants, a bitter crystalline yellow bioactive compound taken as a supplement.

bioimpedance: a process for determining the balance between energy production and energy recovery by looking at body fat, body water, and a measure of regeneration known as the phase angle.

blood lipids: various lipids in the blood, mainly fatty acids and cholesterol.

coenzyme Q10 (CoQ10): a compound of humans and most other mammals that possesses antioxidant properties and is part of an important cofactor in electron transport that helps the mitochondria work better.

cortisol: a hormone that is released by the adrenal gland in response to physical or psychological stress and that also regulates various metabolic processes and has anti-inflammatory and immunosuppressive properties.

dihydroepiandrosterone (DHEA): a hormone secreted by the adrenal gland that is involved in the biosynthesis of testosterone; known as the antiaging hormone.

docosahexaenoic acid (DHA): an omega-3 fatty acid generally found in cold-water fish.

dopamine: a neurotransmitter in the brain that is involved in the biosynthesis of epinephrine.

eicosapentaenoic acid (EPA): an omega-3 fatty acid generally found in cold-water fish oil.

electrodermal testing: testing related to electrical activity in or electrical properties of the skin that facilitates an individualized assessment of what nutrients or medications are recommended for someone.

embryonic stem cells: stem cells harvested from embryos.

endocannabinoid system (ECS): a biological system composed of any of several naturally produced chemical compounds that bind to the same brain receptors as compounds derived from cannabis.

enhanced external counterpulsation (EECP): a fast-acting nondrug protocol that enhances blood circulation to the heart and collateral blood flow.

estriol: a natural estrogenic hormone found in the body that is the main estrogen secreted by the placenta during pregnancy.

estrogen: any of various natural steroids that are secreted chiefly by the ovaries, placenta, and testes, and that lead to the development of female secondary sex characteristics and promote the growth of the female reproductive system.

epigenetics: the study of heritable changes in gene function that do not alter the DNA sequence.

fisetin: a yellow pigment obtained from the wood of various trees or shrubs.

fulvic acid: a water-soluble organic acid derived from humus.

gastroesophageal reflux disease (GERD): a highly chronic condition that is characterized by periodic reflux often accompanied by heartburn.

genomics: a branch of biotechnology that applies the techniques of genetics and molecular biology to the mapping of DNA sequencing of selected organisms.

Heidelberg test: a diagnostic test in which a person swallows an electronic device about the size of a vitamin capsule to help determine the level of hydrochloric acid in the stomach.

hesperidin: a sugar derivative found especially in orange peels and other citrus fruits.

human growth hormone (HGH): the naturally occurring hormone that spurs growth in children and adolescents helps maintain tissues and organs throughout a person's life.

humic acid: an organic acid derived from decomposing plants.

hydrochloric acid (HCl): an acid found in the stomach that is necessary for proper digestion.

hyperlipidemia: when excess fat or lipids are present in the blood.

hyperthyroidism: excessive activity of the thyroid gland that can result in increased metabolic rate, enlargement of the thyroid gland, rapid heart rate, and high blood pressure.

hypothyroidism: deficient activity of the thyroid gland that can result in lowered metabolic rate and general loss of energy.

immunosenescence: gradual deterioration of the immune system due to aging.

lipids: various substances that with proteins and carbohydrates constitute the principal structural components of living cells.

insulin: a protein hormone that is essential for the metabolism of carbohydrates, lipids, and proteins, that regulates blood sugar levels, and that when produced in insufficient quantities results in diabetes.

insulin-like growth factor 1 (IGF-1): the juvenile form of insulin-like growth factor that declines after puberty and is produced by the liver in response to growth hormone.

interleukin-6: an inflammatory immunoregulatory protein that induces growth of myeloma cells, causes excessive bone breakdown, activates the spread of T cells, and stimulates the synthesis of plasma proteins.

lipoproteins: a large class of conjugated proteins composed of a protein and lipid complex.

lymphoid stem cells: stem cells responsible for the production of immunity including lymphocytes, lymphoblasts, and plasma cells.

melanocyte-stimulating hormone (MSH): either of two hormones of the pituitary gland that darken the skin by stimulating melanin dispersion.

melatonin: a hormone derived from serotonin that is secreted by the pineal gland and has been linked to the regulation of circadian rhythms.

metformin: an antidiabetic drug used to treat type 2 diabetes in patients unresponsive to approved sulfonylurea drugs.

methylation: a vital metabolic process that occurs when the methyl group is introduced into a chemical compound.

mammalian target of rapamycin (mTOR): a protein that helps control several cell functions, including cell division and survival, and binds to rapamycin and other drugs.

nicotinamide adenine dinucleotide (NAD+): a coenzyme that occurs in most cells and plays an important role in all phases of metabolism.

nutrigenomics: the study of how DNA expression is influenced by foods and supplements consumed.

oxytocin: a hormone secreted by the pituitary gland that plays a role in social bonding, sexual reproduction, and the period after childbirth.

peptides: chains of two or more amino acids combined through peptide bonds.

pregnenolone: a hormone made by the adrenal gland that plays an important role in the production of steroid hormones including progesterone, DHEA, and estrogen.

progesterone: a female steroid sex hormone that prepares the endometrium for implantation and is later secreted by the placenta during pregnancy to prevent rejection of the developing embryo or fetus.

prolotherapy: an alternative therapy for treating pain that involves injecting an irritant into a ligament or tendon to promote the growth of new tissue.

proton pump inhibitors: a group of drugs that inhibit the activity of proton pumps and are used to inhibit gastric acid secretion.

quercetin: a yellow pigment that often occurs in various plants in the form of sugar derivatives known as glycosides.

regenerative medicine: a branch of medicine that is concerned with therapies that replace injured, diseased, or defective cells, tissues, or organs to restore function.

relaxin: a sex hormone that facilitates birth by causing the pelvic ligaments to relax.

senolytics: interventions aimed at selectively inducing death in senescent cells.

taurine: a colorless acid that is similar to amino acids but is not a component of proteins, and is involved in various physiological functions, including acting as an electricity regulator in the brain and heart.

telomere: composed of a usually repetitive DNA sequence, it is the natural end of a eukaryotic chromosome that stabilizes the chromosome.

testosterone: a male hormone largely produced primarily by the testes that is the main androgen responsible for inducing and maintaining male secondary sex characteristics.

theaflavins: a compound found in black tea that has senolytic properties.

thyroid-stimulating hormone (TSH): a hormone that regulates secretion of the thyroid hormone and is secreted by the pituitary gland.

thyrotropin-releasing hormone (TRH): a hormone that regulates secretion of the thyroid hormone and is secreted by the pituitary gland.

SUGGESTED READING

Blackburn, Elizabeth, Ph.D., and Elissa Epel, Ph.D. *The Telomere Effect: A Revolutionary Approach to Living Younger, Healthier, Longer.* New York: Grand Central Publishing, 2017.

Blaylock, Russell L., M.D. *The Blaylock Wellness Report Archive.* West Palm Beach, Fla.: Newsmax Media, 2009.

———. *Excitotoxins: The Taste That Kills.* Santa Fe: Health Press, 1994.

Bowden, Johnny, Ph.D., C.N.S., and Stephen Sinatra, M.D., F.A.C.C. *The Great Cholesterol Myth: Why Lowering Your Cholesterol Won't Prevent Heart Disease—and the Statin-Free Plan That Will.* Beverly, Mass.: Fair Winds Press, 2012.

Campbell-McBride, Natasha, M.D. *Gut and Psychology Syndrome: Natural Treatment for Autism, Dyspraxia, A.D.D., Dyslexia, A.D.H.D., Depression, Schizophrenia.* Cambridge, U.K.: Medinform Publishing, 2010.

Dean, Carolyn, M.D., N.D. *The Magnesium Miracle.* New York: Ballantine Books, 2007.

Galitzer, Michael, M.D. *Outstanding Health: The 6 Essential Keys to Maximize Your Energy and Well Being.* Los Angeles, Calif.: AHI Publishing, 2015.

Galitzer, Michael, M.D., and Larry Trivieri Jr. *A New Calm.* Columbus, Ohio: Gatekeeper Press, 2016.

Hall, Prudence, M.D. *Radiant Again & Forever: With Bioidentical Hormones and Other Secrets.* Austin, Tex.: Readers Legacy Incorporated, 2017.

Hertoghe, Thierry, M.D. *Atlas of Endocrinology for Hormone Therapy*. Luxembourg: International Medical Books, 2010.

———. *The Hormone Solution: Stay Younger Longer*. New York: Harmony Books, 2002.

———. *Reversing Physical Aging: Volume 1: Head & Senses*. Luxembourg: International Medical Books, 2017.

Kekich, David. *Master Life: The Most Complete Guide to Achieving Your Goals and Aspirations . . . From a Man Who Beat the Odds*. CreateSpace Independent Publishing Platform, 2017.

Keown, Daniel, M.C.E.M., M.B.Ch.B., Lic.Ac. *The Uncharted Body: A New Textbook of Medicine*. Tunbridge Wells, UK: Original Medicine Publications, 2018.

Kresser, Chris. *Unconventional Medicine: Join the Revolution to Reinvent Healthcare, Reverse Chronic Disease, and Create a Practice You Love*. Austin, Tex.: Lioncrest Publishing, 2017.

Kyriazis, Marios, M.D. *The Peptide Bioregulator Revolution: The Use of Bioactive Peptides for Aging and Health*. Dunstable, UK: Profound Health Publishing, 2018.

MacLeod, Kent. *Biology of the Brain: How Your Gut Microbiome Affects Your Brain*. Columbus, Ohio: Ultimate Publishing House, 2018.

Magaziner, Allan, D.O. *The All-Natural Cardio Cure: A Drug-Free Cholesterol and Cardiac Inflammation Reduction Program*. New York: Avery, 2004.

———. *Chemical-Free Kids: How to Safeguard Your Child's Diet and Environment*. New York: Kensington, 2003.

———. *The Complete Idiot's Guide to Living Longer & Healthier*. New York: Alpha Books, 1999.

———. *Total Health Handbook: Your Complete Wellness Resource*. New York: Kensington, 2000.

Morgentaler, Abraham, M.D. *Testosterone for Life: Recharge Your Vitality, Sex Drive, Muscle Mass, and Overall Health*. New York: McGraw-Hill, 2008.

Ober, Clinton, Stephen T. Sinatra, M.D., and Martin Zucker. *Earthing: The Most Important Health Discovery Ever*, 3rd ed. North Bergen, N.J.: Basic Health Publications, 2014.

Pedersen, Gordon, N.D., Ph.D. *The Most Precious Metal: Why Silver Is*

More Valuable than Gold, Platinum, or Money. CreateSpace Independent Publishing Platform, 2013.

Perlmutter, David, M.D. *Grain Brain: The Surprising Truth about Wheat, Carbs, and Sugar—Your Brain's Silent Killers.* New York: Little, Brown and Company, 2013.

Rosa, Tommy, and Stephen Sinatra, M.D. *Health Revelations from Heaven and Earth: 8 Divine Teachings from a Near Death Experience.* New York: Rodale Books, 2015.

Sinatra, Stephen T. M.D., F.A.C.C., F.A.C.N., C.N.S. *The Sinatra Solution: Metabolic Cardiology.* North Bergen, N.J.: Basic Health Publications, 2015.

Smith, Robin L., M.D., and Max Gomez, Ph.D. *Cells Are the New Cure: The Cutting-Edge Medical Breakthroughs That Are Transforming Our Health.* Dallas, Tex.: BenBella Books, 2017.

Tennant, Jerry, M.D., M.D.H., PSc.D. *Healing Is Voltage: The Handbook.* Self-published, CreateSpace, 2010.

INDEX